Clinical Medicine and the Nervous System
Consulting Editor: Michael Swash

Syndromes that have an underlying neurological basis are common problems in many different specialties. Clinical Medicine and the Nervous System is a series of monographs concerned with the diagnosis and management of clinical problems due primarily to neurological disease, or to a neurological complication of another disorder. Thus the series is particularly concerned with those neurological syndromes that may present in different contexts, often to specialists without special expertise in neurology. Since the range of clinical practice embraced by neurologists is wide, the books in this series will appeal to many different specialists in addition to neurologists and neurosurgeons. It is the aim of the series to produce individual volumes that are succinct, informative and complete in themselves, and that provide sufficient practical discussion of the issues to prove useful in the diagnosis, investigation and management of patients. Important advances in basic mechanisms of disease are emphasized as they are relevant to clinical practice. In particular, individual volumes in the series will be useful especially to neurologists, neurosurgeons, physicians in internal medicine, oncologists, paediatricians, neuro-radiologists, rehabilitationists, otorhinolaryngologists and ophthalmologists, and to those in training in these specialties.

Michael Swash, MD, FRCP, MRCPath
The Royal London Hospital

Titles in the series already published:

Headache
Richard Peatfield

Epilepsy: Electroclinical Syndromes
Edited by Hans Lüders and Ronald P. Lesser

The Heart and Stroke
Edited by Anthony J. Furlan

Hierarchies in Neurology
Christopher Kennard and Michael Swash

Imaging of the Nervous System
Edited by Paul Butler

Guillain-Barré Syndrome
Richard A.C. Hughes

Vertigo: Its Multisensory Syndromes
Thomas Brandt

Forthcoming titles in the series:

Diseases of the Spinal Cord
Edited by Edmond Critchley and Andrew Eisen

Malignant Brain Tumours
Edited by David G.T. Thomas and D.I. Graham

Motor Neuron Disease
Edited by Nigel Leigh and Michael Swash

Treatment of Multiple Sclerosis:

Trial Design, Results, and Future Perspectives

Edited by

Richard A. Rudick and Donald E. Goodkin

With 37 Figures

Springer-Verlag
London Berlin Heidelberg New York
Paris Tokyo Hong Kong
Barcelona Budapest

Richard A. Rudick, MD
Cleveland Clinic Foundation, Mellen Center for Multiple Sclerosis Treatment and Research, 9500 Euclid Avenue, Cleveland OH 44195-5244, USA

Donald E. Goodkin, MD
Cleveland Clinic Foundation, Mellen Center for Multiple Sclerosis Treatment and Research, 9500 Euclid Avenue, Cleveland OH 44195-5244, USA

Consulting Editor

Michael Swash, MD, FRCP, MRCPath
Consultant Neurologist, Neurology Department, The Royal London Hospital, Whitechapel, London E1 1BB, UK

The illustration on the cover, drawn by the editors, illustrates the relationship between central nervous system myelin and the oligodendrocyte (the two round cells at the upper left and lower left corners of the illustrations). The illustration shows central nervous system myelin surrounding the nerve fibers in the normal (top of figure) and disrupted (bottom of illustration) state. The irregularly shaped cell at the bottom of the figure represents a macrophage ingesting disrupted myelin.

ISBN 3-540-19683-8 Springer-Verlag Berlin Heidelberg New York
ISBN 0-387-19683-8 Springer-Verlag New York Berlin Heidelberg

British Library Cataloguing in Publication Data
Treatment of multiple sclerosis: trial design results and future perspectives. – (Clinical medicine and the nervous system)
I. Rudick, Richard A., *1950–* Goodkin, Donald E., *1946–* IV. Series
616.83406
ISBN 3-540-19683-8

Library of Congress Data available

Printed in Germany

Typeset by Best-set Typesetter Ltd., Hong Kong
2128/3830-543210 Printed on acid-free paper

Consulting Editor's Foreword

Multiple sclerosis is one of the major current problems in neurological practice. It remains incompletely understood, yet is a common cause of chronic disability in developed Western societies. Patients with the disease have difficulty understanding what has happened to them and become bewildered by the contrast between the evidently large body of knowledge concerning the clinical manifestations and course of the disease, and the conflicting views they so often receive from different specialists as to the best current management of their disease. As in so many disorders for which treatment is only partially effective, at best, "alternative" therapies abound.

Dr. Rudick and Dr. Goodkin have extensive experience in the day-to-day management of multiple sclerosis at the Mellen Center for Multiple Sclerosis Treatment and Research, attached to the Cleveland Clinic. In this book they have assembled a group of experts from several countries and have provided a comprehensive review of the results of different treatments of the disease. Each treatment is considered in the light of its proposed scientific basis or mode of action, and in relation to ethical and trial design issues. This information deserves to be made widely available. As the treatment of multiple sclerosis enters a new era as a result of the new understanding of the cellular mechanisms of demyelination and the molecular biology of the immune response, this information about current treatments assumes additional importance. The book is of interest to all physicians concerned with the management of patients with the disease.

The Royal London Hospital, London — Michael Swash
May 1991

Preface

Multiple sclerosis (MS) is a common crippling neurologic disease that affects people beginning in their young adult years. The disease takes many phenotypic forms, encompasses a wide range of severity, and once established, lasts a lifetime. In many MS patients symptoms fluctuate without apparent pattern, neurologic impairments accumulate, secondary effects on family, job, and economic status multiply, and interactions with health-care providers are characterized by short-term trial-and-error responses to current symptoms. Truly effective therapies seem perpetually just around the corner. In fact, enormous progress has been made in the field of experimental therapeutics for MS in the past 20 years. Many of us believe that these increasingly sophisticated efforts will result in truly effective therapies – treatments that will predictably slow or stop the downhill course of a person afflicted with MS. There is to date no single resource available to clinical investigators, clinical neurologists, internists, primary-care providers or biostatisticians that systematically reviews experimental therapies in MS. We organized this volume to summarize this field.

The book is organized around the following themes: the history of therapeutic trials in MS (Chap. 1); the natural history of MS and the available methods for measuring disease severity (Chaps. 2 and 3); current concepts about study design and statistical analysis (Chap. 4); current concepts of MS pathogenesis (Chap. 5); immunotherapies of recent and current interest (Chaps. 6–13); relevant lessons from immunotherapy of experimental allergic encephalomyelitis (EAE) (Chap. 14); and specific immunotherapeutic strategies in MS (Chap. 15).

We thought it appropriate to begin with a historical perspective of clinical trial design in MS – where had we come from, where are we now, and where are we going? George Ellison has many years of experience with MS clinical trials; he provided a substantive and interesting chapter. A review of the natural history of untreated MS patients allows the reader to place clinical trial results in proper perspective. Donald Goodkin's work with a large cohort of MS patients followed longitudinally enabled him to review this topic with considerable personal experience. Clinical, imaging, and laboratory outcome measures are reviewed in a comprehensive chapter by Donald Paty, Ernest Willoughby, and John Whitaker, all experts in this area. The unique problems in the design and statistical issues related to testing experimental therapy in MS are presented by William Weiss and Emmanuel Stadlin. William Weiss has participated in 10 MS clinical trials, and Emanuel Stadlin has chaired the monitoring committees for all of the collaborative clinical trials supported by the NINDS that have been completed to date. They are uniquely qualified to review this topic.

Richard Ransohoff reviews our current understanding of MS pathogenesis, presenting a cohesive picture that provides the rationale for nonspecific immune suppression protocols and points toward more specific forms of therapy. Since there were a number of relevant experimental therapies, none clearly superior to the others, chapters on promising therapies are presented in alphabetical order. ACTH and corticosteroids are reviewed by Lawrence Myers, whose experience with these therapies is widely appreciated. Azathioprine is discussed by Richard A.C. Hughes, who directed the largest double-blind study of azathioprine to date. Murray Bornstein and Kenneth Johnson present experience with copolymer 1. Cyclophosphamide is discussed by Howard Weiner and colleagues, who have considerable experience with the use of this drug for progressive MS. The cyclosporine experience is clearly presented by Jerry Wolinsky who played a major role in an American multicenter study. The use of interferon for MS is presented by Lawrence Jacobs and Fredrick Munschauer. Dr. Jacobs has been involved in the experimental use of beta interferon throughout the 1980s and is leading a multicenter trial of recombinant beta interferon. John Noseworthy was chosen to discuss the role of plasma exchange in light of his lead role in the Canadian Cooperative Trial of Cyclophosphamide and Plasma Exchange. Stuart Cook, along with his colleagues, presents his own extensive experience with total lymphoid irradiation.

Experience with myelin basic protein-induced EAE has raised hopes for more specific immunotherapy in humans. Robert Bell and Lawrence Steinman present this complex material clearly. Finally, David Hafler and colleagues present their experience to date with relatively specific forms of immunotherapy in MS patients.

We believe that further progress in this field will be greatly facilitated by careful reflection on the experience summarized within this book. This is a propitious time for critical discussions about major areas of controversy. Such reflection and discussion could lead to consensus about a number of critical questions:

1. What is the best way to measure the effect of therapy, how can we incorporate newer and perhaps more sensitive methods

in our efficacy analyses, and can we shorten our clinical trials so that we can test putative therapies more efficiently?

2. What is the optimal trial design that will be maximally efficient and sensitive, yet broadly representative of the at-large MS population afflicted with the disease?
3. Do we know enough about pathogenesis to design effective *specific* immunotherapies rationally? Will the elegant animal experiments described in Chap. 14 prove to be relevant to the design of future therapies in MS patients?
4. To what extent do the experimental approaches described herein change the natural progression of MS? Does one approach appear more effective than others at the present time? Can the best direction be discerned from the experience summarized in this book?
5. Have we considered adequately the ethical aspects of MS therapeutic trials? Can we justify a placebo control group at the present time? How can we reconcile the requirements of clinical care with the often conflicting demands of clinical research?
6. How can we finance clinical trials at a time of constraints on insurance reimbursement for medical care and tight budgets for research?

It should be noted that the contents of this book reflect our concept of MS as a tissue-specific immunologically-mediated autoimmune disease. Should the actual etiology of MS be contrary to this view, future therapeutic trials will move in a different direction. Furthermore, we focused on immunotherapies of current and future interest as well as the best approaches to conducting MS trials and measuring an effect. We did not cover an important area in MS therapeutics – trials of drugs aimed at ameliorating symptoms of the disease – nor have we exhaustively covered every individual therapeutic modality of potential interest. We did not attempt to develop consensus within the field by dealing directly with areas of controversy, of which there are many. We have not dealt with the economics of therapeutic trials, nor the many ethical problems that arise. We hope in future revisions of this book to deal with some of these additional important issues.

We are gratified that so many busy professionals, all experts in their fields, were willing to provide comprehensive summary chapters, submitted on time, for this effort. We hope that this volume will serve to summarize succinctly the current state in a rapidly progressing field and, most importantly, to provoke the types of discussions necessary to facilitate future progress.

Acknowledgements

We wish to acknowledge the courage and conviction of MS patients participating in clinical trials.

We greatly appreciate the expertise and hard work of Amy Guild, who compiled the manuscript for this book.

Cleveland, Ohio
April 1991

Richard A. Rudick
Donald E. Goodkin

Contents

Contributors

Robert B. Bell, MD
Departments of Neurology and Neurological Sciences, Pediatrics and Genetics, Stanford University School of Medicine, Stanford CA 94305-5235, USA

Murray Bornstein, MD
Albert Einstein College of Medicine, 1410 Pelham Parkway South, New York NY 10461, USA

Staley A. Brod, MD
Center for Neurologic Diseases, Brigham and Women's Hospital, 75 Francis Street, Boston MA 02115, USA

Stuart D. Cook, MD
Department of Neurosciences (H-506), New Jersey Medical School, 185 South Orange Avenue, Newark NJ 07103-2757, USA

David M. Dawson, MD
Center for Neurologic Diseases, Thorn 12, Brigham and Women's Hospital, 75 Francis Street, Boston MA 02115, USA

Corrine Devereux, MD
Department of Neurosciences (H-506), New Jersey Medical School, 185 South Orange Avenue, Newark NJ 07103-2757, USA

Peter C. Dowling, MD
Department of Neurosciences (H-506), New Jersey Medical School, 185 South Orange Avenue, Newark NJ 07103-2757, USA

George Ellison, MD
Reed Neurological Research Center, Departments of Neurology, 10833 Le Conte Avenue, Los Angeles CA 90024-1769, USA

Donald E. Goodkin, MD
Cleveland Clinic Foundation, Mellen Center U-10, 9500 Euclid Avenue, Cleveland OH 44195-5244, USA

David A. Hafler, MD
Center for Neurologic Diseases, Brigham and Women's Hospital, 75 Francis Street, Boston MA 02115, USA

Richard A. Hughes, MD
Department of Neurology, Guy's Hospital London SE1 9RT, UK

Lawrence Jacobs, MD
Buffalo General Hospital, 100 High Street, Buffalo NY 14203, USA

Kenneth P. Johnson, MD
Department of Neurology, Room N4W46, University of Maryland Hospital, 22 South Greene Street, Baltimore MD 21201, USA

Annette Jotkowitz, RN
Department of Neurosciences (H-506), New Jersey Medical School, 185 South Orange Avenue, Newark NJ 07103-2757, USA

Glenn A. Mackin, MD
Center for Neurologic Diseases, Thorn 12, Brigham and Women's Hospital, 75 Francis Street, Boston MA 02115, USA

Frederick Munschauer, MD
Buffalo General Hospital, 100 High Street, Buffalo NY 14203, USA

Lawrence W. Myers, MD
Department of Neurology, UCLA School of Medicine, Reed Neurological Research Center, 10833 Le Conte Avenue, Los Angeles CA 90024-1769, USA

John H. Noseworthy, MD
Department of Neurology, Mayo Clinic, 200 First Street SW, Rochester MN 55905, USA

Donald Paty, MD
Division of Neurology, 222-2775 Heather Street, Vancouver General Hospital, Vancouver BC V5Z 3J5 Canada

Richard M. Ransohoff, MD
Cleveland Clinic Foundation, Mellen Center for Multiple Sclerosis, 9500 Euclid Avenue, Area U-10, Cleveland OH 44195-5244, USA

Christine Rohowsky-Kochan, PhD
Department of Neurosciences (H-506), New Jersey Medical School, 185 South Orange Avenue, Newark NJ 07103–2757, USA

Richard A. Rudick, MD
Cleveland Clinic Foundation, Mellen Center for Multiple Sclerosis Treatment and Research, 9500 Euclid Avenue, Cleveland OH 44195-5244, USA

Amiram Sheffet, PhD
Department of Neurosciences (H-506), New Jersey Medical School, 185 South Orange Avenue, Newark NJ 07103-2757, USA

Emanuel M. Stadlan, MD
National Institute of Neurologic Disorders and Stroke, NIH, 7550 Wisconsin Avenue, Room 812, Bethesda MD 20892, and Kennedy Institute of Ethics, Georgetown University, USA

Lawrence Steinman, MD
Departments of Neurology and Neurological Sciences, Pediatrics and Genetics, Stanford University School of Medicine, Stanford CA 94305-5235, USA

Raymond Troiano, MD
Department of Neurosciences (H-506), New Jersey Medical School, 185 South Orange Avenue, Newark NJ 07103-2757, USA

Howard Weiner, MD
Center for Neurologic Diseases, Thorn 12, Brigham and Women's Hospital, 75 Francis Street, Boston MA 02115, USA

William Weiss, PhD
609 Jerry Lane NW, Vienna VA 22180, USA

John N. Whitaker, MD
The University of Alabama at Birmingham, School of Medicine, Department of Neurology, UAB Station, Birmingham AL 35294, USA

Ernest Willoughby, MD
Auckland Hospital Board, Auckland Hospital, Park Road, Auckland 1, New Zealand

Jerry S. Wolinsky, MD
University of Texas, Health Science Center, Department of Neurology, 6431 Fannin, Room 7.044, Houston TX 77030, USA

George Zito, MD
Department of Neurosciences (H-506), New Jersey Medical School, 185 South Orange Avenue, Newark NJ 07103-2757, USA

Abbreviations

ACE	acute disseminated encephalomyelitis
ACTH	adrenal cortical trophic hormone
AI	ambulation index
AZA	azathioprine
BBB	blood–brain barrier
CP	chronic/progressive
CNS	central nervous system
ConA	concanavalin A
CopI	copolymer I
CPMS	chronic progressive multiple sclerosis
CSF	cerebrospinal fluid
CT	computerized assisted tomography
DDS	disability status scale
DMPA	depotmethylprednisolone acetate
EAE	experimental allergic encephalomyelitis
EDSS	expanded disability status scale
ER	exacerbating/remitting
FSS	functional systems score
GCS	glucocorticosteroids
HPLC	high pressure liquid chromatography
IFMSS	International Federation of Multiple Sclerosis Societies
IFN	interferon
IgG	immunoglobulin gamma
IgG,A,B	immunoglobulin gamma, alpha, beta
IL-1	interleukin 1
IL-2	interleukin 2
IL-3	interleukin 3
IT	intrathecal
IV	intravenous
LP	lumbar puncture
MAbs	monoclonal antibodies
MBP	myelin basic protein
MHC	major histocompatibility complex
MIF	migration inhibitory factor
MLR	mixed lymphocyte response

MP	methylprednisolone
MRD	minimal record of disability
MRS	magnetic resonance spectroscopy
MS	multiple sclerosis
NK cells	natural killer cells
NMSS	National Multiple Sclerosis Society
P	progressive
PCR	polymerase chain reaction
PHA	phytohemagglutin
RA	rheumatoid arthritis
RBL	radiographic baseline
RIA	radioimmunoassay
RP	relapsing/progressive
RS	natural suppressor
SLE	systemic lupus erythematosus
TCR	T-cell receptor
TFSS	Troiano functional status scale
TLI	total lymphoid irradiation
WBC	white blood cell
WHO	World Health Organization

Chapter 1

Experimental Therapies for Multiple Sclerosis: Historical Perspective

George W. Ellison

My task is to describe the evolution over the past 20 years of clinical trial designs in multiple sclerosis to their current state; to list major milestones as I see them; and to point out past, present, and future difficulties. From other chapters of the book, I have selected examples of milestones reached, and of problems solved and to be solved by future clinical trialists.

Therapeutic trial designs have evolved to fulfill desiderata simply stated in 1970 by Tore Broman (Broman 1970). They are:

1. Complete cure of the patient
2. Success in preventing further relapses
3. Success in preventing further progress
4. An acceptable risk that the treatment will be less harmful than the disease

After multiple sclerosis was described, investigators treated individuals and characterized the patient's clinical course before and after the treatment; for example, IFMSS (1982), and Sibley (1988). This is a pretreatment and post-treatment, or "repeated measures", design wherein the patient has the same measures (observations) recorded before the treatment is started and again during or after the treatment. The workers counted exacerbations and tried to define the more gradual "progression" by documenting changes in neurologic examinations as time passed. We still use this design in "preliminary" trials done to determine if a proposed treatment is safe and tolerable. Improvement in the patient's course compared to the course before the intervention is interpreted as a "hint of efficacy". Unfortunately, spontaneous remissions can be falsely attributed to the experimental treatment.

Later, in trials done before the 1970s, descriptions of the natural history in groups of patients served as the foil for comparison (McAlpine and Compston 1952). Investigators compared individual patient's (or a group of patients') course(s) before and after treatment to a series of patients, such as an entire clinic population (historical controls) – still a variant of the repeated measures, pre- and post-treatment, or "growth curve" design (Ellison et al. 1988).

A panel led by George Schumacher summarized many of the problems with therapeutic trials in MS and suggested a new approach (Schumacher et al. 1965). They stated "The difficulties inherent in judging the effects of therapy have been stressed. These are: (1) Lack of precision in the diagnosis. (2) The erratic and unpredictable course . . . (3) Lack of a direct method for investigating activity of the disease. (4) The existence of only crude parameters for quantitating and recording the clinical course of the disease. (5) The irreversibility of gliosis and its masking effect on disease activity elsewhere in the nervous system. (6) Psychological disturbances, including hysterical tendencies, in some patients. (7) Problems of keeping large groups of patients under standard conditions of therapy or control for long periods (necessary because of the chronicity and erratic nature of the disease)."

The panel tried to define terms, "relate established principles of scientific investigation and control" and "to provide guidelines" for interested people. They emphasized exacerbations (relapses, bouts, episodes) and remissions. The panel thought four major problems existed: (1) how many patients actually have them, (2) how often do they occur (and do they occur less frequently as the disease advances), (3) the usefulness of retrospective data is suspect when the patient serves as his or her "own control", and (4) imprecise definitions of a "relapse". To avoid "a falsely high numerical score for the relapse rate", the panel recommended counting any worsening within 1 month of the onset of symptoms as part of that episode, even if there was stabilization followed by worsening again.

In the report (which merits repeated readings by all interested in MS therapeutic trials), the panel considered designs for comparison of treatments, calculation of sample size, two "patterns for the treatment contrast" (patient as own control (pre- and post-test), or "physically distinct sets of patients on different treatments" (random assignment of treatment) (parallel groups)), the "double-blind" method where neither the observer nor the subject knows which treatment has been taken, the merits and demerits of matched-pairs designs, inclusion and exclusion criteria, observations (measures, outcome variables), the difficulties in handling dropouts and incomplete follow-up, attention to the use of confidence intervals and if there is no statistically significant difference, "the power of comparison". The panel did not favor using the patient as her own control or the matched-pairs design. Unfortunately, the panel did not give a clear operational definition of "chronic progression".

Now we think the most satisfactory solution is to study two or more groups of patients at the same time (VAMS Study Group 1957; Kurtzke 1986, 1987). Rather than using the patient's course before and after treatment, the average courses of the groups of patients are compared during the treatment period (a comparative or parallel design). One group gets the experimental treatment, the other takes a placebo or a treatment with known efficacy (positive control). The treatments are assigned randomly. Neither the patient nor the person assessing the course should know which treatment is being taken. This technique (double-blind, or as is now preferred by the truly blind, double-masked) helps prevent bias. After 1954, double-blind (masked), placebo-controlled, random treatment assignment trials began (VAMS Study Group 1957). They became the "gold standard" after the publication of the "ACTH Cooperative Trial" (Rose et al. 1970).

During the 1970s and 1980s "endpoint analysis" such as testing differences in proportions of patients changing by one or more grades or steps in a scale became the primary statistical approach (Kurtzke 1986, 1987).

In the late 1980s, investigators found life table or "survival analysis" useful (Bornstein et al. 1987).

Table 1.1. Milestones in therapeutic trial designs in MS over the past 20 years

1970	Cooperative study in the evaluation of therapy in multiple sclerosis: ACTH vs placebo: final report (Rose et al. 1970)
1974	National Advisory Commission on Multiple Sclerosis, report and recommendations (DHEW 1974)
1977	General considerations for the clinical evaluations of drugs (DHEW 1977)
1979	The design of clinical studies to assess therapeutic efficacy in multiple sclerosis (Brown et al. 1979)
1979	Report of the Panel on Inflammatory, Demyelinating, and Degenerative Diseases to the National Advisory Neurological and Communicative Disorders and Stroke Council (DHEW 1979)
1982	Therapeutic claims in multiple sclerosis (IFMSS 1982)
1983	New diagnostic criteria for multiple sclerosis: guidelines for research protocols (Poser et al. 1983)
1983	Rating neurologic impairment in multiple sclerosis: an expanded disability status scale (EDSS) (Kurtzke 1983)
1983	Proceedings of the International Conference on Therapeutic Trials in Multiple Sclerosis (Herndon and Murray 1983)
1984	Early experience in nuclear magnetic resonance imaging of multiple sclerosis (Li et al. 1984)
1984	Magnetic resonance imaging: serial observations in multiple sclerosis (Johnson et al. 1984)
1986	Neuroepidemiology. Part II: assessment of therapeutic trials (Kurtzke 1986)
1987	A pilot trial of COP 1 in exacerbating-remitting multiple sclerosis (Bornstein et al. 1987)
1988	Rationale for immunomodulating therapies of multiple sclerosis (Myers and Ellison 1988)
1988	Double-masked trial of azathioprine in multiple sclerosis (British 1988)
1989	Double-blind study of true vs. sham plasma exchange in patients treated with immunosuppression for acute attacks of multiple sclerosis (Weiner et al. 1989)
1990	The Canadian Cooperative Study of cyclophosphamide and plasma exchange in progressive multiple sclerosis (The Canadian Cooperative MS Study Group 1991)
1990	Efficacy and toxicity of cyclosporine in chronic progressive multiple sclerosis: a randomized, double-blinded, placebo-controlled clinical trial (The MS Study Group 1990)

Recently, in a potentially major advance, workers found some characteristics that might be predictive of the future clinical course (an explanatory variable). If we know variables which help predict the course, we can select patients with and without the variable and increase the power and efficiency of our statistical techniques. This helps us decrease the number of volunteers needed for a trial (sample size). With logistic regression, a statistical technique for detecting these important predictive variables (such as age, sex, type of clinical course, EDSS at entry, etc.) and for delineating the influence (interaction) of one variable upon another, we have learned the single most important variable is the neurologic score at entry into trial (Bornstein et al. 1987; Weiner et al. 1989).

In Table 1.1, I have listed the year, title, and citation for my choices of the major milestones between 1970 and 1990. If you find your favorite work missing from the list, and especially if your ego is bruised, ring me up. It is highly likely ($p = 0.0001$) that I shall change the list next week.

Although problems were solved in these milestone works, we still face many difficulties in future trials. Generally, I have selected problems from my own experience and from the milestones reached (Table 1.1). I have tried to anticipate future difficulties and organize them using the format of a trial protocol and the table of contents and several pages (e.g., pp 111–127) from a book on clinical research (Hulley and Cummings 1988).

Hypothesis to be Tested

The foremost difficulty remains our lack of knowledge of the cause of MS. We cannot tailor a specific treatment until we know why and how MS comes about (IFMSS 1982, Sibley et al. 1988). Because we now think an environmental factor provokes a destructive immune response in the white matter of a genetically susceptible host, our interventions have become more focused on stopping the immune attack (see Chaps. 4–15). We still worry that MS is a syndrome with several to many causes working through a final common pathway of an immune response against white matter. Some investigators believe that without a cause, we shall never find a cure. Others think a palliative treatment is possible.

In 1974, the National Advisory Commission on Multiple Sclerosis observed "The group recognizes four possible alternative approaches to immunotherapy: general suppression of the immune mechanisms (with, among others, drugs borrowed from the chemotherapy of cancer), administration of specific antigens (a process comparable to desensitization in allergic disorders), and on the other hand, either general or specific stimulation of immune processes," (volume 1, p 30, DHEW 1974). "One of the basic principles in the development of drug therapy needs to be re-emphasized, said the working group on pharmacology: to be effective, the drug must reach the target area in adequate concentration. The blood–brain barrier presents special difficulties in the chemotherapy of MS." (volume 1, p 48, DHEW 1974).

The Highly Variable Natural History (see Chap. 2)

On the one hand, we have been told that patients who receive any "experimental treatment" whatsoever tend to get better. "Prior to 1950 . . . 43 different agents were used on a total of 2226 patients, in groups large enough to permit calculations of the 'percentage improvement.' Improvement was reported in 1138 patients, or 51%. In the few cases where the results in acute and chronic patients were reported separately, 89% of the acute patients and 42% of the chronic patients improved." (p 22, IFMSS 1982). Perhaps these figures describe the natural history of MS. Alternatively, we may have just learned what the "placebo effect" is.

On the other hand, most of the treatments quickly fell from favor when other patients continued to have relapses and progression again became manifest. The treatment really was ineffective.

Ethical Dilemmas Remain

Investigators accept placebos and double-masking. Patients try to avoid them. The fourth desideratum (do no harm) still bothers all of us. Adverse reactions often are not what was expected. Risk may be more or less than estimated. I think that in preliminary and early pilot trials investigators unavoidably focus on benefit/risk when in theory they should be exploring risk/benefit. We are supposed to define regimens and determine safety and tolerance at this stage of development. But in our hearts, we know that if there is no "hint of efficacy", we and the patients will not go on.

Design and Statistical Issues (see Chap. 3)

In 1974, the "National Advisory Commission on Multiple Sclerosis" agreed with the Schumacher Panel that therapeutic trials were feasible (DHEW 1974). In volume 2, page 28, they echoed Broman, "The Working Group believes, and with this the Commission concurs, that the primary goal of therapy directed to the multiple sclerosis process should be the prevention of exacerbations and the arrest of progression of the disease." Furthermore, "It recommends the following sequence of steps for the evaluation of any therapeutic agent: (1) Preliminary Study . . . (2) Pilot Study . . . (3) Full Study . . ." (vol. 2, pp 36–37). This progression is similar to the movement through phase I, II, III trials recommended by the Food and Drug Administration (DHEW 1977).

By 1979 the 'Panel on Inflammatory, Demyelinating, and Degenerative Diseases" was doubtful (DHEW 1979). The Panel declares "Given the variable natural history of multiple sclerosis, however, it is difficult to evaluate any proposed treatment. Since there is no effective laboratory marker for disease activity, and no predictor of whether or not another attack will occur, evaluation of treatment necessarily involves expensive and time-consuming controlled double-blind studies. Such studies should only be undertaken when there is pressing evidence that treatment will be effective." How are we to achieve that "pressing evidence"?

In the same year, another Committee gave us some of the answers (Brown et al. 1979). Their report is especially authoritative on the design and organization of trials for the experimental treatment of exacerbations or upon their prevention. The Committee concluded that although the diagnosis of MS remains clinical, ancillary tests could tip the interpretation to a more certain classification (see Chap. 4). They emphasized protection of human subjects. When selecting what to measure, the Committee considered not only exacerbating/remitting but also progressive courses. ". . . , the rate of progression or the frequency of improvement or of inactivity in patients with progressive disease would be the characteristic to measure. For the category of progressive disease to be assigned in such instances, the period of worsening should be at least 1 year" (p 7, column 2, paragraph 3, Brown et al. 1979).

I think the Copolymer I trial not only met all Brown's criteria but extended them (see Chap. 12). In my opinion, "A Pilot Trial of COP 1 in Exacerbating-Remitting Multiple Sclerosis" is the major milestone over the past 20 years in trial design for MS (Bornstein et al. 1987). Cop 1 (Copolymer 1) a random polymer simulating myelin basic protein (but suppressive rather than encephalitogenic for experimental allergic encephalomyelitis) or placebo was given to people with exacerbating/remitting MS in a matched-pairs, double-blind trial. The primary endpoint was the proportion of exacerbation-free patients. "In the 22 matched pairs, there were 12 discordant pairs: 2 patients in the placebo group had no exacerbations, whereas their matches in the Cop 1 group did; 10 patients in the Cop 1 group had no exacerbations, whereas their matches in the placebo group did". By McNemar's statistic such a result by chance alone would have happened only 39 times out of 1000 trials (p = 0.039). In the 25 patients given Cop 1, 14 were free of exacerbations (56%); only 6 of the 23 taking placebo were free of relapses (26%). There were 12 placebo recipients with three or more exacerbations and only 1 in the Cop 1 group. There were borderline differences between the groups for the number of steps change in the Disability Status Scale score with those taking Cop 1 having less change (p = 0.064).

I think this is the first time multiple logistic regression was used in a therapeutic trial to look for the influence of covariates such as treatment group, sex, duration of disease, prior exacerbation rate, Kurtzke score at baseline or interactions amongst the covariates. Only the treatment group and the Kurtzke score at baseline had a significant effect. Subgroup analysis showed Cop 1 had a beneficial effect on those with a Disability Status Scale score of 0–2 at entry.

This is the first MS trial to use odds ratios to calculate relative risk. The risk of having a relapse was 4.6 times greater for the placebo recipients than the Cop 1-treated patients.

I think this also is the first trial where survival analysis was used. Progression was defined as an increase of one step in the DSS maintained over 3 months. Patients in the placebo-treated group reached the milestone of "progressed" (had an increase in their DSS score) sooner than the Cop 1-treated group (p = 0.05). In the placebo-treated group 50% had progressed after 18 months of treatment; only 20% of the Cop 1-treated had progressed at 24 months into the trial. Chap. 13 also contains examples of very effective use of survival analysis.

Blinding (masking) was broken by the patients and the physicians since they equated worsening with the placebo treatment. The risk seemed minimal. The investigators were circumspect and concluded the "pilot" study justified a "full" trial. The only problem seems to be that no one knows how Cop 1 "works". Unfortunately, Cop 1 did not confer such dramatic benefit on patients with the "chronic progressive" type of MS (Miller et al. 1989).

Despite such advances, statistical issues continue to bedevil us. I think we would recognize a completely effective treatment as one which stabilized or improved the course, returned the cerebrospinal fluid IgG to normal, and stopped new magnetic resonance imaging "lesions". Such a therapy would not require a "full" trial and the treatment might well be accepted if the first 5–10 patients were so benefited. We would not require any statistical tools.

However, a very difficult dilemma arises when we seek a partially effective rather than a completely effective treatment (see Chap. 3). We must not underestimate the natural tendency toward improvement – remember, spontaneous "Improvement was reported in 1138 patients, or 51%." (p 22, IFMSS 1982). Thus, the magnitude of the average difference between patients treated with ineffective agents but who improve because of the natural history and placebo effect and the new experimental intervention may be small. For small treatment effects (say a 20% improvement), we need large sample sizes to detect such a small difference when the variance of our sample and measures is as high as it is in MS. Costs escalate. Even if we detect statistically significant differences between our groups, we question the clinical meaning of differences strained so hard to find (British 1988; The MS Study Group 1990). Is it worth it for anything less than "the winner"?

So we must try to minimize the sample size while maintaining statistical power to detect a clinically meaningful effect if it really is there. There are techniques that might make it possible to achieve both goals. Hulley and Cummings recommend using continuous variables, more precise variables, paired measurements, unequal group sizes, and a more common outcome to minimize sample size (p 146 ff, Hulley and Cummings 1988). MRI scans may provide us with the continuous, precise variable which changes more often than clinical scales (see Chap. 4). Also we might enroll subjects with a greater risk of developing the outcome (use an explanatory variable), liberalize our definitions of what constitutes an outcome, and extend the follow-up period (but that increases the costs of the trial).

Perhaps now that we have explanatory variables with which to match patients, we might reconsider the matched-pairs designs or at least stratify our patients. Detels et al. (1982) showed that being male in southern California, having weakness at onset, and using a cane to walk into the doctor's office are bad prognostic indicators. These results agree with those from logistic regression studies in actual therapeutic trials that suggest entry scores are important indicators of who will respond well in a trial (a Kurtzke EDSS grade of 6 corresponds to intermittent use of a cane) (Bornstein et al. 1987; Weiner et al. 1989).

I think we should change our conceptual approach to MS therapeutic trial designs. Rather than start with the neurologist's or patient's point of view "I want worsening stopped", start with the statistician's. Decide what statistical test is the most powerful and most efficient (e.g., probably a parametric test) for supporting the inference that the group differ by chance alone. Decide what groups distribution of the data will optimally satisfy the assumptions of the statistical test. Decide on the experimental unit; e.g., patient or relapse. Craft a "primary" measurement that improves the efficiency of the statistical test (e.g., aim for a continuous variable rather than a categorical or ordinal one; aim for a variable that is precise (low variance); aim for a variable that is sensitive). Do not allow more than 6 measurements in toto. Organize a slightly different approach to confirm your primary test (e.g., also use survival analysis).

Diagnosis

Now we can better define inclusion and exclusion criteria for study subjects. The Schumacher Panel and Dr. Brown's Committee report gave us clinical criteria for diagnosis (Schumacher et al. 1965; Brown et al. 1979). Charles M. Poser and colleagues described "paraclinical" laboratory tests which increased the accuracy of diagnosis and encouraged classification of patients into definite and probable MS (Poser et al. 1983).

Specification

We must decide whether or not the type of clinical course is an important variable. Earlier investigators described not only relapses and remissions but also "chronic progression" (see Chap. 2) and we and others focussed on this phase of illness for our therapeutic trials (Ellison and Myers 1980; Hauser et al. 1983). We thought there was more predictable deterioration by such patients.

Unfortunately, the operational definitions of "chronic progression" are ambiguous. In 1952 McAlpine and Compston declared "It has long been recognized that the course of disseminated sclerosis may be characterized by relapses or remission, or by chronic progression either from the onset or after a number of remissions . . .". By 1955 they codified their definition. ". . . (1) A small number with a course progressively downhill from the onset; (2) a larger number with a course becoming progressively downhill after an initial relapsing pattern of events." (McAlpine et al. 1955). However, by 1972 a subtle shift had occurred when they defined chronic progressive phase as secondary to "(1) relapses of increasing severity and duration and (2) progressive from the onset" (p 207, McAlpine et al. 1972).

Can we accept historical information as a definition of progression, or must we have examined and recorded clinical scores for years before entry? In our trial of azathioprine and methylprednisolone, we accepted the patient's opinion about changes in signs (e.g., walking distance 2 years ago compared to today, need for a cane 1 year ago compared to today, etc.) and defined progression as "A steady gradual deterioration of neurologic signs between visits . . ." (Ellison et al. 1989; Hommes et al. 1975). Consider the specification used by Hauser et al. (Hauser et al. 1983). "All patients had severe progressive disease with worsening in the nine months before entry. Worsening, defined as a decrease in one or more points on the functional-status or disability scale, consisted of either a continuous decline or a continuous decline with superimposed exacerbations." The use of change in grades is important, but the patients from whom we select the sample would have to have been known to the investigators. That implies they were evaluated for some time before entry into the trial. Not all centers do this. If they do, costs increase dramatically. Will not randomization at the time of entry equalize the risk factors?

After all the above, and with the passage of time, I have concluded that this separation of types probably is not essential (see Chap. 2 for inconstancy of clinical type, and Chap. 4 for laboratory and MRI evidence for "activity" that cannot be detected clinically). Perhaps more important are the risks related to the treatment. Younger people with a benign course should avoid high-risk interventions. Those with more rapid deterioration, whatever the type of clinical course, might take more risk. Patients self-select. They do not volunteer early in a benign course; they will "do anything" if deterioration is rapid whatever their classification.

Outcome Measures

Deciding on the observations for a therapeutic trial is difficult (see Chap. 4). We do want accurate and precise measurements. However, they need only be "good enough" to detect change that is pertinent to the question asked in the trial. Moreover, since it is relatively easy to detect worsening, the anguish over the measurements for efficacy may be overdone. I think that the reason we eventually know that a treatment is not effective is that people with MS tell us what happened. They and those around them know they have deteriorated despite the intervention. Everyone looks elsewhere for a more effective treatment.

Parenthetically, such deterioration, even of one person's course, in a preliminary trial or pilot study mandates that we should remain quite skeptical that the intervention has any promise whatsoever.

Sample Sizes

Estimating sample size (the number of subjects in each group that we need to decide confidently that the experimental treatment differs from the control intervention more than by chance alone and that we would have detected a real difference if it were there) is straightforward mathematically, but fraught with practical problems. We must have enough subjects to achieve a believable study. Yet, we want the smallest number possible because it seems like the costs in suffering, effort, time, and money increase geometrically while the gain in power to detect an effect increases arithmetically.

Until the late 1980s, many of us probably were guilty of overestimating treatment effect and underestimating sample size (Detsky 1985). In our trial of steroids and azathioprine we estimated that we would be able to enroll rapidly deteriorating patients in progression phase. At the end of the trial, the rate of deterioration was about one third that calculated. Depending upon the real standardized treatment effect (expected effect size divided by the standard deviation of the outcome variable), our group sizes could have been 16, 44, or 393 to meet the requirements of a two-tailed alpha error of 0.05 and a beta error of 0.8 (p 215, Hulley and Cummings 1988). We may have achieved sufficiently large group size for our proposed treatment effect, but not for the observed one (Ellison et al. 1989).

I think standardized effect size is a great problem in MS because of the enormous natural variation in the course of the disease from person to person. Furthermore, our outcome measures (variables) are inaccurate surrogate estimates of "black box" nervous system chemistry, physiology, and pathology compounded by imprecision from definitions which are difficult to apply consistently, not mutually exclusive, and not all inclusive. I am amazed that we can accomplish a trial with them. We have no choice but to increase our sample sizes even more to deal with their variation.

Also, with ordinal scales (Kurtzke 1986), we must use nonparametric statistical tests rather than the usually much more efficient parametric tests. For example, if the Disability Status Scale is not interval, then perhaps the best we can do is use a nonparametric test like the chi-square test on the proportion of patients changing from one grade to another (Kurtzke 1986, 1987; Weiner et al. 1989). This is not necessarily bad. But, by using proportions rather than average changes in an interval variable we may have tripled the size of the cohort we need for the trial! Although a winner may not require a full trial with 300–500 subjects, we may not be able to detect a treatment that is 20% better than the natural history of the disease with anything less

Will we run out of patients for therapeutic trials? People are receiving powerful immunosuppressive treatments which may make them ineligible for future trials. This makes it even more important to use efficient designs and measurements. If we can obtain the truth with 100 people rather than 300, we have just made our trial three time more efficient. Or, we can do two more trials of promising agents.

Another reason to have the optimal sample size is that when we have large sample sizes we may achieve statistical significance with dubious clinical importance. The cyclosporine A trial is such an example of "a statistically significant but clinically modest delay of progression of disability in a group of patients with multiple sclerosis selected for moderately severe and progressive disease" (The MS Study Group 1990).

Implementing the Study

Beware of recruitment problems. Bornstein et al. found how difficult it is to recruit enough patients to pass the inclusion and exclusion criteria and actually join a trial. They screened 932 volunteers for a total sample size of 50 patients (Bornstein et al. 1987). We screened 1118 for a sample size of 98 (Ellison et al. 1983). Do not underestimate the length of time required. The average change in course may be less than you think and the time to recruit your cohort may be much greater than you planned.

Variables

Outcome measures remain a difficulty (see Chap. 4). In Volume 2, page 37 of the "National Advisory Commission on Multiple Sclerosis, Report and Recommendations", the Commission responded ". . . there is agreement that trials of therapy should focus upon readily demonstrable and substantive changes in neurological functions and not become bogged down in subtle changes which require meticulous scoring procedures and statistical validation" (DHEW 1974). It has not worked out that way.

Although the cyclosporine A trial is an example of redundancy of measures, from it we may have learned a simple way to determine the outcome – ask the patient or the physician (The MS Study Group 1990). With the patient global assessment of benefit, 59.7% of the cyclosporine recipients rated themselves an average of 20% worse (deteriorated) compared to 69% of the placebo-treated who rated themselves 25% worse ($p = 0.01$). The physician raters thought 58.6% of the cyclosporine-treated worsened by 17.5% and 67.9% of those taking placebo deteriorated by 27.5% ($p = 0.009$).

The opinions compare favorably with "objective" measures. With the designed primary outcome measure "At the time of exit from the study (whether by completion of 24 months as planned or at the time of withdrawal from the study for any reason) the cyclosporine-treated patients displayed a mean deterioration of neurological function, as measured by the EDSS, of 0.39 (1.07) compared to a deterioration of EDSS of 0.65 (1.08) by their placebo-treated counterparts (p = 0.002)". Change in the "collapsed EDSS" score between baseline and exit (cyA, 0.33 ± 0.55; and placebo, 0.50 ± 0.51) was statistically significant (p = 0.001). A composite score of "activities of daily living" (dressing, feeding, grooming items from the Incapacity Status Scale of the Minimal Record of Disability) and "time to sustained progression of neurological disability" were not different statistically between the groups. Survival analysis for "time to becoming wheelchair bound" slightly favored the cyclosporine-treated group (p = 0.038).

Perhaps further analysis of the cyclosporine A trial will enable us to settle upon a few suitable "objective" clinical measures. As noted before, neurological disability at entry had an effect on the outcome – those who did best on lower extremity tests in the Quantitative Examination of Neurologic Function at entry did best in the trial whatever treatment they received.

We may have found the long-sought quantitative, accurate, interval, reproducible measure of disease activity – serial magnetic resonance images (see Chap. 4). Because MRI "events" are more frequent than clinical relapses and slow progression, they might allow therapeutic trials with fewer patients (smaller sample size). We shall see.

Attrition

Keeping large groups of patients in trials remains difficult. Attrition from withdrawals because of adverse drug effects may be great. The modern trial most affected by this problem was the cyclosporine A trial (The MS Study Group 1990).

A dilemma is whether to allow adrenal steroid therapy, to prevent dropouts because of deterioration and thus to keep patients in the trial. In the cyclosporine A trial, treatment failure, defined as the use of adrenal cortical steroids, resulted in the withdrawal of 47 (17%) of the cyclosporine-treated and 59 (22%) of the placebo-treated patients (The MS Study Group 1990). We kept patients in after ACTH treatment but I am sure it decreased the IgG synthesis rate in the placebo-treated patients (unpublished data, Ellison 1989).

Analysis

Analysis by "intention-to-treat" means we include all subjects in their group whether or not they completed the treatment regimen. I cannot accept that the results of a patient who takes 3 weeks of a treatment has the same scientific implications as one who completes 3 years exactly according to protocol. Nevertheless, I aim to include everyone who should be included. I guess the way out is to analyze the data both ways.

How to handle attrition from patients withdrawn or study dropouts? Losses may destroy the balance achieved with randomization and if severe, may diminish the sample size to an intolerable level. In the cyclosporine A trial there was a drastic difference in attrition between the cyclosporine-treated (44% by 2 years) and the placebo-treated (32%). Such a disparity casts doubt on the entire study.

Do survival analyses help? With small numbers of dropouts, it probably does (Bornstein et al. 1987). With larger numbers, it may not (The MS Study Group 1990). I think survival analysis is based upon random loss of subjects. What happens when the attrition is dependent upon one of the interventions (adversities from taking cyclosporine) but not the other?

The difficulties of cross-over designs in MS are typified in the trials of the interferons (see also Chap. 9). The "wash out" may not remove all the pharmacologic effects of the intervention; e.g., alpha interferon (Knobler et al. 1984). I am worried that trials of systemic interferon designed to prevent relapses have used the same cross-over design (Johnson 1983).

Also, in cross-over designs where treatment occurs over several years, the natural history of a gradual decrease in exacerbation rate over time is superimposed upon the treatment intervention. This naturally-occurring decrease is even more of a worry in considering the claim from anecdotal trials that azathioprine given long enough (5–10 years) decreases the relapse rate (Ellison and Myers 1980).

Generalization of the Trial Results

What do we do when the trial results are "statistically significant" but we are uncertain of the usefulness of the treatment? The cyclosporine A treatment is an example of this problem (see Chap. 8). Adverse drug effects made the treatment too dangerous. What if the adversities are tolerable and the true benefits minor? Who should make the decision about the treatment – the physician, the patient, significant others, society?

I think trials with azathioprine also are good examples (see Chap. 7). In a pilot trial of azathioprine with and without methylprednisolone in patients with "chronic progressive" multiple sclerosis, we tried to induce immunosuppression with methylprednisolone and maintain it with azathioprine (Ellison et al. 1989). We did not succeed in stopping chronic progression. We did find a decrease in the number of patients having relapses and in the average relapse rate for anyone taking azathioprine. We did not think much of this result since the British and Dutch trial did not find such an effect in a much larger number of patients (British 1988). Then, Goodkin et al. (1991) showed a decrease in the exacerbation rate in early relapsing/remitting patients given azathioprine. I am receiving telephone calls from colleagues in practice who want to know if they should give azathioprine to their relapsing/remitting patients. What should I advise them? What should the practitioner actually do?

High Costs of Therapeutic Trials

Can we reduce the costs associated with studies? I think the orderly progression through the different levels of trial as recommended by the "National Advisory Commission on Multiple Sclerosis" would be less costly in the long run than jumping to a full trial as was done with cyclosporine A (DHEW 1974; The MS Study Group 1990). The objectives of a preliminary trial are different from those of a pilot or full trial (Weiner 1983a,b). However, how many relapses or people who "progress" are necessary before you give up? What does it mean: "Do not progress to a pilot trial unless there is a strong hint of efficacy"?

Once committed to a pilot or full trial we certainly could decrease costs. If we knew the minimal number of measures absolutely necessary, we might delegate simple measures to less high-cost personnel than neurologists, nurses, physical therapists, etc. If we reduce the number and frequency of clinical measures we decrease time and effort for all concerned.

Conclusions

Multiple sclerosis clinical trialists face several apparently conflicting themes: (1) no matter what treatment is used, most patients get better over the short term; (2) "proving" that improvement actually came from the intervention may be quite difficult if the treatment is "partially" rather than "completely" effective; (3) over a longer time, many, but not all, patients worsen. Over the past 20 years we have learned that, because the natural history of MS is so highly variable, parallel-group comparative designs are more effective than "pre- and post-treatment" repeated measures designs for pilot and full trials. I am sure we would recognize, probably without any statistics needed, a completely effective treatment in a trial with a small sample size if all participants improved clinically, relapses ceased, cerebrospinal fluid normalized, there were no new "lesions" in magnetic resonance images, and the intervention had minimal adversities. However, to distinguish trial results with partially effective therapies from the natural history of MS, I strongly believe we must resolutely proceed stepwise through preliminary, pilot, and full trials. Endpoint analysis with change in frequency of exacerbations or of end-minus-beginning scores or slopes continues to be useful in parallel group designs. Survival analysis to important milestones is a major addition to MS therapeutic trial statistical techniques. I think we should change our conceptual approach to MS therapeutic trial designs and think like statisticians rather than neurologists. We are still learning how best to do preliminary (phase I and II) trials, what and how many measurements are really necessary, what variables help predict the outcome, and how to distinguish between "statistically significant" and "clinically meaningful" results. We must continue doing trials. We may find a palliative treatment even if we do not completely know the etiology(s) or pathogenesis of the syndrome of multiple sclerosis.

Acknowledgments. This review was partially supported by the People of the State of California, the Conrad N. Hilton Foundation, the Joe Gheen Fund, and Various Donors to the UCLA Multiple Sclerosis Research and Treatment Program.

References

Bornstein MB, Miller A, Slagle S et al. (1987) A pilot trial of Cop 1 in exacerbating-remitting multiple sclerosis. N Engl J Med 317:408–414

British and Dutch Multiple Sclerosis Azathioprine Trial Group (1988) Double-masked trial of azathioprine in multiple sclerosis. Lancet 2:179–183

Broman T (1970) Management of patients with multiple sclerosis. In: Vinken PJ, Bruyn GW (eds) Multiple sclerosis and other demyelinating diseases. North-Holland Publishing Company, Amsterdam, pp 408–425 (Handbook of clinical neurology, vol 9)

Brown JR, Beebe GW, Kurtzke JF, Loewenson RB, Silberberg DH, Tourtellotte WW (1979) The design of clinical studies to assess therapeutic efficacy in multiple sclerosis. Neurology 29:1–23

Detels R, Clark VA, Valdiviezo NL, Visscher BR, Malmgren RM, Dudley JP (1982) Factors associated with a rapid course of multiple sclerosis. Arch Neurol 39:337–341

Detsky AS (1985) When was a negative clinical trial big enough? How many patients you needed depends on what you found. Arch Intern Med 145:709–712

DHEW 1974 – US Department of Health, Education, and Welfare (February 11, 1974) National Advisory Commission on Multiple Sclerosis, Report and Recommendations. HEW, Public Health Service, National Institutes of Health, Washington DC, Publication # (NIH) 74-534:36–38

DHEW 1977 – US Department of Health, Education, and Welfare, Food and Drug Administration (September 1977) General considerations for the clinical evaluation of drugs. US Government Printing Office, Washington DC, HEW (FDA) 77-3040:6–11

DHEW 1979 – US Department of Health, Education, and Welfare. Public Health Service, National Institutes of Health. National Institute of Neurological and Communicative Disorders and Stroke (1979) Report of the panel on inflammatory, demyelinating, and degenerative diseases to the national advisory neurological and communicative disorders and stroke council. Washington DC, NIH Publication No. 79-1916:24–30

Ellison GW, Myers LW (1980) Immunosuppressive drugs in multiple sclerosis: pro and con. Neurology 30 (7 Pt 2):28–32

Ellison GW, Myers LW, Mickey MR et al. (1983) Multiple sclerosis: patient accrual problems in a therapeutic trial. Neurology 33 (suppl 2):71

Ellison GW, Mickey MR, Myers LW (1988) Alternatives to randomized clinical trials. Neurology 38 (7 Suppl 2):73–75

Ellison GW, Myers LW, Mickey MR et al. (1989) A placebo-controlled, randomized, double-masked, variable dosage, clinical trial of azathioprine with and without methylprednisolone in multiple sclerosis. Neurology 39:1018–1026

Goodkin DE, Bailly R, Teetzen M, Hertsgaard D (1991) The efficacy of azathioprine in relapsing-remitting multiple sclerosis. Neurology 41:20–25

Hauser SL, Dawson DM, Lehrich JR et al. (1983) Intensive immunosuppression in progressive multiple sclerosis. A randomized, three-arm study of high-dose intravenous cyclophosphamide, plasma exchange, and ACTH. N Engl J Med 308:173–180

Herndon RM, Murray TJ (1983) Proceedings of the international conference on therapeutic trials in multiple sclerosis. Arch Neurol 40:663–710

Hommes OR, Prick JJG, Lamers KJB (1975) Treatment of the chronic progressive form of multiple sclerosis with a combination of cyclophosphamide and prednisone. Clin Neurol Neurosurg 78:59–72

Hulley SB, Cummings SR (1988) Designing clinical research. Williams and Wilkins, Baltimore

IFMSS (International Federation of Multiple Sclerosis Societies) (1982) Therapeutic claims in multiple sclerosis. National Multiple Sclerosis Society, New York

Johnson KP (1983) Systemic interferon therapy for multiple sclerosis. Design of a trial. Arch Neurol 40:681–682

Johnson MA, Li DKB, Bryant DJ, Payne JA (1984) Magnetic resonance imaging: serial observation in multiple sclerosis. AJNR 5:495–499

Knobler RL, Panitch HS, Braheny SL et al. (1984) Systemic alpha-interferon therapy of multiple sclerosis. Neurology 34:1273–1279

Kurtzke JF (1983) Rating neurologic impairment in multiple sclerosis: An expanded disability status scale (EDSS). Neurology 33:1444–1452

Kurtzke JF (1986) Neuroepidemiology. Part II. Assessment of therapeutic trials. Ann Neurol 19:311–319

Kurtzke JF (1987) Problems and pitfalls in treatment trials of multiple sclerosis. Neuroepidemiology 6:17–33

Li D, Mayo J, Fache S, Robertson WD, Paty D, Genton M (1984) Early experience in nuclear magnetic resonance imaging of multiple sclerosis. Ann NY Acad Sci 436:484–486

McAlpine D, Compston N (1952) Some aspects of the natural history of disseminated sclerosis. Q J Med 21:135–167

McAlpine D, Compston ND, Lumsden CE (1955) Multiple sclerosis. Livingstone, Edinburgh, p 139

McAlpine D, Lumsden CE, Acheson ED (1972) Multiple sclerosis, a reappraisal. Williams and Wilkins, Baltimore, pp 197–223

Miller AE, Bornstein M, Slagle S et al. (1989) Clinical trial of Copl in chronic-progressive multiple sclerosis. Neurology 39 (suppl 1):356–357

Myers LW, Ellison GW (1988) Rationale for immunomodulating therapies of multiple sclerosis. Neurology 38 (7, Suppl 2):4–89

Poser CM, Paty DW, Scheinberg L et al. (1983) New diagnostic criteria for multiple sclerosis: Guidelines for research protocols. Ann Neurol 13:227–231

Rose AS, Kuzma JW, Kurtzke JF, Namerow NS, Sibley WA, Tourtellotte WW (1970) Cooperative study in the evaluation of therapy in multiple sclerosis: ACTH vs. placebo. Final Report. Neurology 20:1–59

Schumacher GA, Beebe G, Kibler RE et al. (1965) Problems of experimental trials of therapy in multiple sclerosis: report by the panel on evaluation of experimental trials of therapy in multiple sclerosis. Ann NY Acad Sci 122:552–568

Sibley WA, and the Therapeutic Claims Committee of the International Federation of Multiple Sclerosis (1988) Therapeutic claims in multiple sclerosis (2nd edn). Demos Publications, New York, pp vii–x, 1–198

The Canadian Cooperative Multiple Sclerosis Study Group (1991) The Canadian cooperative trial of cyclophosphamide and plasma exchange in progressive multiple sclerosis. Lancet 337:441–446

The MS (Multiple Sclerosis) Study Group (1990) Efficacy and toxicity of cyclosporine in chronic progressive multiple sclerosis: randomized, double-blind, placebo-controlled clinical trial. Ann Neurol 127:591–605

VAMS (Veterans Administration Multiple Sclerosis) Study Group (1957) Isoniazid in treatment of multiple sclerosis. Report on Veterans Administration Cooperative Study. JAMA 163:168–172

Weiner HL, Ebers GC (1983a) Development of simple trial protocols. Arch Neurol 40:700–703

Weiner HL, Ellison GW (1983b) A working protocol to be used as a guideline for trials in multiple sclerosis. Arch Neurol 40:704–710

Weiner HL, Dau P, Khatri B et al. (1989) Double-blind study of true versus sham plasma exchange in patients being treated with immunosuppression for acute attacks of multiple sclerosis. Neurology 39:1143–1149

Chapter 2

The Natural History of Multiple Sclerosis

Donald E. Goodkin

Introduction

It is necessary to understand the natural history of multiple sclerosis (MS) so that the results of clinical trials of experimental therapies can be interpreted. It is, in the final analysis, natural history studies that provide us with the data for rates of progression of disability and of survival in untreated patients, to which therapeutic trials are ultimately compared. Natural history data are used to determine sample sizes and provide us with the disability progression rates in untreated patients from which the magnitude of "placebo effects" in controlled clinical trials can be ascertained. For example, if we knew that 50% of an untreated population of relapsing MS patients deteriorated by a specified amount on an accepted measure of disability over 2 years, the sample size required to demonstrate confidently a designated percentage reduction (e.g., 50%) in this rate by a promising therapeutic agent could be calculated (see Chap. 4). Similarly, an estimate of the placebo effect could be made if the placebo-treated patients deteriorated less than otherwise properly matched and monitored untreated controls from natural history studies.

Numerous reports of the natural history of MS have been published. Our goal in this chapter is to review selected relevant studies and determine to what extent the answers to the following questions in untreated MS patients are known: (1) what are the cross-sectional descriptions of published cohorts of MS patients? (2) what is the prospect for survival in MS patients? (3) what is the outcome of a single exacerbation of MS? (4) what is the frequency of exacerbations over time? (5) can we predict the eventual functional status of MS patients? (6) what are the newer or non-traditional methods of determining the natural history of MS? To address these questions most meaningfully, we need initially to consider a number of methodological issues that influence published and future studies on MS natural history.

Methodologic Considerations

Methodologic aspects of frequently-cited natural history studies are listed in Table 2.1. The major concerns will be discussed below. However, many

Table 2.1. Methodologic considerations: selected clinical course studies

	Case ascertainment					Patient follow-up			Operational definition of terms available				
	Retrospective	Prospective	Mixed	Clinic-based	Hospital-based	Frequency	Mean duration	Examined by author(s)	Meet current diagnostic criteria[e]	Exacerbation	Relapsing/remitting	Relapsing/progressive	Chronic/progressive
Muller (1949)	Yes	No	No	Yes	No	Na[a]	9.3 Yr	Yes	No	Yes Subj[c]	Yes Subj	Yes Subj	Yes Subj
McAlpine and Compston (1952)	Yes	No	No	Yes	No	6 Mos	Na	Yes	No	Yes Subj	No	No	No
Kurtzke (1956)	No	No	Yes	No	Yes	1 Visit	17 Mos	Yes	No	Yes Obj[d]	No	No	No
McAlpine (1961)	Yes	No	No	Yes	Yes	12 Mos	>10 Yr	Yes	Yes	Yes Obj	No	No	No
Leibowitz et al. (1964)	Yes	No	No	Yes	No	Na	Na	Yes	Yes	Yes Subj	Yes Subj	Yes Subj	Yes Subj
Panelius (1969)	Yes	No	No	Yes	Yes	Na	Na	Cbd[b]	Yes	Yes Subj	Yes Subj	Yes Subj	Yes Subj
Fog and Linnemann (1970)	No	No	Yes	Yes	No	3 Mos	9 Yr	Yes	Yes	Yes Subj	Yes Obj	Yes Obj	Yes Obj
Kurtzke et al. (1977)	Yes	No	No	Yes	Yes	Na	>7 Yr	Yes	Yes	Yes Obj	Yes Obj	Yes Obj	Yes Obj
Broman et al. (1981)	No	No	Yes	Yes	No	Na	13–27 Yr	Yes	Yes	No	No	No	No
Wolfson and Confavreux (1987)	Yes	No	No	Yes	No	Na	Na	Cbd	Yes	Yes Subj	Yes Subj	Yes Subj	Yes Subj
Minderhoud et al. (1988)	Yes	No	No	Yes	No	Na	Na	Cbd	Yes	No	No	No	No
Goodkin et al. (1989)	No	No	Yes	Yes	No	6 Mos	2.6 Yr	Yes	Yes	Yes Obj	Yes Obj	Yes Obj	Yes Obj
Weinshenker et al. (1989a)	No	No	Yes	Yes	No	12 Mos	1–12 Yr	Yes	Yes	Yes Subj	Yes Subj	Yes Subj	Yes Subj

[a] Na = Not available.
[b] Cbd = Cannot be determined.
[c] Subj = Subjective criteria provided.
[d] Obj = Objective criteria provided.
[e] Schumacher et al. (1965).

methodologic issues become intuitively evident with an example. Assume that you are the principal investigator of a natural history study or clinical trial and that you plan to use data obtained retrospectively and prospectively during the study. You are examining a patient to determine the accuracy of diagnosis, date of onset, date and type of first symptom, exacerbation frequency, history of treatments, and clinical course of the disease.

Dr.: I understand that you have been diagnosed as having MS. When did this occur?
Patient: I think it was 1978 . . . (patient turns to wife).
Wife: No dear it was 1967 when you lost vision in your eye.
Dr.: Was the diagnosis made by a doctor in 1967?
Wife: The doctors said they were suspicious in 1967 because he had also experienced some numbness and incoordination in his right arm in 1965 which resolved. In 1978 they said they were sure.
Dr.: How were they sure in 1978?
Patient: My legs got weak for about 2 months. The doctor did a spinal tap and said I had MS after the results came back.
Dr.:How have you been since that diagnosis was given? Do you think you have improved, stayed the same, or gotten worse?
Patient: (confidently) I'm pretty much the same.
Wife: (more confidently) I think he is worse.
Dr.: Can you explain . . . you seem to have differing opinions.
Patient: I can do everything I used to do. I still can walk and I'm still able to work as an insurance salesman.
Wife: Yes honey but you are using a cane now.
Patient: I use a cane just to help me balance and I really don't need it.
Dr.: OK . . . Let's assume for the moment that you have worsened just a little because you are using a cane for your balance problem. Have you worsened slowly or do you feel you have had attacks?
Wife: (confidently) Slowly and steadily . . . I can see it every day.
Patient: (tenderly) She worries about me. I always get better after an attack.
Dr.: (surprised) Attack!?
Patient: Yes attack . . . like the last one in 1982 or 1983 when my legs were weak for 2 weeks and I did have to use a cane all the time.
Dr.: Did you see a doctor?
Wife: Yes we did but Jim was already better by the time we were able to get an appointment 2 weeks later.
Dr.: (looking at medical records) Yes I see in his records here that the doctor thought you might be a little unsteady walking and he thought you had an attack. He treated you with prednisone.
Patient: No . . . that one was in July of 1984 . . . I'm talking about the one in 1982. . . .
Dr.: Well the medical records I have here indicate you also received prednisone in 1984. Are you sure you were treated in 1982?
Patient: Yes because that was the year of my daughter's wedding and I had to be treated so I could walk down the aisle with her!
Dr.: I guess we don't have the records for that treatment. How have you been since the treatment in 1984?
Patient: Pretty much the same.
Wife: (with assurance) I think his walking is worse.
Dr.: Have you had any more attacks?
Patient: I have had an attack every spring.
Dr.: Did you see a doctor when you experienced those attacks?
Patient: No. The doctor would call in a prescription for prednisone for me and I'd get better in a week or two.
Dr.: Well I'd like to examine you and compare my examination to the other doctor's done in 1984. . . . (after the exam) You are correct about the spinal tap results. The IgG level was abnormally elevated. It appears you have done quite well with the exception of your walking. This is due to a moderate loss of coordination in your right leg. You are able to walk 25 feet in 9 seconds with or without the cane (pauses to look at the medical records). Let's look at the other doctor's notes from 1984. Everything was normal then except a mild decrease in coordination in your right leg. I guess he didn't record the amount of time it took you to walk 25 feet when he

watched you but I'd say it seems like your right leg is worse. The right leg problem I see today is moderate instead of mild. Give me just a moment to fill out these forms for our natural history study on MS and then we can discuss the potential experimental therapy protocols that you may be eligible for.

While some of the uncertainties raised in this example can be clarified with proper medical records, it should be clear that much of the data to be collected for the natural history study requires highly subjective judgements on the part of the examiner or designated data collector. Brief descriptions and discussion of the most relevant methodologic issues follow to assist in the design of natural history studies and to help the reader interpret many of the studies presented later in this chapter.

Diagnostic Accuracy. The patients studied should meet established diagnostic criteria that have both widespread acceptance and acceptable performance characteristics. This is important since there is no accurate diagnostic test for MS and the rate of incorrect diagnosis is significant. It should be noted that diagnostic criteria have undergone significant changes since the first reports of natural history were published.

Case Ascertainment. The methods of case ascertainment should be described so that potential for bias can be assessed, since some cohorts may not be representative of the full clinical spectrum of MS. An inception cohort – patients followed from disease onset – is ideal for natural history studies, but is difficult to assemble for a relatively uncommon illness like MS that may have had symptoms or insidiously progressive signs long before the diagnosis is suspected or established. Cases can be ascertained retrospectively (e.g., medical records) or prospectively (e.g., during longitudinal follow-up). Both methods have potential limitations (Sackett et al. 1985). Diagnostic accuracy and assessment of disease activity in retrospectively ascertained cases may be suspect because of inadequate objective documentation found in medical records. MS cases may be missed when ascertained from medical records, particularly when multiple diagnoses coexist and the cause of death is listed as another illness. This may exclude either benign forms of the disease without much documented in the record, or more advanced cases with overwhelming terminal disease such as bacterial septicemia. Hospital-based studies may include more severe cases, or those experiencing acute disabling exacerbations. Cohorts derived from community hospitals serving an indigent population may have greater levels of disability or lower average levels of education. A study with only males or only females may not be representative of the clinical spectrum of the illness. Studies based in MS clinics may preferentially follow only cases meeting the entry criteria for special-interest studies that are ongoing at that site.

Patient Follow-up. The observation period should continue to a defined outcome, such as death due to the illness or absence of measurable change in clinical activity for a specified period, after which clinical reactivation is considered extremely unlikely. The extended period of observation required to detect functional change late in the course of MS may be difficult to achieve, since the disease spans decades. Nevertheless, clinical assessments during the period of observation should consist of reliable measures of the subjects' functional status. These measures are practically useful only when they are adequately defined, standardized, sufficiently sensitive, and used often to detect relevant changes in disease.

The follow-up interval for patients differs considerably between published series. Additionally, follow-up frequency within a single series may be inconsistent across patients. The accuracy of outcome measures such as "time to progression of disability score" may, therefore, be uncertain. When progression was observed, was a second examination required to insure that it was not a "fluctuation" in clinical status that might be attributable to a cause other than MS?

Large numbers of patients are typically "lost to follow-up" in long-term prospective studies. This may result from migration away from study centers, increasing disability that makes it difficult or impossible to visit an outpatient clinic, institutionalization, lack of perceived benefit, and death. The fate of patients "lost to follow-up" is important to determine insofar as is possible. Prospective study cohorts may become less representative of the general MS population as cases are lost. For example, those "lost to follow-up" may have been only those who were more severely disabled or who died during the course of the study.

Measurements of disability or clinical disease activity are rarely defined and standardized so that they can be used in the same manner by different examiners. Inter- and intrarater variability of disability scoring systems may not be considered when determining change in functional status and may diminish the validity of calculated rates of exacerbation or disability progression.

Interventions. The population being observed should ideally not be subjected to therapeutic interventions that could alter clinical disease activity. It is recognized, however, that most patients are treated empirically with steroids and increasing numbers of patients are treated with immunosuppressive drugs. Few patients remain untreated.

Definition of Key Terms Relevant to Characterizing the Cohort. It may be difficult to compare studies with one another because of imprecisely defined terms. Consider the definitions of the following terms when reviewing natural history studies and clinical trials.

Diagnostic criteria. Are the diagnostic criteria specifically stated? Do the criteria demand objective verification of subjective complaints? For example, if a patient reported an attack, was an examination required to substantiate a deterioration in functional status? Are the criteria in different studies sufficiently similar to permit a comparison of the data?

Initial disease site. Was the site assigned based upon subjective or objective information? Which site was assigned if the patient experienced more than one complaint or had more than one finding? Were the initial sites defined in such a way that we are reasonably certain of accuracy? For example, are sensory symptoms of spinal or brainstem origin? Is ataxia attributable to cerebellar or brainstem disease?

Disease duration. Is this determined from the time of first symptoms or the time of diagnosis? This may substantially affect the mean disease duration of a cohort. If it is from the time of first symptom was objective verification available or required?

Exacerbation. Is this term defined subjectively or objectively? How long must signs or symptoms last to count as an exacerbation and how long can worsening continue and still be considered an exacerbation as opposed to chronic progression? For example, what if worsening continues for 6 months as opposed to 1 month? What happens if a patient worsens, is stable for a week and then worsens again? Is this one or two exacerbations? Do the authors consider an exacerbation has occurred if worsening is associated with a fever or urinary tract infection? Were these possibilities considered? Exacerbation rates may also vary within a single study if exacerbations were determined retrospectively for a portion of the disease course and prospectively for another.

Disease type: relapsing/remitting, relapsing/progressive, stable, chronic progressive. How are the relapsing/remitting and relapsing/progressive patients distinguished? Is an objective or subjective measure of change in level of disability required to assign a disease type? Are the magnitude and duration of change required clarified? If an objective measure is used in assigning a disease type, does the required change exceed the variability of the scoring system when used by a single examiner (intrarater variability) or by multiple examiners (interrater variability)?

Indices of disease progression. Scoring systems often employ poorly-defined terms such as "mild" or "moderate", may be insensitive to some types of functional change (e.g., weighted heavily towards ambulation instead of upper extremity function or activities of daily living), or may detect functional changes that are not directly attributable to disease activity (e.g., they may detect changes due to medication, fatigue, or infection). It is important to define precisely the terms related to impairment scales, and to determine and state the operating characteristics of whatever test instrument is used. What are the *statistical* characteristics of the disability scoring system that was used? Are disability grades ordered but of unequal steps (ordinal scale) or ordered with equal intervals between the disability grades (equal interval or ratio scale). Comparing an average change in DSS score over 1 year for patients with mild disability (e.g., DSS = 1–3) and moderate disability (DSS = 4–6) may be misleading since it has been shown that "staying times" are longer at higher disability levels using the Kurtzke Expanded Disability Status Scale (EDSS) (Kurtzke 1983; Weinshenker 1991a,b). Failure to recognize this might result in a false impression that patients at lower EDSS levels were progressing more rapidly than patients at higher levels.

Mortality rates. Mortality rates are most informative when indicating the number of deaths attributable to the disease within a specified unit of time (e.g., year) per 100 000 population. Figures may be imprecise when the cause of death is multiple or uncertain, undocumented, diagnostically inaccurate or miscoded, or when cases are lost to follow-up. Survival times obtained by including cases from "onset' will be longer than those obtained from the date they first entered a designated period of observation. Rates determined by analysis of life tables take into account only those patients who were evaluated at the beginning of an observation period. This corrects for withdrawals or additions to the population during the time of observation (Kurtzke 1984). An adjustment of these rates for the distribution of age groups in a standard population (age-adjusted death rates) insures that the observed differences are not due to different age distributions of the study populations. These factors undoubtedly explain some of the discrepancies in death rates reported in different studies.

Selected Descriptions of MS Cohorts

Most published series report retrospective cross-sectional data for selected samples of MS patients gathered at tertiary care centers. Muller published the first carefully detailed cross-sectional data for 810 patients in 1949 (Muller 1949). Fifty-six percent of his population was female. The age of disease onset was less than 25 years in 51% of his population. Thirty percent experienced the onset of symptoms between the ages of 25 and 34 years and 17% after the age of 35 years. The onset symptoms were distributed as follows: balance disturbance 23%, impaired sensation 22%, optic neuritis 20%, paraparesis 14%, monoparesis 14% and diplopia 13%. The percentages of his population requiring assistance for ambulation (EDSS equivalent of ⩾6.0) were 44% at 5 years, 56% at 10 years, and 66% at 15 years. Of his population 6% were dead 5 years after disease onset, and 33% 15 years after disease onset.

McAlpine et al. (McAlpine and Compston 1952) reported cross-sectional data for 475 patients, 65% of whom were female. The age of onset was analyzed according to disease type in this study. A younger age of onset was observed in relapsing/remitting (RR) than in chronic/progressive (CP) patients. Fifty-four percent of RR and 21% of CP patients experienced symptom onset at age 29 years or younger whereas 10% of RR and 28% of CP patients experienced symptom onset after age 40 years. The percentage of CP patients in the total population increased with patient age from 3.5% at ages 20–24 to 33% at ages 50–54. A characterization of onset symptoms was not reported for this population. The percentage of patients requiring assistance to ambulate was 18% at 5 years, 32% at 10 years and 43% at 15 years. Mortality was reported as 13%, 17% and 19% at 5, 10, and 15 years respectively after symptom onset.

Panelius et al. (Panelius 1969) reported cross-sectional data for 146 patients of whom 62% were female. The percentage of patients was 11%, 48%, 29% and 1% for ages of onset below 20, 20–29, 30–39, and above 50 years respectively. Symptoms at onset were recorded as motor or coordination in 33%, brainstem in 24%, sensory in 22% and visual in 21% of patients. The percentages of patients requiring assistance to ambulate were 15%, 31%, and 39% at 5, 10, and 15 years respectively. Mortality data were not reported.

Weinshenker et al. reported cross-sectional data for 1099 patients, 66% of whom were female, in a geographically-based population study in 1989 (Weinshenker 1989a). The median age of onset was 29 years. Initial symptoms were reported by patients as follows; sensory 45%, motor 20%, optic neuritis 17%, diplopia/vertigo 13% and limb ataxia/loss of balance 13%. The disease course was described as relapsing/remitting in 65%, relapsing/progressive in 15%, and chronic/progressive in 19% at final analysis. The median time to reach DSS 3.0 was 7.7 years and DSS 6.0 was 15 years for the total population

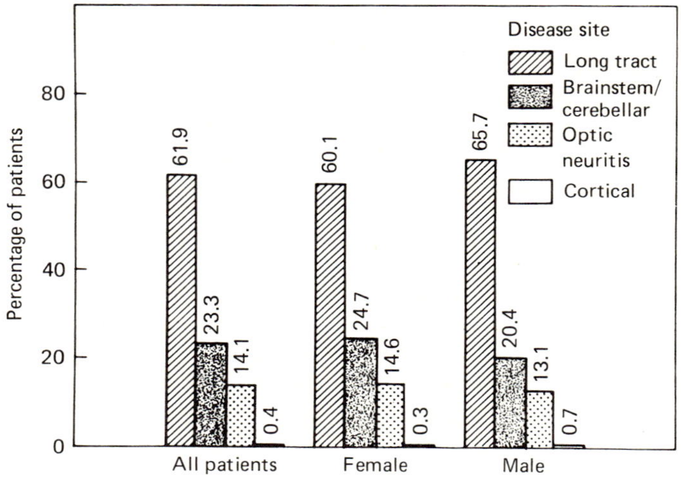

Fig. 2.1. Initial disease site (n = 425). Reproduced with permission, Arch Neurol 46:1008–1112 (1989). Copyright 1989, American Medical Association.

studied. A subgroup of patients followed since disease onset reached DSS 3.0 in 6.3 years and DSS 6.0 in 9.4 years.

Goodkin et al. (1989) published cross-sectional data obtained at initial visit for 425 clinically definite or clinically probable MS patients (Poser et al. 1983). These patients lived in a well-demarcated geographical area (population 550 000) in which there were limited alternatives for neurological care. The case ascertainment rate was ≥77% of the patients registered from North Dakota by The North Star Chapter of The National Multiple Sclerosis Society (NMSS) in 1987. The patients were examined by a single neurologist every 6 months over a period of 1–5 years (mean 2.6 years) using operational definitions of terms relevant to their clinical course. The "initial disease site" for patients in this study was defined using the patient's history and findings on neurological examination at the time of initial presentation. Where presentation antedated intake to the clinic, old neurological examination records were required to assign the initial site. Where multiple symptoms occurred, the first noted by the patient was taken as the initial site. "Optic neuritis" was defined as monocular decrease in visual acuity with central or centrocecal scotoma lasting longer than 5 days. "Brainstem/cerebellar" was defined as cranial nerve deficits with or without motor and/or sensory long tract findings or internuclear ophthalmoplegia or ataxia or crossed sensory findings involving face and body. "Long tract motor/sensory" was defined as weakness or sensory deficit without associated ataxia or cranial nerve findings. "Cortical/cerebral" was defined as higher cognitive dysfunction manifest by impairment in memory, confusion, deteriorating job performance or interpersonal relationships without accompanying focal weakness or sensory disturbance or alternative explanation, or as a visual field deficit referable to optic radiation or tract.

The percentages of patients experiencing specific initial disease sites are presented in Fig. 2.1. The definitions of disease-course types at *study entry* are

Table 2.2. Definition of disease type at entry, based on patient and family history and record review at study entry

	Objective exacerbation	Time period (yr)	Worsening activities of daily living	Improve to baseline
Stable	No	2	No	NA
Relapsing/remitting stable	Yes	2	Yes	Yes
Relapsing/remitting progressive	Yes	2	Yes	No
Chronic/progressive	No	2	Yes	No

Table 2.3. Expanded disability status score (EDSS) and disease duration according to initial disease site

Disease site	n = 425	EDSS[a] Mean ± SD	Disease duration[b] Mean ±SD (years)
Long tract	265	4.35 ± 2.58	13.88 ± 11.45
Brainstem/cerebellar	100	4.76 ± 2.28	12.21 ±9.36
Optic neuritis	60	3.35 ± 1.89	13.62 ± 11.01

Reproduced with permission Arch Neurol 46:1008–1112 (1989). Copyright 1989, American Medical Association.

[a] The EDSS score for female patients with optic neuritis was significantly lower than the scores for other initial disease sites ($p = 0.002$; $F = 6.433$).

[b] No significant difference was found in disease duration (years) for differing initial disease sites ($p = 0.571$; $F = 0.570$).

Table 2.4. Disease duration and EDSS according to disease type

Disease type	n = 425	EDSS[a] Mean ± SD	Disease duration[b] Mean ±SD
Stable	80	3.83 ± 2.51	15.97 ± 13.09
Relapsing/remitting stable	155	2.63 ± 1.71	8.69 ± 8.22
Relapsing/remitting progressive	48	4.49 ± 2.13	9.59 ± 6.17
Chronic/progressive	142	6.38 ± 1.74	18.58 ± 10.84

Reproduced with permission Arch Neurol 46:1008–1112 (1989) Copyright 1989, American Medical Association.

[a] Mean EDSS values significantly differ between disease types ($p = 0.0001$; $F = 94.714$).

[b] The mean disease durations were significantly different when compared by types ($p < 0.0001$; $F = 28.37$).

summarized in Table 2.2. The relationships between disease course, site of first symptom, disease duration and level of disability as measured by Kurtzke EDSS score are presented in Tables 2.3 and 2.4. In summary, greater disability was observed with increasing disease duration and chronic progressive course. Optic neuritis, as the initial disease site, was associated with a lower EDSS score in female patients when controlling for disease duration.

What Is the Prospect for Survival for MS Patients?

It is important to know what percentage of MS patients will die from MS or related problems and to be able to predict those patients who are at high risk to do so. A significant reduction in survival time is frequently reported in earlier studies. These data are difficult to interpret because of retrospective data acquisition (Muller 1949), small sample size (Allison 1950) or hospital- rather than clinic-based data collection (McAlpine 1961). Additionally, these studies were performed during the pre-antibiotic era.

Kurtzke et al. (1977) estimated a mean survival period exceeding 30 years in US male armed service veterans. Weinshenker et al. (1989a) reported a median survival time of 15.1 years for their total population of 1099 patients. A subgroup of their total population followed since onset of disease sustained only one death in 197 patients followed a mean of 4.2 years.

Phadke (1987) presented data on 1055 patients who had been followed for more than 10 years as part of an epidemiological investigation. A centralized record-keeping system of death certificates for the region enabled continuous monitoring of the entire population for recorded deaths. Between 1970 and 1980, 216 deaths occurred and the mean survival time was 24.5 years. Information was recorded for sex, age at onset, initial symptoms, course of disease, and survival calculated from the year of first symptom. Initial symptoms and course of disease were clearly defined. There was no difference in time of survival between sexes. The life expectancy of the patients compared to the Scottish general population using life table analysis demonstrated only a slight reduction in short-term (<10 years) survival in all age groups with the exception of those with onset age above 50 years. A 44% reduction in survival for males and 22% for females was observed in the latter age group. Long-term (≥10 years) life expectancy was markedly reduced in all age groups compared with controls. In the 40–49-year-old disease-onset group, only 26% of females and 5% of males were alive at 30 years after onset compared to 70% of females and 60% of males for age-matched general population controls. Survival time also correlated with level of disability at the time of the initial examination. A mean of 94% of those without significant disability survived 10 years compared to 28% of those who were no longer functional ambulators. Similar results have been reported by others (Hyllested 1961; Gudmendsson 1971). Survival was significantly shorter for those patients in all age groups who sustained a relapse within 6 months of disease onset, compared to those whose relapse occurred later than 6 months, and for those who had a progressive course since onset as opposed to a relapsing course. Patients with cerebellar symptoms at onset had a significantly shorter survival, and those with optic neuritis or isolated brainstem initial symptoms had longer survival than those with other presentations. Sixty-two percent died of causes directly related to MS (pneumonia, sepsis), 12% from hematological or malignant disease, and 19% from coronary artery disease.

The possibility that additional illnesses might contribute to death rates in MS patients has also been considered. Zimmerman et al. reported an uncontrolled series of 41 autopsied MS cases in which an insignificant increase in the prevalence of coexistent malignant disease was noted (Zimmerman and Netsky 1950). This trend has not been seen by others (Kurtzke et al. 1970; Allen et al. 1978).

In summary, survival is reduced in MS patients compared to age-matched population controls. Data suggest that survival is predominantly influenced by older age of onset, male sex, and advanced level of disability at initial examination.

What Is the Outcome of a Single Exacerbation?

The data available to answer this question are limited. Definitions of exacerbation, course of onset and progression, frequency of examinations, stabilization, resolution or chronic-progression are generally lacking.

In 1949 Muller reviewed 1850 case records from which 810 (44% male) were felt to have a verifiable diagnosis of MS (Muller 1949). All patients received treatment at one of four different hospitals or the private practice of one neurologist between 1920 and 1945. Seventy-one percent of the patients were followed for more than 5 years (mean 9.7 years). Approximately 50% of the patients were seen within 2 years of symptom onset and 11% of the patients had experienced symptoms for more than 15 years prior to neurological assessment. Definitions of exacerbation were subjective, and antedated the current era of widely accepted diagnostic criteria and disability scoring scales. Nonetheless, Muller's data remain important and first established the notion that recovery rates from initial symptoms were inversely related to symptom duration (Table 2.5).

Kurtzke (1961) published data regarding the clinical course following a single bout of MS. This hospital-based study of clinically definite MS patients (Schumacher et al. 1965) included predominantly male US army recruits who demonstrated objective deterioration in their neurological status. Patients experienced either an "acute attack superimposed on a previously healthy or stable individual, or onset of accelerating deterioration in an individual with chronic progressive MS". In the hospital 220 patients were observed for more than 104 days. None of the patients was treated with steroids or immuno-

Table 2.5. Patients experiencing complete recovery from initial symptoms[a]

Initial symptom	Percent recovery by duration of symptom	
	<2 months	≥2 months
Diplopia	94	16
"Giddiness"	86	NA[b]
Paresthesia	83	25
Hemiparesis	57	NA
Optic neuritis	56	12
Monoparesis	45	33

Adapted from Muller (1949).
[a] Less than 5% of patients who completely recovered had symptoms that lasted more than 6 months.
[b] Data not available.

Table 2.6. Clinical course of patients during hospitalization: effect of pre-hospital episode duration

	Improved (%)	Same (%)	Worse (%)
Group B[a]	0	82	12
Group A[b]	33	50	17

Adapted from Kurtzke (1961).
[a] Pre-hospital episode duration >2 years. Mean hospitalization 7.7 months.
[b] Pre-hospital episode duration ≤2 years. Mean hospitalization 104 days.

Table 2.7. Correlation of clinical course after discharge and during hospitalization

	Course after discharge (% of patients) (mean follow-up period 17 months)		
	Better	Same	Worse
After discharge	39	46	15
In hospital course			
improved	24	33	43
unchanged	12	20	68
worse	0	63	37

Adapted from Kurtzke (1961).

suppressant therapy. The patients were divided into two groups. Group A consisted of 175 patients whose "admitting episode was of ≤2 years duration prior to hospitalization". The mean disease duration of this group was 4.5 years. Group B consisted of 45 patients whose "admitting episode was of >2 years duration prior to hospital admission". Their mean disease duration was 9.6 years. All patients were examined and assigned a DSS at admission and again at discharge. All attacks were accompanied by objective changes on neurological examination. A change of condition (better, worse) between admission and discharge required an appropriate change of 1 or more points on the DSS. Patients with a shorter pre-hospital episode duration (Group A) experienced a greater chance of clinical improvement during hospitalization (Table 2.6).

Clinical follow-up for 2–80 months (mean 17 months) after discharge from the hospital was maintained for 172 patients from Kurtzke's study. The post-hospitalization clinical course correlated positively with their clinical course in the hospital. More patients who improved during hospitalization showed continued improvement after discharge than those who failed to show improvement while in the hospital (Table 2.7). The clinical course of patients during hospitalization or after discharge did not correlate with age, initial signs on examination (e.g., pyramidal, cerebellar), age of disease onset by symptom, history of prior remission following attack, severity of disease on admission by DSS score, disease duration prior to admission, or cerebrospinal fluid (CSF) protein, cells or colloidal gold curve. There was, however, a striking inverse correlation between percentage improved and the duration of the episode

Table 2.8. Clinical course during hospitalization: influence of episode duration prior to hospitalization

Duration of episode	% Improved
<7 days	86
8–14 days	64
15–31 days	38
>1 month	14
>2 years	<2

Adapted from Kurtzke (1961).

prompting hospitalization (Table 2.8). Higher rates of remission from attacks (85%) have been reported by other authors (McAlpine and Compston 1952) but this may reflect the inclusion of patients whose first episodes of neurologic dysfunction was attributable to one locus (e.g., optic neuritis). Kurtzke's population consisted predominantly of patients who experienced more than one symptom at onset.

What Is the Frequency of Exacerbations in MS Patients?

Exacerbation rates are calculated by determining the number of exacerbations each year of retrospective or prospective follow-up. Clearly the rate depends upon the definition of exacerbation. There is a general notion that the frequency of exacerbations decreases with time although the evidence for this is conflicting. Muller used data derived from reviewing retrospective records and reported decreasing frequency of "bouts" with increasing duration of disease (Muller 1949). Although Thygessen examined patients prospectively for 18 months, his determination of declining yearly exacerbation rates was also based upon comparison to retrospective data for that cohort (Thygessen 1955). Fog and Linnemann (1970) followed patients longitudinally with yearly examinations for an average of 9 years. They defined exacerbations subjectively as "... episodic exacerbations which have either been observed by the patient as being so pronounced that they have altered his condition ... in the form of a deficit symptom, or have been observed by his family." Interestingly, exacerbation rates did not decline during that 9-year observation period.

Authors most frequently refer to McAlpine (McAlpine and Compston 1952) and Leibowitz (Leibowitz et al. 1964) when quoting declining exacerbation rates with increasing disease duration. McAlpine's data were based on a review of medical records undertaken between 1948 and 1950 from patients seen predominantly at the Middlesex Hospital from 1930 to 1950. He also followed a subgroup of patients prospectively. The exacerbations in his material were defined subjectively and the extent to which objective correlation was present cannot be determined. Calculated exacerbation rates were determined from a mixture of retrospective and prospective data. Although a tendency for decreasing exacerbation rates with time was reported, it was not recognizable for more than 10 years after disease onset. Leibowitz et al. completed a country-wide survey of patients with MS in Israel in 1961. Cases were obtained by record review but those patients with "probable or possible" MS were personally examined. Although exacerbations were defined, patients were examined infrequently and data regarding the exacerbations were largely retrospective. Leibowitz et al. stated the exacerbation rates were "inexact" and at best "an approximation".

Decreasing exacerbation rates were also reported in a more recent study by Broman et al. (1981). This study also compared rates obtained retrospectively and prospectively. Exacerbation was not defined and it is unclear how frequently patients were reexamined.

Goodkin et al. (1989) determined yearly operationally defined exacerbation rates in prospectively followed patients. These patients were examined every 6 months or sooner upon report of functional deterioration. Objective change in examination rather than subjective report was required for exacerbation. Patients received ACTH or prednisone for 2 weeks if clinically indicated for exacerbation. No patient received immunomodulatory medications. There was no significant change in yearly total or individual patient exacerbation rates during 3 years of prospective follow-up, even when patients were stratified by disease duration (Table 2.9). In contrast, Goodkin et al. (1991) did demonstrate a significant decline in identically defined exacerbation rates over 2 years in placebo-treated patients participating in a funded clinical trial of azathioprine in relapsing MS. Exacerbations in these patients were also treated with ACTH or prednisone for 2 weeks when clinically indicated.

Table 2.9. Prospectively determined total exacerbation rates in patients stratified by disease duration

Year of follow-up	No.	Disease (duration in years)	Rate[a] (mean ±SD)
1	34	1–3	0.68 ± 0.84
	22	4–8	0.64 ± 1.09
	32	>8	0.67 ± 0.87
Total	88	–	0.65 ± 0.91
2	23	1–3	0.57 ± 0.73
	14	4–8	0.86 ± 0.86
	20	>8	0.50 ± 0.89
Total	57	–	0.61 ± 0.82
3	11	1–3	0.73 ± 1.01
	5	4–8	0.80 ± 0.84
	10	>8	0.50 ± 0.85
Total	26	–	0.65 ± 0.89

Reproduced with permission, Arch Neurol 46:1008–1112 (1989). Copyright 1989, American Medical Association.

[a] No significant difference in mean total exacerbation rates for years 1 through 3 ($p = 0.9573$; $F = 0.03$). No significant differences in total exacerbation rates within years when stratified by disease duration: year 1 ($p = 0.9603$; $F = 0.03$); year 2 ($p = 0.4339$; $F = 0.85$); and year 3 ($p = 0.7903$; $F = 0.24$).

In summary, with the notable exception of Fog and Linnemann (1970), investigators report that the frequency of subjectively defined exacerbations decreases with increasing disease duration. This rate reduction is most noticeable several years after disease onset. The decline in exacerbation rates observed in some retrospective studies may in part be an artifact of definition. For example, the definition of exacerbation within a single study might be determined retrospectively for the early years after diagnosis and prospectively for the later years after the patient is being followed longitudinally. The decline in rate may also be a reflection of conversion to chronic progressive disease course rather than clinical stabilization over time. The frequency of objectively defined exacerbations in an untreated cohort of longitudinally followed MS patients was reported to be relatively constant during a 3-year observation period, even when patients are stratified by disease duration (Goodkin et al. 1989). The frequency of exacerbations in these untreated patients for longer periods of time remains unknown. Placebo-treated patients participating in a clinical trial do, on the other hand, experience a reduction in identically defined exacerbation rates (Goodkin et al. 1991). The extent to which this represents a placebo effect or regression to the mean (Weinshenker et al. 1989b, 1991a) is uncertain. This finding must be taken into account in the design of clinical trials of experimental therapeutic agents and is more fully discussed in Chap. 3.

Can We Predict the Eventual Functional Status of MS Patients?

The first comprehensive assessment of functional status over time was reported by Muller in 1949 (Muller 1949). A loss of independent ambulation or a complete loss of ambulatory status, equivalent to an EDSS score ⩾6.0, was reported for 44%, 56%, and 66% of this population at 5, 10, and 15 years disease duration. In this series of 810 personally-examined cases, patients who retained their ambulatory status were more likely female, younger than age 25 at disease onset, had relapsing/remitting disease type, or experienced sensory or cranial nerve symptoms at onset. Lower levels of disability at 5 years predicted milder disability at time points thereafter. Motor or cerebellar symptoms at onset were associated with greater disability after 10 or more years.

McAlpine (1961) reported a mixed clinic/hospital-based cohort of 241 cases of MS seen within 3 years of disease onset. All cases had clinically-definite or probable MS, 62% were female, and all cases were examined annually by the author. Exacerbations were defined subjectively. The mixed retrospective and prospective "observation" period for each patient exceeded 10 years. The authors reported that 58% and 66% of patients were no longer ambulatory or required assistance to ambulate 10 years and 15 years after disease onset. One-third of their patients at both 10 and 15 years experienced no "impairment in their work or domestic activities". These patients were considered to represent a subgroup with a "benign" form of MS. Poser (1978) similarly found that 33%

of her 812 MS patients were still working and 40% still walking 15 years after disease onset. Patients with a "benign" course in McAlpine's series were more likely to have a relapsing course, optic neuritis or monosymptomatic onset, and absence of lower extremity weakness or pyramidal signs within 3 years of disease onset. Disability level at 5 years predicted disability level at time points thereafter.

Leibowitz et al. (1964) reported a retrospective, clinic- and hospital-based cohort of 262 cases in Israel. The authors included clinically "possible" in addition to clinically definite, and probable cases in this study. Exacerbations were defined subjectively. The authors reported that 34%, 47%, and 56% of the patients required assistance to ambulate or had lost ability to ambulate by 5, 10 and 15 years after disease onset. Patients with relatively minor disability experienced a relapsing/remitting course. No correlation between sex, optic neuritis or initial motor or cerebellar symptoms was found.

Fog and Linnemann (1970) reported a population of 70 clinically-definite or probable MS patients characterized by precisely defined criteria for disease course. Exacerbations were defined subjectively. Every patient was examined by the author every 3 months for an average of 9 years. Objectively-measured disability was found to worsen at varying rates in more than 90% of his patients with passing time and failed to correlated with sex, or age of onset. Relapsing/remitting patients and those presenting with optic neuritis experienced less severe disability with passing time.

Kurtzke et al. (1977) extended his earlier study (Kurtzke 1956) of US army recruits who were hospitalized with MS by obtaining follow-up data for 476 clinically-definite and 51 clinically-probable (Schumacher et al. 1965) MS patients. In contrast to his initial study in which patients were examined by Kurtzke or his staff, follow-up data were obtained by reviewing the records of neurological examinations performed by many different neurologists throughout the United States. The temporal relationship of these follow-up examinations and clinical stability or exacerbation is not clear, nor is their use of steroids or other treatments at the time of examination. Examinations for 293 patients who experienced their initial bout before army entry and 234 patients who experienced their initial bout in the army were abstracted and functional system scores (FSS) and Kurtzke DSS scores were assigned and recorded for 5, 10, 15, and 20 years after onset and 10 and 15 years after diagnosis. Twenty percent of the patients experienced a benign course, defined as a DSS = 0–2 over 15 years of longitudinal follow-up. No relationship between socioeconomic status, education, DSS score, brainstem, sensory, sphincter, cerebral FSSs, age of disease onset from first symptom, CSF findings (total protein, cell count or colloidal gold curve), severity (DSS) of the onset bout, or frequency of bouts during the first 5 years after diagnosis and DSS score at 10 and 15 years was found. A weak relationship (r = 0.19–0.41) was evident at those times for cerebellar and pyramidal FSSs, and the total number of FSSs involved at the time of first examination. A strong relationship was found for the patients' DSS score at 5 years after symptom onset and their DSS score recorded later at 10 and 15 years. A DSS score of 0–2 at 5 years after symptom onset predicted a DSS score of 0–2 at 10–15 years and a DSS score above 6 at 5 years predicted a DSS score of above 6 at 10–15 years (r = 0.61–0.81) (Table 2.10). A similar but less striking relationship was seen for the pyramidal and cerebellar FSSs at 5 years.

Table 2.10. Predicting DSS score at 15 years from DSS score at 5 years

DSS at year 5	DSS at year 15 (%)	
	0–2	>6
DSS 0–2	66	11
3–5	14	40
>6	1	99
FSS 0–2	72	5
>3	0	88

Adapted from Kurtzke (1977).

Sibley (1985) followed 170 serial MS patients from 1976 to 1984. These patients were interviewed monthly by telephone and examined every 3 months or whenever worsening was reported and assigned FSS and DSS scores. Patients did not receive any immunomodulatory drug during the mean follow-up period of 5.3 years. Exacerbations were treated with ACTH for 10–14 days. Baseline DSS scores correlated positively with increasing age and disease duration. All patients experienced an increase in DSS score during the observation period. The increases were of greater magnitude in patients who were younger, had shorter disease durations and had relatively lower disability scores. This superficially suggests that disease activity was greatest in patients at the lower end of the DSS scale. The significance of disproportionately greater progression at the lower end of the DSS becomes moot when the non-linear nature of the DSS is taken into account (Kurtzke 1989; Weinshenker et al. 1991a). It is, therefore, difficult to translate the observed differences in magnitude of DSS score change at specific scale levels to degree of disease activity.

Wolfson and Confavreux (1987) and Confavreux and Wolfson (1989) developed mathematical models to predict the clinical course of patients based upon sex, mode of onset, and length of first remission. Inconsistent results observed with these mathematical models limit their predictive value in individual patients. Multivariate mathematical models have similarly been shown to have limited predictive value to individual MS patients (Weinshenker et al. 1991b).

Weinshenker et al. (1989b) reported the natural history of a geographically-based study of 1099 consecutive cases of MS. The data in this study were analyzed for the total population (TP) of patients, a subgroup of 196 patients from Middlesex county (MC) that represented a population-based group for which case ascertainment was 90% complete, and a separate subgroup of 197 patients who were "seen from onset" (SO). The SO group consisted of 114 patients seen within 12 months of onset, 34 seen between 1 and 2 years of onset and 49 seen more than 2 years after onset (range not reported). With the exception of the SO subgroup, the TP were mainly institutionalized patients with advanced levels of disability. Retrospective record review was used to characterize the early phase of the illness in those patients. Quantitation of disability (DSS) during that phase of the illness was done by medical record review rather than by patient examination. Diagnostic criteria were defined (Poser 1983) but descriptive terms such as relapsing/remitting, relapsing/progressive, chronic/progressive were not. Exacerbations were defined subjectively and did not require an objective change in functional assessment. The duration of an attack or interval required between episodes to qualify as separate attacks as opposed to a prolonged single attack was not provided. Attack frequency was determined retrospectively and prospectively in all patients except those in the SO group who were actually seen since onset. Mean disease duration in the total population was 11.9 years and 4.2 years in the SO subgroup. Age of onset was approximately 30 years in both groups. The authors found that the frequency of conversion from remitting to progressive MS was positively correlated with disease duration for the TP, MC, and SO subgroups. Over half of the initially remitting patients entered a progressive phase within 10 years of onset. Forty percent of the SO patients followed for more than 5 years also developed progressive disease. In contrast, only 10.3% of SO subgroup patients followed for less than 5 years had converted from remitting to progressive course.

Weinshenker et al. (1989b) also compared the longitudinal progression of disability in a population of previously diagnosed MS patients to that of a recently diagnosed ("since onset") patient population. The mean time from onset of disease to a progressive phase was 5.8 years for the total population and 1.8 years for the since onset (SO) subgroup. Of the total population 33% had reached DSS 6 (walking with unilateral assistance at 10 years from onset, as did 55% of the SO group. The SO patients experiencing three or more subjectively defined attacks during the first 2 years of their illness reached DSS 3–6 more frequently, and in a significantly shorter time than those with ≤2 attacks (Table 2.11). Other authors using objective as opposed to subjective criteria to define exacerbations did not find that attack frequency predicted future disability levels in MS patients during mean observation periods exceeding 9 years (Kurtzke et al. 1977; Fog and Linnemann 1970).

Goodkin et al. (1989) also reported increasing mean EDSS score with increasing disease duration from first symptom for a population of 425 MS patients (Fig. 2.2). The highest EDSS scores were found in the relapsing/progressive and chronic/progressive disease types (Table 2.2). The other relevant clinical and demographic characteristics at the time of first examination for this population are presented in Figs 2.1–2.4. The relative lack of patients at the EDSS 4.0–5.5 has been noted in other populations

Table 2.11. Percentage of patients reaching designated DSS by disease duration and attack frequency

Disease duration	Attacks during study year 0–2	Number	Percentage reaching	
			DSS3	DSS6
2–3 years	≤2	22	13	0
	≥3	22	27	23
4–5 years	≤2	22	23	9
	≥3	17	53	47

Adapted from Weinshenker (1989a).

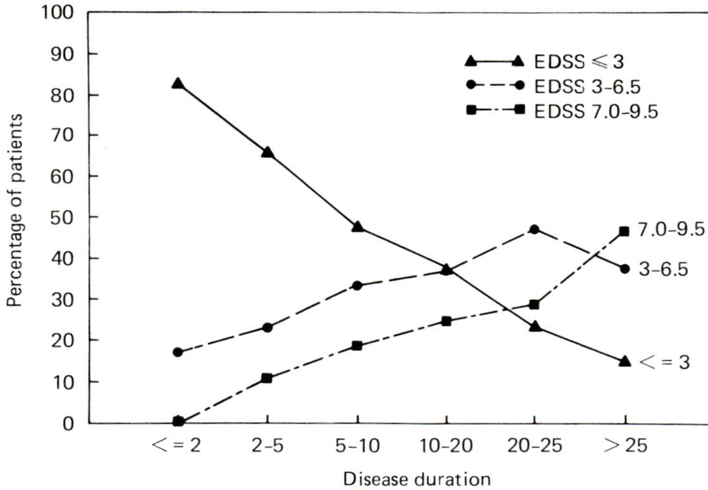

Fig. 2.2. Average EDSS score and disease duration (n = 425). Reproduced with permission, Arch Neurol 46:1008–1112 (1989). Copyright 1989, American Medical Association.

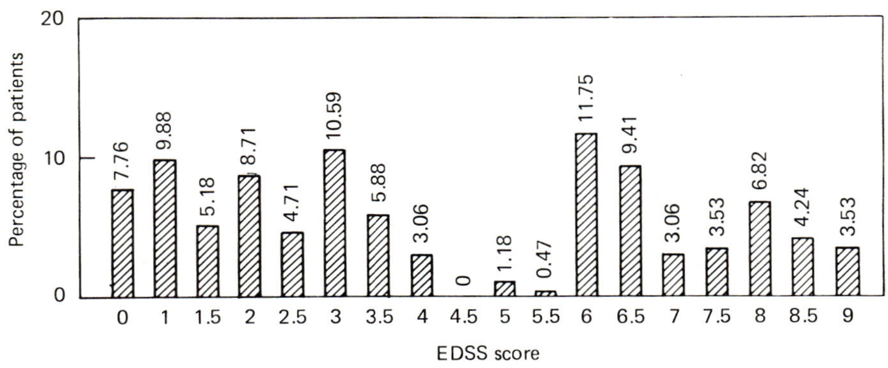

Fig. 2.3. Current EDSS scores (n = 425). Reproduced with permission, Arch Neurol 46:1008–1112 (1989). Copyright 1989, American Medical Association.

(Weinshenker et al. 1989a) (for further discussion of EDSS see Chap. 4). The patients in this study were all examined and assigned EDSS scores by the same neurologist every 6 months. Disease was defined using the Washington Panel criteria (Poser et al. 1983) and operational definitions were employed for initial disease sites, clinical course and exacerbation. The authors found that relapsing/remitting disease course and initial symptom of optic neuritis in females predicted relatively lower disability levels with time (Tables 2.3 and 2.4). No correlation between sex, age of onset, or initial disease site (excluding optic neuritis in females), and level of disability was noted.

Goodkin et al. (1989) also monitored adherence to operationally-defined disease types during a mean longitudinal follow-up period of 2.6 years. Each

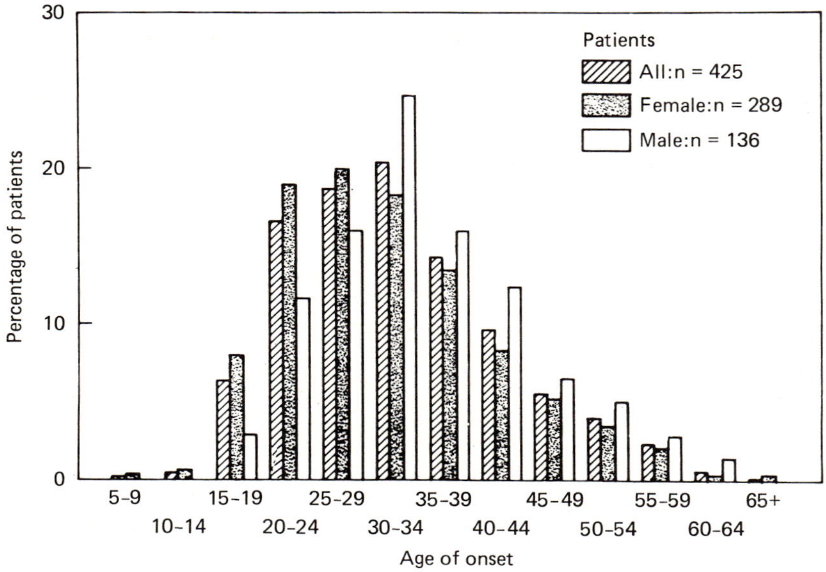

Fig. 2.4. Age of onset of MS (n = 425). Reproduced with permission, Arch Neurol 46: 1008–1112 (1989). Copyright 1989, American Medical Association.

patient was assigned a disease type at study entry according to their disease course during the prior 2 years and was recharacterized each year thereafter while maintaining longitudinal follow-up. The distributions of disease types for those patients entering the study (n = 425) and those choosing not to maintain follow-up (n = 262) were similar, suggesting that disease type did not contribute to patient attrition (Fig. 2.5). Ninety-two percent of the subgroup that did not return for follow-up responded to a standardized questionnaire designed to assess reasons for discontinuing clinic visits. The most frequently cited reasons were (1) lack of perceived benefit, 39%, (2) distance from clinic or level of disability, 35%, (3) seeking a second opinion or diagnosis confirmation, 13%, (4) cost, 8%, (5) other, 5%.

The 2-year longitudinal follow-up was completed by 163 patients. A significant change in the proportion of disease types was noted in these patients as compared to those lost to follow-up (Fig. 2.6). Exacerbation in these patients was originally defined as a change of 0.5 or more points on the EDSS or 1.0 or more points on the Ambulation Index (AI) lasting between 5 and 60 days (Goodkin et al. 1989). This data was reanalyzed increasing the required change for exacerbation to 1.0 EDSS point to account for the intra-rater variability associated with serial EDSS determinations. These revised definitions for disease types are summarized in Table 2.12. The authors found that when reapplying these definitions only 43% of chronic/progressive patients remained chronic/progressive after 2 years of longitudinal follow-up. Over 44% of these chronic/progressive patients spontaneously stabilized during that same follow-up period. These data and rates of adherence to the other disease types are listed in Table 2.13. Data from 131 of the 163 patients were available for

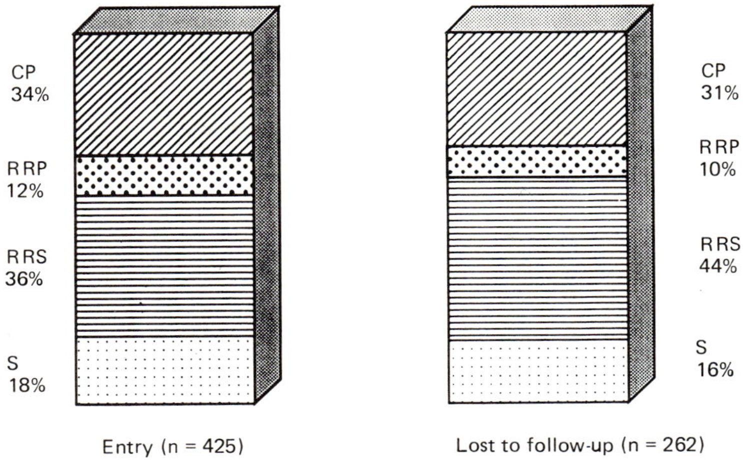

Fig. 2.5. Comparison of disease types with patients lost to follow-up. Entry, n = 425 lost to follow-up, n = 262. The difference between the disease types is not significant, Chi-square = 3.504, $p = 0.3076$.

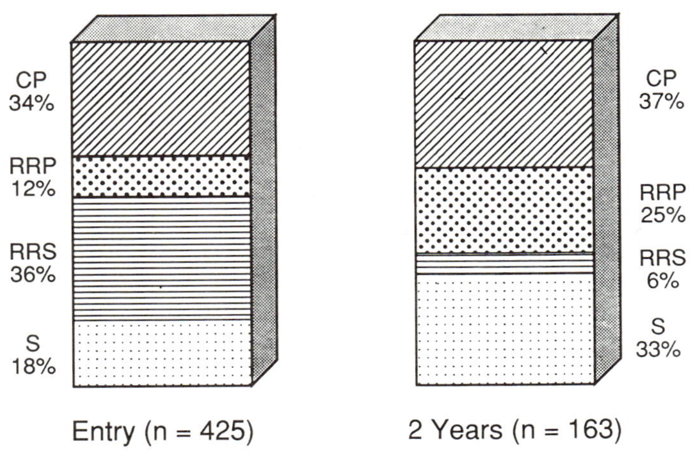

Fig. 2.6. Comparison of disease types at entry (baseline, n = 425) and at 2 years (n = 163). The difference between the disease types is significant, Chi-square = 65.70, $p = 0.0001$.

Table 2.12. Definition of disease type after entry, based on serial neurologic examinations

	Objective exacerbation	Time period (yr)	Change		Improvement to baseline
			EDSS	AI	
Stable	No	2	0	0	NA
Relapsing/remitting stable	Yes	2	⩾1.0	⩾1.0	Yes
Relapsing/remitting progressive	Yes	2	⩾1.0	⩾1.0	No
Chronic/progressive	No	1	⩾1.0	⩾1.0	No

Table 2.13. Adherence to disease type: 2-year longitudinal follow-up. (EDSS change = 1.0)

Disease type at entry	Number of patients	Disease type at 2-year longitudinal follow-up[a] (no. (%) of patients)			
		Stable	Chronic/ progressive	Relapsing/ remitting stable	Relapsing/ remitting progressive
Stable	37	27 (73.0)	7 (18.9)	0 (0)	3 (8.1)
Chronic/progressive	61	27 (44.3)	26 (42.6)	1 (1.6)	7 (11.5)
Relapsing/remitting stable	41	13 (31.7)	6 (14.6)	4 (9.8)	18 (43.9)
Relapsing/remitting progressive	24	5 (20.8)	2 (8.3)	4 (16.7)	13 (54.2)

[a] The percentage of patients adhering to different disease types was significantly different. Chi-square = 56.84; $p = 0.0001$.

analysis after 3 years of longitudinal follow-up in this study. Rates of adherence to disease type in these 131 patients during year 3 compared to year 2, as well as during year 4 compared to year 3 for those 67 of 131 patients who underwent 4 years of follow-up are presented in Table 2.14. In summary, adherence to chronic/progressive disease type during years 3 and 4 was 59% and 36%.

These findings have the following important implications for clinical trials. Some previous clinical trials restricted enrollment to patients with chronic/progressive disease because it was believed these patients had a "predictable" relentlessly progressive course during periods of longitudinal follow-up (Goodkin et al. 1989; Hauser et al. 1983). The validity of this notion is rejected by data in Tables 2.13 and 2.14 reporting that EDSS or AI stabilize in a substantial number of chronically progressive patients each year. This finding re-emphasizes the importance of proper control groups in randomized clinical trials. Additionally, data in Tables 2.13 and 2.14 illustrate that a substantial number of relapsing patients will either spontaneously stabilize or become progressive with time. Relapse rates, therefore, will not necessarily reflect disease activity since rates will fall when patients enter the chronic/progressive category. Relapse rate should not be used as a primary outcome measure in clinical trials for this reason.

We should be mindful that published data for disability progression and survival rates of MS patients may be overly pessimistic since they fail to account for the unsuspected cases that exist in the general population. These cases tend to have less evident disability. The incidental detection of clinically

Table 2.14. Adherence to disease type: 3-and 4-year follow-up. (EDSS change = 1.0)

Disease type 2 years after entry (n = 163)	n	Years	Disease type after three (n = 131) and four (n = 67) years of follow-up			
			Stable n (%)	Chronic/progressive n (%)	Relapsing/remitting stable n (%)	Relapsing/remitting progressive n (%)
Stable	66	3	41 (62.1)	21 (31.8)	0 (0)	4 (6.1)
	32	4	12 (37.5)	15 (46.9)	0 (0)	5 (15.6)
Chronic/progressive	39	3	4 (10.3)	23 (59.0)	5 (12.8)	7 (17.9)
	22	4	10 (45.5)	8 (36.4)	1 (4.5)	3 (13.6)
Relapsing/remitting stable	7	3	2 (28.6)	1 (14.3)	4 (57.1)	0 (0)
	2	4	0 (0)	0 (0)	1 (50)	1 (50)
Relapsing/remitting progressive	19	3	9 (47.4)	4 (21.1)	1 (5.3)	5 (26.3)
	11	4	2 (18.2)	6 (54.5)	3 (23.3)	0 (0)

Table 2.15. Potential prognostic markers of later disease course: selected natural history studies

			Initial symptom							Disease type		Early disability
	Female sex	Age at onset <25 yr	Optic neuritis	Sensory	Motor	Cerebellar	Cranial nerve	No. of exacerbations	Monosymptomatic onset	Relapsing	Chronic progressive	Mild disability level at 5 yr
Muller (1949)	B[a]	B	Nd	B	W	W	B	Nd	Nd	B	W	B
McAlpine and Compston (1952)	NPEF[b]	B	B	B	W	W	Nd	W	Nd	B	W	B
Kurtzke (1956)	Nd[c]	NPEF	Nd	NPEF	NPEF	NPEF	NPEF	NPEF	Nd	B	W	Nd
McAlpine (1961)	Nd	NPEF	B	Nd	W	Nd	Nd	Nd	Nd	B	W	B
Leibowitz et al. (1964)	W[d]	Nd	NPEF	NPEF	NPEF	NPEF	NPEF	Nd	Nd	B	W	Nd
Panelius (1969)	B	B	Nd	Nd	Nd	Nd	Nd	Nd	Nd	Nd	Nd	Nd
Fog and Linnemann (1970)	NPEF	NPEF	B	NPEF	W	NPEF	W	NPEF	Nd	B	W	Nd
Kurtzke et al. (1977)	NPEF	NPEF	NPEF	NPEF	W	W	NPEF	NPEF	Nd	NPEF	NPEF	B
Broman et al. (1981)	B	B	Nd	Nd	Nd	Nd	Nd	Nd	Nd	Nd	Nd	Nd
Wolfson and Confavreux (1987)	B	B	NPEF	NPEF	NPEF	NPEF	NPEF	NPEF	W	B	W	Nd
Minderhoud et al. (1988)	W	NPEF	B	NPEF	W	NPEF	NPEF	NPEF	NPEF	B	W	Nd
Goodkin et al. (1989)	NPEF	NPEF	B	Nd	Nd	NPEF	Nd	Nd	Nd	B	W	Nd
Weinshenker et al. (1989b)	B	B	B	NPEF	NPEF	W	W	W	Nd	B	W	B

[a] B = Better prognosis found as potential marker.
[b] NPEF = No prognostic effect found as potential marker.
[c] Nd = Not determined by author.
[d] W = Worse prognosis found as potential marker.

unsuspected MS found at autopsy suggests that this may not be rare (Gilbert and Sadler 1983).

A summary of selected natural history studies that report clinical prognostic markers in MS is presented in Table 2.15.

Summary

Certain demographic and disease-related features have been reported to be associated with a favorable prognosis in selected cohorts of MS patients. Female gender (Muller 1949; Weinshenker et al. 1989b; Broman et al. 1981; Wolfson and Confavreux 1987) has been associated with a more benign course in some studies and male gender in others (Leibowitz et al. 1964; Minderhoud et al. 1988). Other studies have failed to detect this correlation (Goodkin et al. 1989; Fog and Linnemann 1970; McAlpine 1961). A younger age of onset has been found to be favorable by some (Muller 1949; McAlpine and Compston 1952; Weinshenker et al. 1989b; Thygessen 1955; Broman et al. 1981; Wolfson and Confavreux 1987), but not all investigators (Goodkin et al. 1989; Kurtzke et al. 1977; Fog and Linnemann 1970; McAlpine 1961; Minderhoud et al. 1988; Alexander et al. 1958). Relapsing/remitting disease course has been associated with favorable prognosis and chronic/progressive disease has been associated with unfavorable prognosis in most series (Muller 1949; Weinshenker et al. 1989b; Goodkin et al. 1989; Kurtzke et al. 1977; Thygessen 1955; Fog and Linnemann 1970; Leibowitz et al. 1964; McAlpine 1961; Wolfson and Confavreux 1987; Minderhoud et al. 1988). A favorable prognosis has also been observed when the presenting symptom is optic neuritis by some (Weinshenker et al. 1989b; Goodkin et al. 1989; Fog and Linnemann 1970; McAlpine 1961; Minderhoud et al. 1988), but not all investigators (Kurtzke et al. 1977; Leibowitz et al. 1964; Wolfson and Confavreux 1987). Similarly, initial sensory symptoms have also been considered favorable by some (Muller 1949; McAlpine 1961) but not by others (Weinshenker et al. 1989b; Goodkin et al. 1989; Fog and Linnemann 1970; Leibowitz et al. 1964; Minderhoud et al. 1988; Kurtzke 1956). More recent studies have shown that patients with a monosymptomatic onset (e.g., optic neuritis) who also have abnormal cerebrospinal fluid oligoclonal banding or cranial magnetic resonance imaging are more likely to develop MS than similar patients with normal CSF (Moulin et al. 1983; Salmaggi et al. 1987; Kostulas et al. 1986; Miller et al. 1989; Ormerod et al. 1987). Selected cohort studies suggest that young female MS patients with a relapsing/remitting disease course who have presented to a physician with optic neuritis or sensory symptoms and have recovered fully from an initial attack are most likely to experience a benign clinical course. It is important, however, to remember that these "predictors" have only been determined in published cohorts and no reliable early prognostic marker for individual patients has yet been convincingly identified. The same caution should include individual patients with relatively mild disability 5 years after diagnosis even though they appear as a group to have a more favorable prognosis in selected cohort studies. Our inability to provide a reliable prognosis at the time or shortly after diagnosis in individual MS patients remains a frustrating reminder of our limited understanding of the pathogenesis of this disease.

Non-Traditional Methods of Determining the Natural History of MS

The definition of the natural history of any illness is restricted to some extent by the measures of clinical activity that are used. In this regard, the progression of disability in MS has traditionally been measured by scoring systems that depend predominantly on ambulatory status or survival (Kurtzke 1961; Hauser et al. 1983; Kurtzke 1983). The natural history of MS might be found to be significantly different if more sensitive measures of detecting significant changes were available. Additional measures of disability have, therefore, recently been developed in an effort to increase sensitivity of detecting clinical change in MS patients. Potvin and Tourtellotte (1985) have suggested a battery of functional status measures, parts of which have gained increasing acceptance as outcome measures in funded clinical trials. Rapidly administered tests of upper extremity function have been demonstrated to detect deteriorating function in 15% of patients who show no change on EDSS or AI (Goodkin et al. 1988).

Magnetic resonance imaging of the head and spine have shown changes in patients who have not experienced clinical activity or measurable change on EDSS (Willoughby et al. 1989; Koopmans et al. 1989). Though there is a growing consensus that MRI changes do in some way reflect disease activity this is not yet accepted by all investigators. Even though preliminary data demonstrate a correlation of MRI changes with immunologic function (Oger et al. 1987) and post-mortem areas of demyelination on brain sections (Noseworthy et al. 1985), the relationship between MRI changes and disease pathology in vivo remains largely uncharacterized. A comprehensive discussion of this topic is presented in Chap. 4.

Neuropsychological testing is an additional non-traditional method of measuring functional (cognitive) status changes in MS patients. An assessment of the comparative efficacy of neuropsychological testing, cranial MRI, and T-cell subset perturbations to predict or monitor traditionally measured functional status change is also under way in funded clinical trials by the NMSS. Preliminary data suggest that cognitive function is relatively stable over 2 years in a cohort of well characterized MS patients (Rao 1986; Filley et al. 1990). Similar stability of cognitive functioning has also been reported by Jennekens-Schinkel et al. (1989) after 4 years in a carefully characterized cohort from the Netherlands. Some individuals in this cohort deteriorated and others actually improved on test/retest performance over the 4-year period, indicating considerable variability between patient performances. Recent data demonstrates that cognitive impairment correlates with the extent of cerebral white matter involvement on cranial MRI. Correlation of neuropsychological testing and cranial MRI white-matter changes appear to be more informative than correlation of cognitive function and EDSS or other more traditional measures of disease activity (Franklin et al. 1988). This finding is intuitive since impairment of ambulatory status may predominantly reflect spinal MS plaque location. The data being collected in ongoing clinical trials should help to determine the relative correlational and predictive values of serial cranial MRI and neuropsychological testing with traditional measures of disability (EDSS).

References

Alexander L, Berkeley AW, Alexander AM (1985) Prognosis and treatment of multiple sclerosis-quantitative nosometric study. JAMA 166:1943–1949

Allen IV, Millar JHD, Hutchinson MJ (1978) General disease in 120 necropsy-proven cases of multiple sclerosis. Neuropathol Appl Neurobiol 4:279–284

Allison RS (1950) Survival in disseminated sclerosis: a clinical study of a series of cases first seen twenty years ago. Brain 73:103–120

Broman T, Andersen O, Bergmann L (1981) Clinical studies on multiple sclerosis. 1. Presentation of an incidence material from Gothenburg. Acta Neurol Scand 63:6–33

Confavreux C, Wolfson C (1989) Mathematical models and individualized outcome estimates in multiple sclerosis. Biomed Pharmacother 43:675–680

Filley CM, Heaton RK, Thompson LL, Nelson LM, Franklin GM (1990) Effects of disease course on neuropsychological functioning. In: Rao SM (ed) Neurobehavioral aspects of multiple sclerosis. Oxford University Press NY, NY 10016, pp 136–147

Fog T, Linnemann F (1970) The course of multiple sclerosis in 73 cases with computer-designed curves. Acta Neurol Scand (suppl) 47:11–175

Franklin GM, Heaton RK, Nelson LM, Filly CM, Seibert C (1988) Correlation of neuropsychological and magnetic resonance imaging findings in chronic/progressive multiple sclerosis. Neurology 38:1826–1829

Gilbert JJ, Sadler M (1983) Unsuspected multiple sclerosis. Arch Neurol 40:535–536

Goodkin DE, Hertsgaard D, Seminary J (1988) Upper extremity function in multiple sclerosis: improving assessment sensitivity with box-and-block and nine-hole-peg-tests. Arch Phys Med Rehab 69:850–854

Goodkin DE, Hertsgaard D, Rudick RA (1989) Exacerbation rates and adherence to disease type in a prospectively followed-up population with multiple sclerosis: Implications for clinical trials. Arch Neurol 46:1107–1112

Goodkin DE, Bailly RC, Teetzen ML, Hertsgaard D, Beatty WW (1991) The efficacy of azathioprine in relapsing remitting MS. Neurology 41:20–25

Gudmendsson KR (1971) Clinical studies of multiple sclerosis in Iceland–a follow-up of previous survey and reappraisal. Acta Neurol Scand 47 suppl (48):1–78

Hauser SL, Dawson DM, Lehrich JR et al. (1983) Intensive immunosuppression in progressive multiple sclerosis: a randomized three-arm study of high dose intravenous cyclophosphamide, plasma exchange, and ATCH. N Engl J Med 308:173–80

Hyllested K (1961) Lethality, duration and mortality of disseminated sclerosis in Denmark. Acta Psychiatr Scand 36:553–564

Jennekens-Schinkel AJ, Laboyrie PM, Lanser JBK, van der Velde EA (1989) Cognition in patients with multiple sclerosis after four years. J Neurol Sci 90:187–201

Koopmans RA, Li DKB, Oger JJF et al. (1989) Chronic progressive multiple sclerosis: serial magnetic resonance imaging over six months. Ann Neurol 26:248–256

Kostulas VK, Henriksson A, Link H (1986) Monosymptomatic sensory symptoms and cerebrospinal fluid immunoglobulin levels in relation to multiple sclerosis. Arch Neurol 43:447–451

Kurtzke JF (1956) Course of exacerbations of multiple sclerosis in hospitalized patients. Arch Neurol 76:175–184

Kurtzke JF (1961) On the evaluation of disability in multiple sclerosis: Neurology 11:686–694

Kurtzke JF (1983) Rating neurologic impairment in multiple sclerosis: an expanded disability status scale (EDSS). Neurology 33:1444–1452

Kurtzke JF (1984) Neuroepidemiology. Ann Neurol 16:265–277

Kurtzke JF (1989) The disability status scale for multiple sclerosis: Apologia pro DSS sua. Neurology 39:291–302

Kurtzke JF, Beebe GW, Nagler B, Nefziger MD, Auth TL, Kurland LT (1970) Studies on the natural history of multiple sclerosis. V. Longterm survival in young men. Arch Neurol 22:215–225

Kurtzke JF, Beebe GW, Nagler B, Kruland L, Auth TL (1977) Studies on the natural history of multiple sclerosis – 8. Early prognostic features of the later course of the illness. J Chronic Dis 30:819–830

Leibowitz U, Alter M, Halpern L (1964) Clinical studies of multiple sclerosis in Israel. 3. Clinical course and prognosis related to age at onset. Neurology 14:926–932

McAlpine D (1961) The benign form of multiple sclerosis. A study based on 241 cases seen within three years of onset and followed up until the tenth year or more of the disease. Brain 84:186–203

McAlpine D, Compston N (1952) Some aspects of the natural history of disseminated sclerosis. Part 1. The incidence, course, and prognosis. Part 2. Factors affecting the onset and course. Q J Med 21:135–160

Miller DH, Ormerod IEC, Rudge P, Kendall BE, Moseley IF, McDonald WI (1989) The early risk of multiple sclerosis following isolated acute syndromes of the brainstem and spinal cord. Ann Neurol 26:635–639

Minderhoud JM, van der Hoeven JH, Prange AJA (1988) Course and prognosis of chronic progressive multiple sclerosis. Acta Neurol Scand 78:10–15

Moulin D, Paty DW, Ebers GC (1983) The predictive value of CSF electrophoresis in possible MS. Brain 106:908–916

Muller R (1949) Studies on disseminated sclerosis with special reference to symptomatology, course and prognosis. Acta Med Scand (suppl) 222:1–214

Noseworthy JH, O'Brien JT, Gilbert JJ, Karlick SJ (1985) Nuclear magnetic resonance (NMR) changes in experimental allergic encephalomyelitis (EAE). Neurology 35:(Suppl 1) 259

Oger J, Willoughby E, Paty D (1987) Serial studies of relapsing multiple sclerosis: Reduced IgG secretion in vitro and reduced suppressor cell function correlate with disease activity as recognized by magnetic resonance imaging. Ann Neurol 22:152

Ormerod IEC, Miller DH, McDonald WI et al. (1987) The role of NMR imaging in the assessment of multiple sclerosis and isolated neurological lesions. A quantitative study. Brain 110:1579–1616

Panelius M (1969) Studies on epidemiological, clinical and etiological aspects of multiple sclerosis. Acta Neurol Scand 45 (suppl) 39:1–82

Phadke JG (1987) Survival pattern and cause of death in patients with multiple sclerosis: results from an epidemiological survey in north east Scotland. J Neurol Neurosurg Psychiatry 50:523–531

Poser S (1978) Multiple sclerosis. An analysis of 812 cases by means of electronic data processing. Springer-Verlag, Berlin, pp 54–66

Poser CM, Paty DW, Scheinberg L et al. (1983) New diagnostic criteria for multiple sclerosis: guidelines for research protocols. Ann Neurol 13:227–231

Potvin A, Tourtellotte W (1985) Quantitative examination of neurologic functions. Vol. 1: Scientific basis and design of instrumented tests. CRC Press, Boca Raton, Florida

Rao SM (1986) Neuropsychology of multiple sclerosis: a critical review. J Clin Exp Neuropsychol 8:503–542

Sackett DL, Haynes GR, Tugwell P (1985) Clinical epidemiology. Little, Brown and Company, Boston and Toronto, pp 159–169

Salmaggi CF, Bortoloam C, La Mantia L et al. (1987) Prognostic value of cerebrospinal fluid electrophoresis in optic neuritis and suspected multiple sclerosis. Ital J Neurol Sci (suppl) 1:77–80

Schumacher GA, Beebe GW, Kibler RF et al. (1965) Problems of experimental trials of therapy in multiple sclerosis. Ann NY Acad Sci 122:552–568

Sibley WA (1985) Semin Neurol 5:134–144

Thygessen P (1955) Disseminated sclerosis; influence of age on the different modes of progression. Acta Psychiatr Scand 30:365–374

Weinshenker BG, Bass B, Rice GPA et al. (1989a) The natural history of multiple sclerosis: a geographically based study. 1. Clinical course and disability. Brain 112:113–146

Weinshenker BG, Bass B, Rice GPA et al. (1989b) The natural history of multiple sclerosis: a geographically based study 2. Predictive value of the early course of the disease. Brain 112:1419–1428

Weinshenker BG, Rice GPA, Noseworthy JH, Carriere W, Baskerville J, Ebers GC (1991a) The natural history of multiple sclerosis a geographically based study 4. Applications to planning and interpretation of clinical therapeutic trials. Brain, in press

Weinshenker BG, Rice GPA, Noseworthy, JH, Carriere W, Baskerville J, Ebers GC (1991b) The natural history of multiple sclerosis: a geographically based study. 3 multivariate analysis of predictive factor and models of outcome. Brain, in press

Willoughby EW, Grocholwski E, Li DKB, Oger J, Kastrukoff LF, Paty DW (1989) Serial magnetic resonance scanning in multiple sclerosis: a second prospective study in relapsing patients. Ann Neurol 25:43–49

Wolfson C, Confavreux C (1987) Improvements to a simple Markov Model of the natural history of multiple sclerosis. Neuroepidemiology 6:101–115

Zimmerman HM, Netsky MG (1950) The pathology of multiple sclerosis. Research Publication of the Assoc Res Nerv Ment Diseases 28:271–312

Chapter 3

Assessing the Outcome of Experimental Therapies in Multiple Sclerosis Patients

Donald Paty, Ernest Willoughby and John Whitaker

Introduction

Some measure of clinical outcome will always be necessary in trials of treatment in MS, even if the efforts to find a laboratory test for measuring disease activity are successful. It is apparent that clinical scoring does not measure the total burden of disease, it measures the impact of the disease. The demonstration of beneficial effects on magnetic resonance scans or in CSF will never be convincing without some indication of changes for the better in the patient's clinical state.

The measures of clinical outcome most often used are those that rate the severity of each patient's neurologic dysfunction on rank order or ordinal scales (see Chap. 4) before and after treatment. A complementary measure in patients with active relapsing/remitting disease is to count the number of acute exacerbations occurring during the period of treatment. The focus is usually on trials of treatment aimed at halting the course of the disease. We will also mention measures of clinical outcome relevant to treatment of chronic symptoms and treatment aimed at speeding recovery from acute exacerbations.

Guidelines for the measurement of clinical outcome have been published by the International Federation of Multiple Sclerosis Societies (IFMSS) in the Minimal Record for Disability in MS (MRD) (National Multiple Sclerosis Society 1985). The guidelines follow the 3-tier classification of dysfunction (impairment, disability, handicap) developed by the World Health Organization (WHO 1980). The scales suggested for the measurement of these components of dysfunction in MS are given in Table 3.1. The obvious problems with terminology reflect the original titles for the MRD clinical scales that predate the WHO terminology.

The EDSS is dependent upon a detailed standard neurologic examination and therefore requires assessment of the patient by a physician. The ISS and ESS can be graded by paramedical personnel. The EDSS gives the most direct measure of changes in a patient's clinical state in response to treatment, but the other scales provide complementary information on the effects of the disorder on the patient's life. To date, the EDSS (or its predecessor the DSS) has been used almost universally in trials of treatment, while the ISS and ESS have been used infrequently, partly because of the extra effort required, and partly because the information provided is a less direct measure of the state of the disease.

Table 3.1. Neurologic dysfunction (WHO classification)

	Impairment	Disability	Handicap
Based on:	Symptoms/signs (neurologic examination)	Limitations of activities of daily living	Social/environmental limitations
MRD Scale:	Expanded disability status scale (EDSS)	Incapacity status scale (ISS)	Environmental status scale (ESS)

Measuring Impairment and Disability

The Expanded Disability Status Scale (EDSS)

The EDSS is the most widely used measure of clinical impairment in MS, although it also contains elements of disability in its grading. This comprehensive system of scoring summarizes all of the major neurologic impairment likely to be seen in patients with MS. It was originally introduced by Kurtzke as the DSS (Kurtzke 1955, 1961), but after a number of modifications, it was extended to form the EDSS (Kurtzke 1983) where each of the 10 DSS steps was divided into 2 to improve sensitivity. The findings on neurologic examination are scored on a set of subscales (functional systems) which are used as guides for scoring the EDSS in combination with extra information about gait dysfunction (Tables 3.2, 3.3).

In practice, the lower EDSS grades (0–3.5) are defined primarily by variations in grades in the functional systems, while grades 4 and above are largely dependent on disturbance of gait.

A number of problems with the EDSS have been discussed in detail in the literature (Willoughby and Paty 1988; Kurtzke 1989). There is a lack of precision of definition of some grades of dysfunction in several of the functional systems. The terms mild, moderate and severe are only loosely defined, and in some functional systems it is necessary to integrate a complex mixture of signs of varying types and extent without clear guidelines. The process of combining the score in the functional systems with extra data based on the patient's general mobility can also be confusing, especially in the middle ranges of the EDSS in patients with high scores in functional systems that do not seriously affect the ability to walk. The key distinctions between some of the grades (e.g., between 4.5 and 4.0, and between 5.5 and 5.0) are the ability to walk different distances that are not practicably observable on routine examination in the clinic. For this purpose it is useful to know the distance a patient has to walk to get from the parking lot to the clinic and various intervals in between.

Because the EDSS is an ordinal scale where the steps between each point on the scale are not necessarily equal, it is necessary to use non-parametric statistics in data analysis (Kurtzke 1986). There are also problems in adding and subtracting EDSS scores to produce means and differences over time. Those issues are covered in Chap. 4.

Table 3.2. The functional systems for the Expanded Disability Status Scale (EDSS). Modified from the Minimal Record for Disability for Multiple Sclerosis (scale for spasticity deleted)

(Descriptors have been added to the Kurtzke items for additional clarification and are in parentheses.)

1. Pyramidal functions
   - 0 – Normal
   - 1 – Abnormal signs without disability
   - 2 – Minimal disability
   - 3 – Mild to moderate paraparesis or hemiparesis (detectable weakness but most function sustained for short periods, fatigue a problem); severe monoparesis (almost no function)
   - 4 – Marked paraparesis or hemiparesis (function is difficult), moderate quadriparesis (function is decreased but can be sustained for short periods); or monoplegia
   - 5 – Paraplegia, hemiplegia, or marked quadriparesis
   - 6 – Quadriplegia
   - 9 – Unknown

2. Cerebellar functions
   - 0 – Normal
   - 1 – Abnormal signs without disability
   - 2 – Mild ataxia (tremor or clumsy movements easily seen, minor interference with function)
   - 3 – Moderate truncal or limb ataxia (tremor or clumsy movements interfere with function in all spheres)
   - 4 – Severe ataxia in all limbs (most function is very difficult)
   - 5 – Unable to perform coordinated movements due to ataxia
   - 9 – Unknown

     Record when weakness (grade 3 or worse on pyramidal) interferes with testing.

3. Brainstem functions
   - 0 – Normal
   - 1 – Signs only
   - 2 – Moderate nystagmus or other mild disability
   - 3 – Severe nystagmus, marked extraocular weakness, or moderate disability of other cranial nerves
   - 4 – Marked dysarthria or other marked disability
   - 5 – Inability to swallow or speak
   - 9 – Unknown

4. Sensory functions
   - 0 – Normal
   - 1 – Vibration or figure-writing decrease only in one or two limbs
   - 2 – Mild decrease in touch or pain or position sense, and/or moderate decrease in vibration in one or two limbs; or vibratory (c/s figure writing) decrease alone in three or four limbs
   - 3 – Moderate decrease in touch or pain or position sense, and/or essentially lost vibration in one or two limbs; or mild decrease in touch or pain and/or moderate decrease in all proprioceptive tests in three or four limbs
   - 4 – Marked decrease in touch or pain or loss of proprioception, alone or combined, in one or two limbs; or moderate decrease in touch or pain and/or severe proprioceptive decrease in more than two limbs
   - 5 – Loss (essentially) of sensation in one or two limbs; or moderate decrease in touch or pain and/or loss of proprioception for most of the body below the head
   - 6 – Sensation essentially lost below the head
   - 9 – Unknown

5. Bowel and bladder functions

   (Rate on the basis of the worse function, either bowel or bladder)
   - 0 – Normal
   - 1 – Mild urinary hesitancy, urgency or retention

Table 3.2. (Continued)

2 – Moderate hesitancy, urgency, retention of bowel or bladder or rare urinary incontinence (intermittent self-catheterization, manual compression to evacuate bladder, or finger evacuation of stool)
3 – Frequent urinary incontinence
4 – In need of almost constant catheterization (and constant use of measures to evacuate stool)
5 – Loss of bladder function
6 – Loss of bowel and bladder function
9 – Unknown

6. Visual (or optic) functions
   0 – Normal
   1 – Scotoma with visual acuity (corrected) better than 20/30
   2 – Worse eye with scotoma with maximal visual acuity (corrected) of 20/30 to 20/50
   3 – Worse eye with large scotoma, or moderate decrease in fields, but with maximal visual acuity (corrected) of 20/60 to 20/99
   4 – Worse eye with marked decrease of fields and maximal visual acuity (corrected) of 20/100 to 20/200; grade 3 plus maximal acuity of better eye of 20/60 or less
   5 – Worse eye with maximal visual acuity (corrected) less than 20/200; grade 4 plus maximal acuity of better eye of 20/60 or less
   6 – Grade 5 plus maximal visual acuity of better eye of 20/60 or less
   9 – Unknown
   Record presence of temporal pallor

7. Cerebral (or mental) functions
   0 – Normal
   1 – Mood alteration only (does not affect DSS score)
   2 – Mild decrease in mentation
   3 – Moderate decrease in mentation
   4 – Marked decrease in mentation (chronic brain syndrome – moderate)
   5 – Dementia or chronic brain syndrome – severe or incompetent
   9 – Unknown

8. Others
   0 – None
   1 – Any other neurological findings attributed to MS: Specify
   9 – Unknown

Table 3.3. Expanded Disability Status Scale, taken from the Minimal Record for Disability for Multiple Sclerosis

Note 1: EDSS steps 1.0 to 4.5 refer to patients who are fully ambulatory, and the precise step number is defined by the Functional System score(s). EDSS steps 5.0 to 9.5 are defined by the impairment to ambulation, and usual equivalents in Functional System scores are provided.
Note 2: EDSS should not change by 1.0 step unless there is a change in the same direction of at least one step in at least one FS. Each step (e.g., 3.0 to 3.5) is still part of the DSS scale equivalent (i.e., 3). Progression from 3.0 to 3.5 should be equivalent to the DSS score of 3.

0 – Normal neurological exam (all grade 0 in FS‡)

1.0 – No disability, minimal signs in one FS‡ (i.e., grade 1)

1.5 – No disability, minimal signs in more than one FS‡ (more than one FS grade 1)

2.0 – Minimal disability in one FS (one FS grade 2, others 0 or 1)

2.5 – Minimal disability in two FS (two FS grade 2, others 0 or 1)

Table 3.3. (Continued)

3.0 – Moderate disability in one FS (one FS grade 3, others 0 or 1) or mild disability in three or four FS (three or four FS grade 2, others 0 or 1) though fully ambulatory

3.5 – Fully ambulatory but with moderate disability in one FS (one grade 3) and one or two FS grade 2; or two FS grade 3; or five FS grade 2 (others 0 or 1)

4.0 – Fully ambulatory without aid, self-sufficient, up and about some 12 hours a day despite relatively severe disability consisting of one FS grade 4 (others 0 or 1), or combinations of lesser grades exceeding limits of previous steps; able to walk without aid or rest some 500 meters

4.5 – Fully ambulatory without aid, up and about much of the day, able to work a full day, may otherwise have some limitation of full activity or require minimal assistance; characterized by relatively severe disability usually consisting of one FS grade 4 (others 0 or 1) or combinations of lesser grades exceeding limits of previous steps; able to walk without aid or rest some 300 meters

5.0 – Ambulatory without aid or rest for about 200 meters; disability severe enough to impair full daily activities (e.g., to work a full day without special provisions) (Usual FS equivalents are one grade 5 alone, others 0 or 1; or combinations of lesser grades usually exceeding specifications for step 4.0)

5.5 – Ambulatory without aid or rest for about 100 meters; disability severe enough to preclude full daily activities; (Usual FS equivalents are one grade 5 alone, others 0 or 1; or combination of lesser grades usually exceeding those for step 4.0)

6.0 – Intermittent or unilateral constant assistance (cane, crutch, brace) required to walk about 100 meters with or without resting; (Usual FS equivalents are combinations with more than two FS grade 3+)

6.5 – Constant bilateral assistance (canes, crutches, braces) required to walk about 20 meters without resting; (Usual FS equivalents are combinations with more than two FS grade 3+)

7.0 – Unable to walk beyond approximately five meters even with aid, essentially restricted to wheelchair; wheels self in standard wheelchair and transfers alone; up and about in wheelchair some 12 hours a day; (Usual FS equivalents are combinations with more than one FS grade 4+; very rarely pyramidal grade 5 alone)

7.5 – Unable to take more than a few steps; restricted to wheelchair; may need aid in transfer; wheels self but cannot carry on in standard wheelchair a full day; may require motorized wheelchair; (Usual FS equivalents are combinations with more than one FS grade 4+)

8.0 – Essentially restricted to bed or chair or perambulated in wheelchair, but may be out of bed itself much of the day; retains many self-care functions; generally has effective use of arms; (Usual FS equivalents are combinations, generally grade 4+ in several systems)

8.5 – Essentially restricted to bed much of day; has some effective use of arm(s); retains some self-care functions; (Usual FS equivalents are combinations generally 4+ in several systems)

9.0 – Helpless bed patient; can communicate and eat; (Usual FS equivalents are combinations, mostly grade 4+)

9.5 – Totally helpless bed patient; unable to communicate effectively or eat/swallow; (Usual FS equivalents are combinations, almost all grade 4+)

Reliability of the EDSS

Only a few studies of the reliability of the EDSS have been reported. Those most relevant for clinical trials have assessed scoring of the EDSS by different examiners after independent examination of the same patients and have shown considerable interrater variability. Amato et al. (1988) found that EDSS scores in 25% of 24 examinations by pairs of examiners differed by 1 or more points. The Kappa coefficient which corrects for the amount of agreement to be expected by chance indicated, at best, moderate agreement (Kappa 0.49–0.56) in the EDSS and most of the functional systems of differences of up to 1.0 scale point. For 3 of the functional systems (pyramidal, sensory and mental) agreement was only fair (Kappa 0.28–0.32). In a larger study of 545 paired examinations, Noseworthy et al. (1988) showed consistently better agreement between examiners for differences of up to 1.0 scale step (Kappa 0.6–0.9). Most of those patients had EDSS scores of 4.5 or greater and Goodkin et al. (1991) have recently shown that interrater variability is greater in patients with EDSS scores below 4.0. The practical point is that differences of up to 1.0 on the EDSS score may be due to examiner inconsistency and do not necessarily indicate significant clinical change.

Future of the EDSS

It is expected that the EDSS will remain the standard measure of neurologic impairment in trials of treatment of MS over the next few years. It should be possible to achieve more consistent results among neurologists using the scale by undertaking 2 measures:

1. Defining more precisely the criteria for allocating different grades in each of the functional systems.
2. Setting out more clearly the criteria for applying the scores for the functional systems to the summary EDSS score. A computer-based system for carrying out these procedures is under development at the University of British Columbia (UBC) where the MS-Costar computerized clinical data system is used to record the results of the neurologic examination for each patient using semi-quantitative scales. This data is used to assign the grade for each functional system in the EDSS automatically. The overall EDSS score is then assigned automatically on the basis of the scores for the functional systems.

Other Comprehensive Impairment Scales

Most of the other suggested scales are now of historical interest only (Willoughby and Paty 1988) but the Neurologic Rating Scale (Sipe et al. 1984) has been used in some recent clinical trials in addition to the EDSS. It has the advantage of a straight-forward system for scoring motor and sensory function in each limb, but still lacks precision in defining the steps on each scale. Reliability studies have not yet been reported. Criteria for a more satisfactory scale have been proposed, but there has not been much enthusiasm for the effort required to change to a system which has not been formally validated or proven in practice (Weiner and Paty 1989).

Complementary Restricted Impairment Scales

The functional systems of the EDSS do not provide separate assessment of impairment in the arms and legs and the scale for measuring mental state is

Table 3.4. Ambulation index. (From Hauser et al. 1983)

0	Asymptomatic; fully active
1	Walks normally but reports fatigue that interferes with athletic or other demanding activities
2	Abnormal gait or episodic imbalance; gait disorder is noticed by family and friends; able to walk 25 feet (8 meters) in 10 seconds or less
3	Walks independently; able to walk 25 feet in 20 seconds or less
4	Requires unilateral support (cane or single crutch) to walk; walks 25 feet in 20 seconds or less
5	Requires bilateral support (canes, crutches, or walker) and walks 25 feet in 20 seconds or less; or requires unilateral support but needs more than 20 seconds to walk 25 feet
6	Requires bilateral support and more than 20 seconds to walk 25 feet; may use wheelchair[a] on occasion
7	Walking limited to several steps with bilateral support; unable to walk 25 feet; may use wheelchair[a] for most activities
8	Restricted to wheelchair; able to transfer self independently
9	Restricted to wheelchair; unable to transfer self independently

[a] The use of a wheelchair may be determined by lifestyle and motivation. It is expected that patients in Grade 7 will use a wheelchair more frequently than those in Grades 5 or 6. Assignment of a grade in the range of 5 to 7, however, is determined by the patient's ability to walk a given distance, and not by the extent to which the patient uses a wheelchair.

very simple. Separate scales for those functions have therefore been suggested. With the exception of the Quantitative Upper Extremity Index, all of these scales, like those above, are ordinal scales which can be handled statistically in the same manner as the EDSS.

Ambulation Index (AI)

Because disturbance of gait is such a frequent cause of long-term disability in MS, separate scales for assessing ambulation have been proposed. The most widely used is the Ambulation Index (Hauser et al. 1983a,b; Table 3.4). It has the advantage of specifying several grades in semi-quantitative terms and probably provides a more precise measure of ambulation than the EDSS in the commonly observed range of EDSS scores between 4.0 and 6.0. However, comment has been made about a wide gap between grades 3 and 4 (Matthews 1991). Doubts have also been expressed about the use of one versus two canes as a criterion of grading. As with the EDSS, it is important to consider what the patient actually needs in the way of mechanical aids for effective ambulation, rather than simply to state what is most convenient at the time. It is also necessary to specify the type of surface on which the patient is tested (usually a smooth, level floor indoors).

Upper Limb Scales

Arm function is not separately described in the functional systems in the EDSS, which distinguishes the neurologic signs on the basis of neurologic pathways. An Upper Extremity Index has been proposed (Weiner and Ellison, 1983) with grades that relate to function in normal activities rather than neurologic signs. This scale therefore overlaps with the ISS. Goodkin et al. (1988) have described a test of upper extremity function which scores the ability to manipulate pegs and blocks rather than the findings on neurologic examination. Quantitative measures of that sort are more objective and should become more widely used in the future, but they complement rather than displace systems for coding the findings on neurologic examination.

Scales of Cognitive Function

It is now recognized that impairment of cognitive function occurs commonly in MS, although its manifestations may be subtle and detailed testing may be necessary to demonstrate it (Peyser et al. 1980; Rao 1986; Franklin et al. 1990). An important aspect is that significant cognitive impairment may occur in patients without substantial motor or sensory impairment. Simple bedside tests of higher mental function such as the Mini-mental State Examination (Folstein et al. 1975) and the Cognitive Capacity Screening Examination (Jacobs et al. 1977) are insensitive to the cognitive deficits in MS, even though they are more detailed than the mental state assessment included in the EDSS (Heaton et al. 1990; Beatty and Goodkin 1990). It has to be accepted that the EDSS provides a very insensitive guide to cognitive impairment. Unfortunately, more sophisticated tests are time-consuming and are often not practicable in trials of treatment as a routine measure especially if other measures such as the ISS are being used in addition to the EDSS.

Intermediate length screening tests for cognitive impairment such as the Neuro-psychological Screening Battery (Franklin et al. 1988; Heaton et al. 1990) may establish a place in treatment trials. They can be administered in 45–60 min, but little information is available to date about their reliability on repeated testing.

Quantitative Measures of Impairment

While the standard neurologic examination provides essential data in the assessment of patients, a strong case has been made for the use of tests carried out with the assistance of instruments that provide more quantitative information, e.g., measurement of muscle strength in selected muscles with a myometer and the time of activities, such as finger or foot tapping or the placing of pegs in holes (Goodkin et al. 1988). Tourtellotte and his colleagues have led the way in the application of this technology in trials of treatment of MS (Potvin and Tourtellotte 1975; Potvin et al. 1981; Tourtellotte and Syndulko 1989). The advantages are that changes in a patient's neurologic function can be measured reasonably precisely and objectively and the results are expressed as numbers on true interval (or ratio) scales. These scales can be handled with standard mathematical and statistical techniques without the need to stretch the underlying concepts to their limits. The disadvantages are that special facilities and a trained technician are necessary and comprehensive tests for all relevant aspects of neurologic impairment are not available, e.g., the usual test battery does not measure impaired eye movements or disturbance of speech or swallowing.

Logistic problems are likely to restrict the use of standard batteries of instrumented quantitative tests in the foreseeable future, but the principle of increasingly defining more precisely the steps used in grading the standard neurologic examination should be applied. Timed tests of rapid movements can be simply carried out in the clinic by a physician or nurse and incorporated into definitions of degrees of clumsiness of the limbs. An established example of this principle is the timed test of walking a fixed distance in the grades of the Ambulation Index.

The Incapacity Status Scale (ISS)

The ISS fills a demand for a measure of disability, i.e., the effect of the disease on the patient's daily activity. It includes the following aspects, each with its separate scale:

1. Stair climbing
2. Ambulation
3. Transfers
4. Bowel function
5. Bladder function
6. Bathing
7. Dressing
8. Grooming
9. Feeding
10. Vision
11. Speech and hearing
12. Medical problems
13. Mood and thought
14. Mentation
15. Fatiguability
16. Sexual function

The MRD sets out a structured questionnaire to assist paramedical staff in compiling the scales. It can be seen that some scales (ambulation, bladder function, vision, mentation) overlap with the EDSS and its functional systems. To some extent, this overlap is inevitable, as the distinction between impairment and disability is blurred.

In practice, in clinical trials changes in the ISS closely parallel changes in the EDSS and doubt has been expressed whether the extra time and effort to complete the ISS is warranted as a routine measure in treatment trials (Poser 1989).

Counting Acute Exacerbations

In patients with relapsing/remitting disease, especially those with little residual disability, a measure complementary to the EDSS is to count the number of clinical acute exacerbations during the treatment period (Bornstein et al. 1987). This measure can be expressed most simply for each patient as the number of exacerbations per year (number of exacerbations experienced by the patient during the trial divided by the length of the trial in years). The results are usually not whole numbers, but they are real numbers that can be handled mathematically in a standard fashion, without the conceptual difficulties posed by the variable interval problem seen in ordinal scales. A method for grading the severity of exacerbations has been described by Millar et al. (1967).

Determining that an acute exacerbation has occurred is not always a simple matter and a clear definition must be established at the beginning of a trial (Schumacher et al. 1965; Weiner and Ellison 1983). Suggested criteria are: new symptoms with objective signs confirmed on neurologic examination, or sudden worsening of old symptoms with objective changes on examination of at least one grade in the relevant functional system in the DSS. The new or increased symptoms and signs must be separated by at least 1 month from the onset of an earlier exacerbation and must persist for at least 24 h. The involvement of an experienced neurologist in this assessment is invaluable in distinguishing acute exacerbations from "pseudo-exacerbations". Pseudo-exacerbations are changes in neurologic function due to increased feelings of fatigue or transient symptoms associated with temporary dysfunction in previously damaged pathways due to fever or intercurrent infection, both of which are common problems in MS. The severity of individual exacerbations at their height can be assessed by changes in scores in the appropriate functional systems, but that measure is less relevant than the amount of residual disability following recovery from an exacerbation, which can be measured by changes in the EDSS over the course of the trial.

Assessing Treatment of Acute Exacerbations

There are many variables in this sort of trial that make comparisons between groups of patients difficult. Apart from the differing types and severity of new symptoms and signs associated with individual attacks, there is also a varying background of preceding impairment and often varying periods over which exacerbations progress, so that treatment may be initiated in different phases of the exacerbation.

The EDSS may be used but more precise assessment of changes in acute attacks in individual patients may be obtained by also analyzing the functional systems primarily affected by the attack. If the numbers of patients are large enough, changes in the different functional systems can be compared separately between the patient groups. It is to be expected that a separate comparison (for example) of improvement in the pyramidal system or of visual acuity in the treated and control groups would be more likely to detect clinically-significant differences than comparisons of the scores on the EDSS as a whole. Separate comparisons of that sort would be particularly useful if many of the patients have exacerbations occurring on a background of substantial chronic neurologic impairment.

Assessing Treatment of Chronic Symptoms

Trials of symptomatic therapy are usually short-term studies in patients with relatively severe disease and disability of moderate or severe degree. Although the background severity of impairment may be of some importance in matching treatment and control groups, it is not usually expected that there will be substantial changes in overall impairment during the course of the study. Changes in the EDSS are not, therefore, of primary interest.

However, improvement in disabling symptoms such as fatigue, pain, or spasticity may lead to important benefits in terms of function, so that measurement of the Incapacity Status Scale may give useful information. The primary measure should be one tailored to the symptom of interest; most commonly spasticity with or without spasms, fatigue, urinary urgency and/or frequency or pain. These areas of function will all be measured on ordinal scales and can be handled statistically in the same way as the EDSS.

MRI as an Outcome Measure

The introduction of MRI into clinical medicine provides a powerful new approach to quantitate objectively the morbid pathology of MS (Paty 1988). MR images, to a considerable extent, reflect the water content of tissue. The images also reflect alterations in local populations of cells and their aggregate biochemically-defined constituents, particularly their lipid content and composition. Differences in water content between cerebral white and grey matter contribute greatly to the exquisite anatomical definition of MR images of brain. lesions (Stewart et al. 1988a; Ormerod et al. 1987; Newcombe et al. 1991) account for the remarkable sensitivity of MRI in this disease.

These changes contribute to the prolonged T_1 and T_2 values obtained from MS lesions. Evolving data from comparative pathologic, biochemical and MRI studies of acute and chronic EAE in animals, post-mortem studies of MS in man, and magnetic resonance spectroscopy (MRS) in man, will likely define the relative contribution of these pathologic changes to the MR image of MS in the near future.

Currently used imaging parameters, which are appropriately T_2-weighted, exquisitely define the location and extent of MS lesions above the level of the mid-cervical cord. Diagnostically-abnormal head scans can be seen in about 90% of patients with clinically definite MS; lesions can be seen less consistently in optic nerve and spinal cord. However, findings on individual MRI scans do not correlate well with clinical status as measured by disability status scales or with the prior clinical course (i.e., relapsing/remitting, chronic/progressive, occult) (Li et al. 1984b). However, serial imaging of individual patients often shows the asymptomatic accumulation of new lesions, lesion enlargement, and striking changes in the blood–brain barrier with time. This MRI activity likely reflects an objective measure of disease progression which occurs at a greater rate and may be independent of changes in clinical neurologic status. *One would anticipate that any therapeutic modality which affects the disease at a fundamental level would arrest or slow the accumulation of new lesions*. Serial MRI would thus provide objective supportive data for clinically documented stabilization or improvement of function. Therefore, clinical trials should include the following studies:

Quantitative Analysis: Quantitative analysis of entry and exit MRI data obtained in blinded fashion on a significant cohort of control and treated patients, and;

Serial MRIs: Serial frequent MRI examinations for determining the rate of development of active lesions.

First, as noted above, in most MRI studies correlation measurements have been poor except in primary and in progressive patients (Thompson et al. 1990). In addition, control imaging for specificity has been done in numerous conditions. However, MRI cannot reliably determine the pathology of individual lesions.

Pathology of MS as Revealed by MRI

The appearance of MRI lesions seen on coronal MRI slices in patients with MS is very reminiscent of the classical appearance of periventricular demyelination seen at autopsy. Several post-mortem cadaver MR and fixed brain studies have been done (Stewart et al. 1984, 1986; Ormerod et al. 1987) (Newcombe, et al. 1991). Post-mortem spin echo (SE) sequences show a remarkable degree of anatomical detail. MRI pathological correlation studies show an extensive degree of abnormality, similar to that seen on scans in severely affected MS patients. There is extensive increased SE signal periventricularly. The differences seen in T_1 and T_2 measurements between grey and white matter and between normal and abnormal white matter are probably due to surrounding molecules modifying the relaxation behaviour of water protons. In fixed brains the SE image contrast persists quite well.

Realizing that MR images reflect volume-averaging over the thickness of the slice, the areas noted as abnormal on the MR image will not correspond exactly to the gross appearance of demyelination seen on the brain sections. The best correlation has been seen at the level just above the lateral ventricles and in the brainstem.

Errors due to inaccurate setting of the plane of imaging, can be reduced as follows:

MRI scans: An MRI scan should be done immediately post-mortem

The brain: The brain is then removed and immediately fixed in formaldehyde. After 3 weeks of fixation an MRI scan of the fixed brain is done

Slicing of brain: Subsequent slicing of the fixed brain in the plane of the MRI slices is done

Slicing alignment: Careful attention should be paid to the alignment of the slices both on the MRI and the pathologic sections. The pathologic slice should be positioned so that the surface of the brain slice corresponds to the middle of the appropriate MRI slice

Photographs: Pathological surfaces can then be photographed and digitized for display on the same TV monitor as is the MRI image. Care should be taken to ensure that the photograph of the brain slices and the MRI slices are size-scaled appropriately

Stewart and her colleagues have reported several pathologic correlation studies (Stewart et al. 1984, 1986). The correlation between the MRI slice and the pathology in her studies (as expected) was not exact. Small lesions, especially in the top slice, can be missed by the MRI. The total "error" in measurement of extent of disease varied between ±13% and ±30% slice by

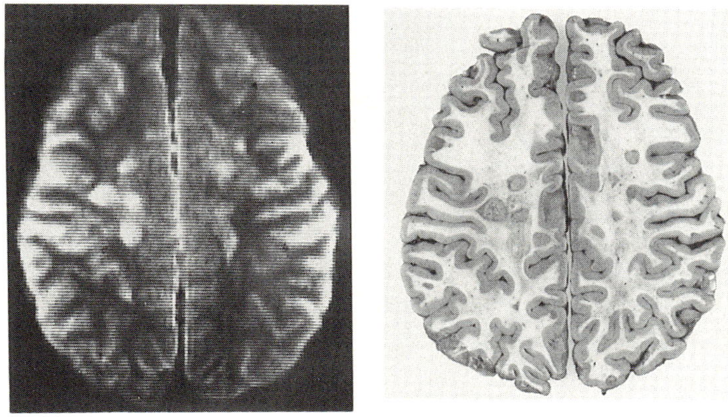

Fig. 3.1. **a.** The MRI slice image of a fixed brain at a level just above the ventricle. **b** The cut brain slice appropriate to the MRI image in **a**.

slice. The fixed-brain digitized images usually had larger areas of demyelination than were seen on the post-mortem MRI scans. The pathological correlation varied, however, with some slices showing greater extent and some smaller extent of pathology than the appropriate MRI slice. In future studies the errors introduced by volume averaging will be minimized by using thin slice or volume MRI techniques.

The qualitative T_1 and T_2 data on the post-mortem and fixed-brains was compared to the histopathology in 4 cases. The comparison was done only on lesions that were seen to extend completely through the MRI slice (10 mm). T_1 and T_2 measurements were then taken from the geographic center of such lesions. This selection method was chosen in order to ensure that the tissue from which the measurements were taken was as homogeneous as possible. The histopathology was done by neuropathologists who were totally unaware of the MRI quantitative data. In several instances it was shown that in completely demyelinated lesions that the more heavily gliotic lesions had the longest T_1 and T_2 values. Fig. 3.1 shows a typical pathologic correlation with the MRI slice.

Omerod et al. (1987) also did pathologic correlation studies on 6 formalin-fixed MS brains. Their analysis showed good concordance between the areas of abnormality on the MR images and the histopathology. They concluded, as did Stewart, that the abnormalities seen on the MRI scan originated from chronic plaques of MS. Some abnormal areas on MRI may not actually represent MS lesions, especially in older patients; however, we have no way of determining such specificity. It is by using age-matched controls that such non-specificity errors can be minimized.

MRI Quantitative Studies

Several studies have compared severity (extent) of disease on the MRI scan, head, with the degree of clinical severity (Franklin et al. 1988; Kiel et al. 1988;

Huber et al. 1988). There is usually poor correlation between the two. A computer-assisted method for measuring the abnormal areas seen on the MRI scan has been developed in order to follow the evolution of the pathologic process over time (Paty 1985). This method of analysis has been shown to be reproducible. In the analysis of the scans a radiologist experienced in serial MRI evaluation indicates the number, size, and distribution of lesions for each subject. The lesions are identified and marked on the MRI film in the following manner:

1. Small solitary lesions (max. dia <10 mm)
2. Large solitary lesions (dia >10 mm)
3. Confluent lesions e.g., those lesions that are relatively large, probably formed by the merging of two or more rounded smaller lesions producing an irregularly shaped (lumpy/bumpy) or thick (>5 mm) linear area of abnormality on the MR image

All lesions are identified, localized and named. All of the lesions are marked on the MRI hard copy film for subsequent quantitation. For quantitation purposes a technician with a known reproducibility record traces the margins of the lesions as displayed on a computer monitor, using the radiologist's marking as a guide. In several studies on the same patient an experienced and skilled technician can trace and measure the MRI lesions with a reproducibility error of about 6%. Therefore, a single technician is used for each study in order to keep variability to a minimum. The lesion borders are outlined using a mouse tracing system. In this way a computer-based description of the slice-by-slice area of lesions in square millimeters can be obtained. The computer is programed to calculate individual lesion area, individual lesion area per slice and total lesion area from all head slices in each patient. At the end of the process all of the areas traced are added up, slice by slice, in order to obtain an overall index of the extent of the disease in mm^2.

Serial studies of the same patient require very careful repositioning. Careful attention is key to the repositioning process remembering that patient comfort is vital. For accurate repositioning we use both internal and external landmarks. The process of repositioning the patient usually takes about 20 min additional time at each study. For the first examination the patient must be positioned as comfortably as possible. The angle of the radiographic baseline (RBL), the canthomeatal line as well as the angle between the tragus of the ear and the nasion are measured. On follow-up examination the patient must be positioned so that these two angles are the same as they were during the first examination. Internal landmarks are also used. We have chosen to use a line from the top of the cerebellum to the anterior superior portion of the sphenoid sinus. In addition the angle of the head is extremely important for repositioning. Even a slight difference (3°–4°) can make a dramatic difference in the scan. If not comfortable the patient will change position during the scan. After the patient has been positioned a trial scan should be done to see if the internal angle varies more than 2° from the baseline. A full scan sequence is then made and compared with the original scan in the series. If the two scans do not match well the entire sequence should be repeated. Fig. 3.2 shows a sample of how the computer tracing of the MRI lesions is done.

This MRI quantitation method has been used for clinical correlation studies

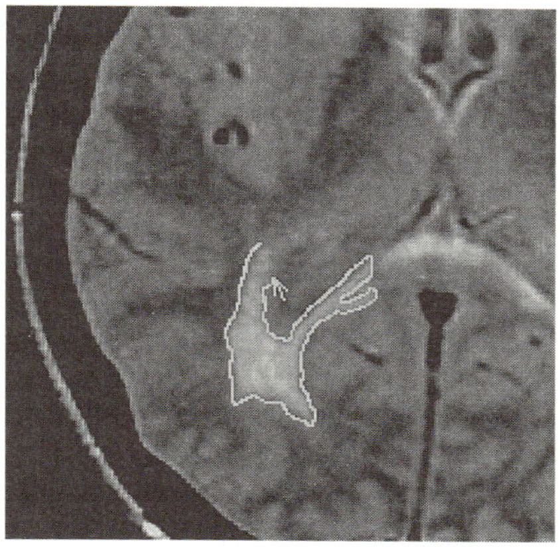

Fig. 3.2. Computer image of MRI slice with one periventricular lesion partially traced for quantitation purposes.

and in clinical trials. Koopmans et al. (1989a) did a careful MRI/neurological correlation study contrasting 32 benign MS patients with 32 relapsing/progressive (RP) disease patients matched for age, sex and duration of disease. The duration of disease was greater than 10 years in all patients. The benign patients (mean EDSS 1.55) varied from 0 to 4661 mm^2 total area of MS lesions (mean: 1162). The RP patients (mean EDSS 6.03) varied from 140 to 11 190 mm^2 total area (mean: 2912). In 6 of the pairs (20%) the benign patient of the pair was measured as having a heavier load of disease by MRI than was the relapsing/progressive member. Correlation between the location of MRI lesions (brainstem and cerebellum) and clinical symptoms showed about 50% concordance. For example, only 50% of the benign patients who had brainstem lesions seen on the MRI had a history of brainstem symptoms.

Honer and colleagues (1987) did a controlled MRI study of 8 patients who had both MS and diagnosed psychiatric disease (mostly depression and bipolar disease). The patients with psychiatric disease had a greater degree of involvement of the temporal lobe than did matched patients without psychiatric diagnoses. Several investigators have attempted to do quantitative evaluations of the extent of abnormality on MRI scans in MS. Baumhefner et al. (1990) used an IBAS interactive image analysis system to trace the abnormal area slice by slice. They found a correlation of disease burden in the cerebral hemispheres with the IgG intra blood–brain barrier synthesis rate. Kapouleus (1989) has developed an automatic detection system for MS lesions, but has not applied the system to longitudinal monitoring.

Several investigators have found weak correlations between the extent of the MS process and the disability of the patient (Huber et al. 1988) while most others have failed to find any meaningful correlation (Franklin et al. 1988; Li et al. 1984b). Even in the better correlations, the correlation coefficient has been low but some have been statistically significant (e.g., $R < 5$, $p = 0.05$). The most consistent correlation has been between corpus callosum involvement on the MRI and neuro-psychological findings (Huber et al. 1987). At the University of British Columbia we have completed three separate studies comparing the burden of disease as measured by MRI with clinical severity, usually the EDSS (Paty et al. unpublished data). The highest r value (correlation coefficient) that we found was 0.5. The other r values range between 0.22 and 0.02. The lack of correlation between neurologically determined (clinical) severity and the extent of MRI lesions should not be surprising. Clinical severity, as measured by the EDSS, is to a great extent determined by the location of lesions, particularly spinal cord ones. However, most MRI studies have not imaged the spinal cord. In addition, the element of severity of the pathologic process must also be considered. The clinical expression of lesion severity is probably due to location plus a combination of additional factors, including the degree of axonal loss within the lesion. MRI has no way of determining such severity. However, MRI does give an accurate measure of the extent of disease process slice by slice which is a clear improvement over previous methods of measurement.

The important application of serial MRI quantitative measurements will be in clinical trials. Clinical trials in MS have long been hampered by the lack of an objective measurement of "burden of disease". As noted above, neurologic findings (impairment) and functional deficits (disability) at best indicate the anatomical localization of some of the MS lesions and give some approximation of the extent of their severity. However, the bulk of MS lesions are probably silent to the neurological examination.

Therefore, in order to have a more objective approach to clinical trials, the MRI quantitation method has been used several times. In a prospective evaluation of 100 patients during a placebo-controlled therapeutic trial of alpha lymphoblastoid interferon (Kastrukoff et al. 1990) 80 of the subjects had quantitative MRI evaluations at entry, at 6 months, and at 2 years. The MRI quantitation technique based to analyze the MRI changes that occurred over that time. The changes in the "burden of MS" ranged from −70% to +221% over 2 years. The mean change in extent was +21%. The results were disappointing in that no significant difference was seen between the treated and placebo groups of patients in either the clinical or MRI measurements. Visual evaluation of the same MRI images gave similar information, though there were instances where there had been major development of new and enlarged lesions that was not well reflected in the total measurement of disease burden or in the clinical measurements. This follow-up experience has shown that both the quantitative measure of disease burden and a visual assessment of individual lesion changes contribute important information to the assessment of outcome and that there is an increase in MRI-detected lesion burden, as expected, in most patients over the 2 years of a clinical trial.

The greatest variability in the MRI measurements was seen in patients with the smallest total lesion load. However, a separate analysis done for patients with large "disease burden" and those with minimal "disease burden" did not change the outcome of the study.

The MRI quantitation method has been used in 2 collaborative therapeutic trials in MS. In order to do the MRI analysis in collaborative studies computer software was developed to read the MRI tape formats from various manufacturers including GE, Siemens, Fonar, Diasonics, Picker, and Phillips. A therapeutic effect was not shown by MRI in the cooperative cyclosporine therapeutic trial (Multiple Sclerosis Study Group 1990). Kappos et al. (1988) had previously used a visual assessment of the MRI in a final 6 months exit evaluation in a 2-year clinical trial of cyclosporine. They found that there was no therapeutic effect on either the MRI or on the clinical status of the patients. The MRI quantitation method is now being used in a cooperative clinical trial of systemically administered Beta interferon (Paty, unpublished results). As part of that trial, the Vancouver cohort of 50 patients is being imaged once every 6 weeks to detect the dynamics of lesions coming and going (see below). These experiences in clinical trials have shown us that MRI can be used as an index measure of the extent and activity of disease over time.

Serial MRI Studies (Natural History)

Early in the experience with MRI, intermittent scans showed that chronic lesions could be seen to increase in size and asymptomatic lesions could be seen to come and go (Li et al. 1984a; Johnson et al. 1984). It quickly became apparent that disease activity as measured by MRI could often be quite dramatic and was often subclinical. Therefore systematic serial studies combining frequent neurological and MRI examinations were done.

At the University of British Columbia, 3 such MRI natural history studies have been completed. Systematic frequent (biweekly or monthly) carefully repositioned MRI scans over 5–6 months' duration were done. For these studies MRI activity events were defined as follows:

1. *New lesions* are those that have never been seen before and develop out of previously normal areas of white matter
2. *Reappearing lesions* are those which reappear at the same site from which an earlier lesion had disappeared
3. *Increasing size (expanding) lesions* are those that increase in size from a previously seen stable appearance. "Significant enlargement" was measured as approximately 70% change in small (<1 cm) lesions or as little as 10% change, which was usually obvious, in larger lesions

Any of the above changes were considered to be signs of increasing disease activity. However, if a lesion was seen to continuously enlarge in repeated scans, for the purpose of these studies, it was counted as only one disease activity event.

In order to contrast the various stages and phases of MS the 3 studies were done as follows (see Table 3.5):

1. The first study was in 7 relapsing patients (Isaac et al. 1988). Some of the patients were disabled, but most were completely independent. The patients were examined by monthly MRI scans, physical examination, and immunologic testing over 6 months. Careful interim neurologic histories were performed at each visit. Five clinical relapses occurred in 3 patients. There were 17 new and enlarging MRI lesions during the study. Of the 36 MRI follow-up examinations, 17 (48%) showed MRI evidence for new and/or increasing disease activity. The mean clinical relapse rate was 1.4 relapses per patient per year. The rate for the appearance of new MRI lesions was 4.9 new lesions per patient per year and the total MRI activity rate was 8.0 activity events per patient per year.

Table 3.5. Serial MRI studies

Author	Year	Type of patient	Activity rate		Comments
			Clin[a]	MRI[b]	
Isaac et al.	1988	RR	1.4	4.9	1.7 Active lesions per active scan
Willoughby et al.	1989	PR	0.4	2.4	
Koopmans et al.	1989a,b	RP	0	11.8	
Miller et al.	1988	RR			MRI activity higher than clinical: all new MRI lesions enhanced
Kermode et al.	1990	RR			Gd enhancement can precede standard MRI lesion
Bastianello et al.	1990	Mixed			All new lesions enhanced
Thompson et al.	1991	Primary CP			Pattern differs from RR and RP; low number of small non-enhancing lesions

[a] Relapses per patient per year.
[b] Active scans per patient per year.
RR = Relapsing Remitting.
RP = Relapsing Progressive.
CP = Chronic Progressive.

Parallel immunologic studies showed that T-cell and NK cell phenotypes did not vary in any predictable fashion. However, immunologic function studies (Oger et al. 1988) showed that suppressor cell activity, NK cell activity and IgG secretion in-vitro changed in parallel with some of the largest lesions. Of the 7 patients, 2 had distinctly large MRI lesions which evolved and then disappeared over several months. In both of those patients there were quite significant changes in immunologic function tests that paralleled the evolution of the large MRI lesions. When the MRI lesions reached their maximal size, striking abnormalities of immune function were seen, that had not been present 1 month earlier. These abnormalities of immune function were not found in simultaneously tested controls. It is possible that the immunologic changes were secondary to the development of large cerebral lesions.

2. The second study included 9 patients with minimally disabling but actively relapsing disease (Willoughby et al. 1989). Each patient had careful interim history, neurologic and MRI examinations done once every 2 weeks for an average of 5 months. Each also had parallel immunologic testing done as in the first study. Clinically-detected activity was minimal with 3 instances in which asymptomatic changes in neurological findings occurred. One patient had 2 minor spinal cord sensory relapses. MRI examination showed that there were 10 instances in which new MRI lesions appeared, and 2 instances in which there were enlargements of pre-existing lesions. All of the MRI activity was asymptomatic. The clinical relapse rate was 0.4 relapses per patient per year. The frequency of MRI activity was 2.6 positive MRI examinations per patient per year. There were 83 follow-up MRI examinations and 10 of those examinations (12%) showed evidence for increasing disease activity. This study, along with the first study, showed that the degree of disease activity as detected by MRI could be as high as 5 times the clinical relapse rate.

3. The third study included 8 severely disabled patients in the progressive

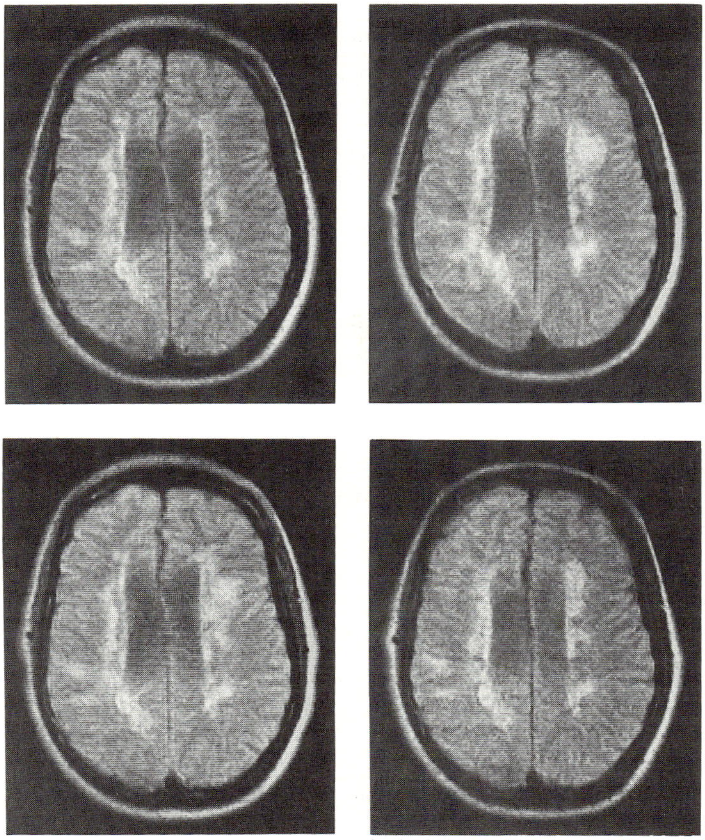

Fig. 3.3a–d. A series of T_2-weighted MRI images showing the evaluation of a new perventricular lesion. This patient was in the study reported by Koopment et al. (1989a).

phase of MS (Koopmans et al. 1989b), who were selected because of documented chronic deterioration over the previous year. Of the 8 patients, 7 had begun with relapsing disease and could be considered relapsing/progressive (RP) or secondarily progressive. The other patient had chronic/progressive (CP) or primarily progressive disease from the outset. All patients, as in the second study, had histories, physical examinations, and MRI examinations, in addition to immunologic tests once every 2 weeks over a period of 6 months.

In this study there were 98 follow-up MRI examinations during which time no clinical relapses were seen. However, 25 new MRI lesions were seen. There were also 61 instances in which previously-seen stable MRI lesions increased in size. There was a total of 86 MRI activity events during the study (remember that a continuous increase in size over several scans was counted as only a single activity event). Of the 98 follow-up scans, 47 (48%) showed evidence for increasing disease activity.

One patient developed a non-specific upper respiratory infection (URI) during the study, followed closely by the appearance of a large left frontal

MRI lesion (Fig. 3.3) that reached a peak within a month and then disappeared before the end of the study. None of the chronic patients showed any neurological deterioration during the 6 months of the study. However, several have worsened considerably since the study was completed (see below).

Other MRI serial studies have been reported, some using gadolinium (Gd) (Miller et al. 1988; Bastianello et al. 1990; Wiebe et al. 1990). Up to 90% of new MRI lesions enhance with Gd, and occasionally an enhancing area can be seen before the standard MRI lesion is seen (Kermode et al. 1990). Spinal cord imaging adds about 20% to the activity seen on the standard head MRI scan. A recent workshop on the use of MRI in monitoring disease activity in MS was held at Queen Square, London, UK, and brought together a number of European and North American investigators to make recommendations for cooperative studies. Miller and his colleagues reported that, in a study with scans every 2 weeks, ⅔ of Gd-enhancing lesions showed enhancement on only one scan. They also found that the optimum time to see enhancement was 20 min after Gd injection; repeat Gd injections were tolerated well by their patients, but they noted that anaphylaxis to Gd has been reported (Miller DA, personal communication).

The Queen Square group (Thompson et al. 1991) also reported some profound differences between several clinical categories of patient. Primary progressive patients had the lowest rate of development of new lesions (very few of which were enhancing) at 3.3 new lesions per patient per year. The next highest rate was for benign patients (<DSS 3 at >10 years) who had 8.8 new lesions per patient per year. The typical relapsing (RR) and relapsing/progressive (RP) patients had 17.2 and 18.2 new lesions per patient per year respectively. Both the Queen Square and the UBC serial data have shown that the rate of lesion activity varies widely between patients. Unfortunately, the rate of development of new and/or otherwise active lesions also varies considerably over time in the same patient. Some patients can be active over a 3-month period and then be totally inactive over the next 2–3 months. Such variability means that a "run in" period of scanning prior to the start of a clinical study does not predict the subsequent activity in that individual patient.

The current data from the 50 patients imaged every 6 weeks from the Beta-interferon trial has shown that the rate of MRI activity (3.0 active lesions/patients/year) is twice the rate of clinical relapses (1.5/patient/year). The patients who are seen to be active by scanning overlap with the patients who are active by clinical activity, but not completely so. Of the patients ⅓ are only active clinically and ⅓ are only active by MRI. An overlapping ⅓ are active both clinically and on MRI.

In summary, 35% of follow-up scans show at least one event that could be considered evidence for increasing disease activity. It is not unusual to see one lesion enlarging while other lesions, in different portions of the brain, are simultaneously becoming smaller. A preliminary study of outcome has been done (Paty, unpublished data). Of the 24 serial patients studied at the University of British Columbia 17 have remained clinically stable and 7 have become much worse. The average rate of MRI activity in the 7 patients who later became worse was higher (9.5 active lesions per patient per year) than in those who remained stable (3.6 active lesions per patient per year) but

Table 3.6. Three serial studies. Clinical follow-up on 24 patients in the original UBC serial studies (about 2-years follow-up)

	Clinically worse	Clinically stable
Number of patients	7	17
Average no. active lesions during study	9.9 (2–26)	3.4 (0–13)
Average no. new lesions	3.1 (1–6)	1.7 (0–5)
Average no. reactive lesions	6.8 (0–20)	1.6 (0–9)

there was so much overlap between the groups that the differences were not statistically significant (see Table 3.6).

Koopmans et al. (1989c) followed 49 enhancing CT lesions by using serial MRI scans. Most of the enhancing CT lesions showed a tendency to enlarge and/or become smaller on MRI follow-up. Additional high volume delayed (HVD) contrast CT scans showed that some of the previously enhancing lesions continued to enhance or reenhanced after 2–7 months. At the same time 13 new enhancing lesions developed. About half of the newly seen CT-enhancing lesions had previously been seen on the serial MRI follow-ups. Of the CT-enhancing lesions, 60% became markedly smaller on MRI follow-up. Some of the lesions eventually disappeared; 25% continued to change actively in size, becoming larger and smaller over time, and 16% eventually merged with neighbouring lesions to develop the appearance of confluence. The average time from initial CT-enhancement to the detection of confluence on MRI was 16 months. Confluent lesions have a very different appearance from that of new lesions. New lesions are usually rounded (spherical) in shape, whereas confluent lesions are irregularly shaped or linear with a lumpy/bumpy appearance.

Miller and his colleagues (1988) have seen similar high rates of asymptomatic changes in their serial gadolinium-enhanced MRI studies in relapsing/progressive patients. As in the UBC experience using serial unenhanced MRI examinations, new lesions reached a maximum size in 2–4 weeks and then faded over the subsequent 6–8 weeks. In contrast to the pattern seen in relapsing (secondarily) progressive (RP) MS by the UBC group and by the Queen Square group (noted above) Thompson et al. (1990, 1991) found primary CPMS to have a different pattern. Their primary CP patients had a low relative

Table 3.7. University of British Columbia studies in multiple sclerosis

Frequency of scans (weeks)	Activity seen with each interval (%)[a]	% of lesion activity seen at each frequency of scanning
2	100	36
4	67	28
6	40	7
8	29	4
Up to 10	–	23

[a] 100% of activity detected was seen, by definition, at the 2 weekly scanning interval. Looking at the scans at less frequent intervals detected significantly less activity.

load of disease, and a markedly lower tendency to develop new MRI lesions than did relapsing patients. In addition, only one of the 20 small new MRI lesions that they saw enhanced. The optimum frequency of scanning (considering the information obtained versus cost) is a question that cannot be answered unequivocally at this point. The protocol most likely to give good detailed information has been to scan once every 2 weeks. Assuming no lesion lasts less than 2 weeks, 100% of new and active lesions are detectable. The UBC experience has been that only 67% of lesion activity is seen with scans performed every 4 weeks and 40% with scans performed every 6 weeks. Conversely 36% of lesions had a duration of activity of <4 weeks, another 28% between 4 and 6 weeks, and another 7% between 6 and 8 weeks (see Table 3.7). It is also not necessary to do enhancement studies on a routine basis, since enhancement only adds 20% to the activity detected, but more than doubles the scanning time and increases the invasiveness.

Magnetic Resonance Spectroscopy (MRS) and Experimental Studies

Studies using magnetic resonance spectroscopy (MRS) techniques to sample the chemical information coming from tissue will be of great help in beginning to understand the evolution of the pathologic process during life. For example, there are several studies that have found changes in spectroscopically detected chemical components of MS/MRI lesions. N-acetyl aspartate (NAA) is decreased in chronic MS lesions (Arnold et al. 1990). This chemical change may be a reflection of the tissue alterations in gliosis and the loss of axons. Similar findings have been noted in cerebral infarction and in Binswanger's disease.

The detection of fat in evolving MS lesions could be critical to the understanding of the sequence of events. In-vitro hydrogen MRS studies (Simon and Fonte 1988) have shown that there is a lipid signal associated with demyelination in animals with acute experimental allergic encephalomyelitis (EAE). In-vivo hydrogen spectroscopy studies on EAE have also detected lipid changes (Richards et al. 1988). Fat signals have also been reported in MS patients (Narayana et al. 1989). Suggestive evidence for the presence of cholesterol and/or fatty acids was seen in 5 of 21 possibly acute MS lesions. The lipid changes that were seen in the MS lesions disappeared after 2 weeks. In collaboration with Dr. Peter Allen of the University of Alberta, we have found that in some new and active lesions detected by serial MRI examinations a hydrogen MR signal that could be neutral fat (Koopmans et al. 1990) can be seen. The fact that no lipid changes were seen in other new MRI lesions suggests that the pathological process in new and evolving lesions is heterogeneous. These limited observations are consistent with the hypothesis that the majority of new lesions are inflammatory ones and do not involve demyelination in the first instance. The Queen Square group have also used a new technique for detecting a fat signal (Hawkins et al. 1990) and have looked at both post-mortem and in-vivo material. Preliminary evidence is that they can detect mobile fat in active lesions.

The ability to detect mobile lipid in both pathological section and in spectroscopy could be a very important investigative tool for markers of demyelination in active MS lesions. Pathological studies show that the appearance of neutral fat in macrophages is a transient phenomenon. The possibility of reliably detecting changes in lipid and perhaps identifying the age and activity of MS lesions in-vivo is very exciting. In the future, the use of combined serial MRI and MRS studies should enable the simultaneous identification of both the morphological and chemical changes that occur in MS lesions during the process of edema, and/or inflammation, demyelination, gliosis, and axonal loss.

Karlik et al. (1986) have looked at the T_1 and T_2-relaxation times in tissue excised from guinea-pigs with EAE. They found that the relaxation times changed with the pathology, but unfortunately the MR changes were not specific to the pathologic changes seen in the tissue. In fact, in some inflammatory lesions, the T_1-relaxation times were long in edematous tissue but when a heavy cellular infiltrate was present the trend was reversed and the T_1 times were normalized.

Stewart and her colleagues (Stewart et al. 1988b) have also studied the pathology in EAE by measuring multi-exponential relaxation times. Her multi-exponential relaxation time techniques show that various degrees of pathology could indeed be identified by NMR methods. In a series of studies in primate EAE Stewart also showed that MR lesions could be seen to develop before the animals became ill. One observation showed that a relapsing and remitting form of demyelination could be produced with a single immunization in the primate EAE model (Stewart et al. 1988a). In one animal bilateral cerebral MRI lesions developed entirely asymptomatically after an unusual delay following low strength inoculation. These lesions disappeared, but subsequent MRI follow-up showed an asymptomatic new lesion to appear spontaneously in a fresh anatomical site. All of the MRI activity came and went away without the appearance of illness in the animal. Subsequent pathology in that animal did not show any evidence for either demyelination or inflammation. Additional attention to this very mild EAE model in the future should help us to understand better the mechanisms involved in the evolution of the acute inflammatory lesion and provide a more realistic model for relapsing MS.

MRI Experience and Changes in MS Pathology

As shown in these serial studies there is a lot of dynamic change going on that is not seen in the measurement of chronic MRI lesions. Serial frequent MRI examinations have shown that the rate of appearance of new lesions is considerably higher than the rate of development of new neurological symptoms. Therefore, the pathology of the acute lesion see on the MRI scan has been the object of considerable speculation. There is now one pathological correlation abstract in the literature showing intense inflammation in what had been an enhancing lesion (Katz et al. 1990).

The first pathologic event that occurs in the evolution of the MS lesions seems to be breakdown in the blood–brain barrier (BBB). The Queen Square group has seen several Gd-enhancing lesions appear before they were detectable on the standard MRI scan (Kermode et al. 1990). After BBB breakdown, intense and spreading inflammation develops. Serial scanning experience has found that new and active lesions evolve to become larger over a period of 1 month or 6 weeks and then gradually become smaller. In the UBC experience, many of the lesions that became smaller actually disappeared. Disappearance is probably related to the low field strength of the machine (0.15T). The pathological change that accompanies the waxing and waning of a lesion is probably pure inflammation. Even though remyelination is known to occur in the central nervous system in MS (Ludwin 1979) most investigators do not think that remyelination accounts for the resolution of the active MRI lesions.

The Queen Square group has shown that 88% of the new MRI lesions are gadolinium-enhancing. As noted above they also found that the gadolinium enhancement can be very short-lived, showing that breakdown of the blood–brain barrier could be a very transient phenomenon. UBC studies have shown, however, that CT enhancement can last, or perhaps reappear many months after the first episode of enhancement. In addition, the Queen Square group found only 10% of old lesions to enhance, though occasionally morphologically stable lesions would develop transient enhancement.

In addition, several preliminary studies of the effect of steroids on MRI and MRI enhancement suggest that, as with CT, IV steroids can reduce the degree of enhancement. Steroids do not, however, affect the number and extent of the standard T_2-weighted MRI lesions seen on T_2-weighted scans.

Evoked Potentials as a Measure of Outcome

Evoked potentials are useful in detecting asymptomatic lesions in the diagnosis of MS. Serial studies of the VEP were reported by Matthews and Small (1979) and Becker and Richards (1984). Matthews and Small found that 9 out of 51 patients who had abnormal latencies returned to normal in follow-up, and 27 had increasing abnormalities over time. They found that their reversion to normal was disappointing in a diagnostic sense in that the abnormality did not always persist.

Becker and Richards found that control patients' VEPs changed very little over time (23 months). MS patients changed quite a bit. A few VEP latencies improved in follow-up. All patients with improvement had a clinical episode of optic neuritis in the appropriate eye within 7 weeks of the initial VEP study. The daily variability in the VEP in MS patients was between 5 and 7 ms. For that reason the authors stated that any change of less than 10 ms was probably not significant. Using those criteria, they found that 18 out of 80 (23%) of eyes has showed significant changes over 2 years, and ⅔ of those changes were asymptomatic. Prolongations were seen most frequently in patients with a chronic/progressive clinical course. Changes were not related to age or disease duration.

Iragui et al. (1986) also did a prospective 4-year follow-up of EP (evoked potentials, not specified) studies as part of a clinical trial of myelin basic protein (MBP). They found that changes were most likely to be seen in the VEP and that many of the changes were asymptomatic. When clinical deterioration occurred, the EP was likely to become more prolonged.

However, when clinical improvement occurred the EP was likely to remain prolonged. The overall correlation between clinical changes and EP changes was not good. There was no overall treatment effect in the trial; the authors felt that EP studies could be useful in future clinical trials.

De Weerd (1987) used EPs over 3.5 months in normal subjects and found less than 12% variability. Of 35 MS patients, however, 23 had greater than normal variability. Twenty patients were treated with ACTH, and changes in EP occurred equally in treated and non-treated patients.

Anderson et al. (1987) monitored the EPs in 57 patients, half of whom were treated with hyperbaric oxygen. They found that half of the patients had ambiguous results. Test/re-test variability was large. The 2-h duration of the testing procedure was possibly a factor in the variability because of fatigue. The authors felt that the reproducibility problem was a significant deterrent to the routine use of EP in clinical trials.

Nuwer et al. (1989) used annual EPs during a 3-year double-blind placebo-controlled therapeutic trial with azathioprine (AZA), with and without steroids, in chronic/progressive disease. All testing was started at 0900h and the testing variables were carefully controlled to minimize variability. They found that the patients treated with a combination of azathioprine and methyl prednisolone had significantly less progression in the EP latency than did patients treated with placebo or AZA alone.

In summary, EP latencies can be seen to prolong over time. There is a problem in consistency and interpretation of the EP results in chronic MS patients. Prolongation of EP probably does reflect new lesions, but just how to weigh the changes seen in the EP is not clear. More data on natural history are necessary, but in the meantime it would be a mistake not to monitor at least the VEP in MS clinical trials. As indicated by Nuwer, very careful attention must be paid to factors which might influence reproducibility, such as time of day, temperature, degree of fatigue, and, of course, technical measurement factors.

Application of MRI and Other Techniques to Clinical Trials

It is very clear that the MRI scan of the cerebral hemispheres detects an extent of disease that is very different from that which is reflected in clinical severity measurements, particularly neurological ones.

Quantitative and serial MRI studies have helped to describe a newly revealed aspect of measurable activity of the pathological process in MS. The degree of activity revealed by serial MRI studies is considerably greater than the degree of activity determined by history and physical examination. In addition, a measurement of the extent of the abnormality can be done by outlining the lesions and summing the areas of abnormality, slice by slice. Frequently repeated scans, with or without Gd enhancement also reveal a markedly dynamic nature to the MS pathologic process that is for the most part asymptomatic.

Careful follow-up studies must be done in order to identify the prognostic implications of the MRI data. In the meantime, however, statistical assessment of the rate of appearance of new MRI lesions has shown that frequent scans can be used as a method of assessing disease activity in therapeutic trials.

A quantitative approach to the MRI scan is complementary to the clinical evaluation and is an important outcome measurement for clinical studies. There are two issues related to the MRI that are important to consider in developing an objective measurement of the burden of disease. The first consideration is to find a measure of the extent and/or severity of the pathological process. MRI can measure the extent of abnormality but it is still not capable of measuring the severity of the pathologic process within lesions. Future developments in 3-D imaging will bring even more new information to bear concerning disease activity.

The second issue relates to the dynamic features of the disease which cannot be measured by a single MRI. Just as with the clinical expression of disease in which patients have relapses and remissions, frequent MRI evaluations provide evidence for waxing and waning of disease activity.

Therefore, in order to do comprehensive studies, these 2 methods of MRI measurement should be combined. First, patients should be imaged frequently enough (every 2–8 weeks) to determine the rate at which new lesions come and go. Second, the extent of abnormality should be measured at entry and at exit, preferably at times during which there is not a lot of reversible disease activity occurring. Entry and exit MRI scans can furnish information on numbers of lesions and the total extent of the process. It is interesting to note that in serial studies, the dynamic changes that are obvious on inspection of the images do not have much impact on the quantitative measurements of disease burden. This lack of impact is because of the large chronic extent of disease present at baseline in most patients. As might be expected, the dynamic changes made the most significant impact on patients with low burden of disease at baseline. The current data from the 50 patients imaged every 6 weeks from the Beta-interferon trial has shown that the rate of MRI activity (3.0 active lesions/patient/year) is twice the rate of clinical relapses (1.5/patient/year). The patients who are seen to be active by scanning overlap with the patients who are active by clinical activity but not completely so. One-third of the patients are only active clinically and one-third are only active by MRI. An overlapping one-third are active both clinically and on MRI.

The same issues apply to the use of evoked potentials. There may be some variability in the technique and also some reversion to normal over time, but the use of EPs in large numbers of patients in both placebo and treated groups should provide adequate controls. Unfortunately the laboratory to laboratory variability in EP latencies means that the changes will have to be analyzed by simple, stable or algorithms of number stable, number worse, and number improved. Parametric methods applied to the actual latency data cannot be used.

Common sense would suggest that, if one could reduce the rate of MRI activity or clinical activity with a new therapy, the ultimate outcome of the disease would be improved. The strategy is the same for relapses as a measure of clinical activity and for MRI as a measure of pathologic activity. That is, one uses the number of relapses or the number of MRI events over time as an outcome measure assuming that those measures have prognostic importance in the long run.

Biological Measures of Outcome

The uncertain natural history, clinically unapparent lesions and the simultaneous phases of central nervous system (CNS) injury and repair of MS have prompted the examination of a number of biological measures that might reflect disease activity. Most of these measures relate to the known CNS tissue changes of demyelination, inflammation and astrogliosis. To be optimal for charting the natural history and determining a change in it effected by therapy, a measurement selected should be objective, quantitative, feasible and meaningful. A number of components of cerebrospinal fluid (CSF), blood and urine have been examined in this regard, but none currently available meets all of these demands. Those pertaining to the appearance of CNS myelin components in body fluids and to the status of the immune system appear to hold the greatest promise.

CNS Myelin Components

The rationale for this approach is based on the expectation that characteristic CNS myelin components, degraded and released at the site of inflammatory demyelination, will be detectable in body fluids at a level proportional to the amount of CNS myelin damage. CNS myelin is composed of 40% water and 60% solid which consists of protein and lipids in a ratio of approximately 20:80 (reviewed in Lees and Brostoff 1984 and Morell et al. 1989). Three different proteins – 2′,3′-cyclic 3′-phosphodiesterase (CNPase), proteolipid and myelin basic protein (MBP) occurring in a ratio of 2:5:3 – account for over 95% of CNS myelin proteins. MBP is a very cationic protein present in several isoforms with one of 18500 daltons (170 amino-acid residues) dominating in adult human CNS. MBP has received particular attention because of its encephalitogenic property of inducing experimental allergic encephalomyelitis. A fourth protein, myelin-associated glycoprotein (MAG), is a minor (<1%) CNS myelin constituent. This 100000-dalton glycoprotein is present in oligodendroglial cytoplasm, notably in that abutting the axon. It is not present in compact CNS myelin. Each of these 4 CNS myelin components has been sought in CSF and other body fluids. The most extensively studied is MBP which at present is the best candidate for a laboratory test for monitoring disease activity in MS.

Myelin Basic Protein

A number of independent studies have shown that, in association with active CNS demyelination, MBP or fragments thereof can be detected by radioimmunoassay (RIA) in CSF (Alling et al. 1980; Cohen et al. 1976, 1980; Gangji et al. 1980; Hemphill et al. 1980; Whitaker et al. 1977, 1980; Biber et al. 1981; reviewed in Whitaker 1982). Different types of RIAs have been utilized in which intact MBP (Cohen et al. 1975) or a peptide of MBP (Whitaker et al. 1977; Biber et al. 1981; Whitaker et al. 1980) serves as the radio-labelled antigen, permitting a sensitivity of 1 ng or less per assay tube. Most of the assays have been validated by the standard criteria used for establishing a RIA, but the identification of the material immunologically measured as MBP has still not been documented by an independent test of biological activity or by determination of its chemical structure. For these reasons, the material being measured must be interpreted presently as cross-reactive with MBP, or MBP-like. Although there are minor differences among these reports, each has shown that MBP-like material is absent in normal human CSF but appears in the range of ng/ml following acute myelin damage, irrespective of cause. Elevated CSF MBP-like material may also be found in acute necrotic lesions of the CNS caused by infarctions, hemorrhage, necrotizing encephalitis, hypoxic brain injury, gross head injury, and surgical brain damage (Palfreyman et al. 1978, 1979). The level of CSF MBP-like material is related to both the mass and time of myelin damage. Large lesions, especially those in the cervical spinal cord and within 5 days of onset, are correlated with high values. CSF from persons with diseases affecting peripheral nervous system (PNS) myelin, such as Guillain–Barré syndrome and chronic inflammatory demyelinating polyneuropathy, rarely contains MBP-like material and, if so, only in small amounts (Whitaker et al. 1980). Only a small number of patients have been serially sampled before, during and after episodes of acute CNS myelin damage (Alling et al. 1980; Cohen et al. 1976, 1980; Ohta et al. 1980). In these serial studies and in studies where single samples of CSF are available and the antecedent episodes precisely dated (Whitaker 1977) it is evident that the MBP-like material rapidly declines and disappears and may do so before the clinical features improve. CSF from MS patients 1 week or more beyond an exacerbation are frequently negative and are nearly always so after the second week. One of the shortcomings of the measurement of CSF MBP-like material is that it does not show changes in parallel with chronic/progressive phases of MS (Whitaker 1977). Low levels may occasionally be detected with the most sensitive assays (Whitaker and Herman 1988). The absence of CSF MBP-like material in MS patients 2 weeks or more after an exacerbation suggests either rapid clearance, degradation or modification of the antigen by some mechanism. In contrast to this temporal profile in MS patients, the MBP-like material in the CSF of persons with surgical brain damage (Alling et al. 1980) or ischemic cerebral infarction (Whitaker et al. 1980) does not rise as predictably or correlate as closely with the onset of CNS tissue damage.

The appearance or level of MBP-like material in CSF has little or no relationship to the imunoglobulin abnormalities commonly noted in the CSF of MS patients (Warren and Catz 1985; Whitaker 1977). The presence of MBP-like material in CSF is not related to changes in total protein or IgG levels (Whitaker 1977); however, striking elevations of protein (>10 g/l) may interfere with the methods utilizing ethanol for precipitating bound antibody (Kohlschutter 1978).

Features of MBP-like Material in CSF

The MBP-like material in CSF appears to exist in a spectrum of molecular sizes, much of it apparently in fragments (Bashir and Whitaker 1980a; Karlsson and Alling 1984). The existence of MBP peptides in CSF is postulated to result from the action of enzymes, in areas of CNS inflammatory demyelination or in CSF, on MBP which is very susceptible to degradation by a number of proteinases (Einstein et al. 1972; Cammer et al. 1978; Whitaker and Seyer 1979). The existence of MBP fragments in CSF may explain why many antibodies to MBP, presumably directed against epitopes of MBP not present in CSF, fail to detect MBP-like material in CSF (Whitaker et al. 1980). CSF MBP-like material, from MS and non-MS patients, may exist as complexes of antigen and antibody (Bashir and Whitaker 1980a; Warren and Catz 1987). Such complexes lower the level of MBP-like material measured and obscure the detection of antibody to MBP.

The exact form(s) of MBP peptides which are presumed to create the MBP-like material in CSF, remains to be structurally ascertained. Immunochemical reactivities suggest the presence of a decapeptide of MBP encompassing the residues 80–89 in a conformation shared with MBP peptide 45–89 and intact MBP (Whitaker et al. 1980, 1986). The conformation and immunochemical behaviour are markedly affected by minor structural changes (Whitaker 1987; Whitaker et al. 1990). The MBP-like material in the CSF of MS patients is probably a result of different fragments of MBP; however, an RIA designed for the detection of material cross-reactive with MBP peptide 69–89 affords the most sensitive assay of MBP-like material in CSF (Whitaker and Herman 1988). Multiple antigenic sites of MBP are represented in CSF after myelin injury (Cohen et al. 1980). Larger forms predominate in patients with cerebral infarction and head injury and smaller sizes in patients with acute MS (Bashir and Whitaker, 1980a; Karlsson and Alling 1984). Large molecular weight forms of MBP-like material in CSF were also noted in necrotic brain damage (Palfreyman et al. 1978). The difference in sizes, plus the differences in temporal appearance (see above) of CSF MBP-like activity in acute MS and cerebral infarctions, suggest differences in the mechanisms of production or disposal of MBP-like material in these two conditions.

Attempts to Measure MBP-like Material in Blood

Successful attempts to detect MBP or MBP peptides in the sera of humans have been reported (Palfreyman et al. 1978, 1979) but technical difficulties have so far precluded the validation of an immunoassay for MBP-like material in blood. This is believed to be a result of proteinases (Pescovitz et al. 1978) and binding proteins (McPherson et al. 1970; Lennon and Mackay 1972; Bernard and Lamoureux 1975), which may interfere with the measurements of MBP. Extraction protocols for removing these interfering materials have not yet been developed.

Urinary MBP-like Material

The demonstrated renal clearance of MBP peptide (Bashir and Whitaker 1980b) led to a series of investigations revealing that human kidney contains a neutral proteinase capable of degrading MBP peptide 45–89 (Whitaker and Heinemann 1983). Utilizing this information plus the known differences in immunochemical reactivity among MBP peptides (Whitaker 1982; Whitaker et al. 1977), MBP-like material was demonstrated in urine (Whitaker 1987). The immunoassay for urinary MBP-like material recognizes a different MBP epitope, one in MBP peptide 80–89 but *not* in intact MBP (Whitaker 1987; Whitaker et al. 1990). Urinary MBP-like material is found in all persons tested, is higher in individuals with MS, is heat-stable, is less than 1000 daltons in size and appears most closely to simulate immunochemically MBP peptide 82–89 or 83–89 (Whitaker 1987). The chemical nature of urinary MBP-like material and its clinical correlation await clarification. Urinary MBP-like material does not mirror acute CNS myelin damage, does not correlate with CSF levels of MBP-like material and is higher in chronic/progressive than relapsing/remitting MS (Whitaker et al. 1989). It is possible that urinary MBP-like material reflects an alteration of MBP turnover after myelin damage or MBP synthesis in excess of incorporation into myelin during attempted remyelination.

Other Myelin Markers

Proteolipid is elevated in the CSF or serum of approximately 50% of persons with acute-phase MS, but it is not as disease-specific and is not as consistently associated with myelin damage as is the level of MBP or MBP peptide (Trotter et al. 1980). Normal CSF contains very little (Raes et al. 1981) or no (Banik et al. 1979) CNPase, but CSF from persons with myelin damage, irrespective of cause, frequently has increased CNPase activity (Sprinkle and McKhann 1978; Banik et al. 1979). In CSF the quantitation of MBP has better sensitivity and specificity for myelin damage than does CNPase (Sprinkle and McKhann 1978). MAG is decreased in MS plaques (Itoyama et al. 1980), and is found in CSF in the range of 2–13 ng/ml in normals and MS patients (Yanagisawa et al. 1985). In the CSF it exists as a 90 000-dalton proteolytic derivative, referred to as DMAG, of the 100 000-dalton MAG. Its CSF level does not correlate with clinical episodes of demyelination (Yanagisawa et al. 1985). Studies of levels of lipids in the CSF of MS patients show a broad variation and no consistent alterations of the general lipid classes (Pedersen 1974).

CSF Proteinases

Both neutral and acidic proteinases show increased activities in the CSF of persons with demyelinating diseases, but without relationship to disease activity in MS (Alvord et al. 1979; Cuzner et al. 1978; Rinne and Riekkinen. 1968; reviewed in Bever and Whitaker 1985). Increased net enzyme activity might result not only from an increase in amount of enzyme, but also an increase in activators or decline in inhibitors. Levels of the CSF a_1-antitrypsin and transferrin are marginally decreased in MS, but show no difference between cases in exacerbation and in remission (Price and Cuzner 1979).

Glial Proteins

Efforts have been made to measure CSF levels of proteins which are uniquely or preferentially localized to certain glia. These might be related to astrogliosis occurring in MS tissue lesions. Glial fibrillary acidic protein (GFAP) (Eng 1980) may appear in the CSF in acute bouts of MS (Lowenthal et al. 1978), but its frequency in such situations is unknown. GFAP in CSF is not specific for myelin injury and may occur in individuals with brain tumors and strokes (Hayakawa et al. 1979). S-100 is usually regarded as a glial marker, but may occur in other cells (Zomzely-Neurath and Walker 1980). The elevation of S-100 in the CSF (Michetti et al. 1979) has been noted in a similar pattern to that of GFAP and is elevated in acute phases of MS as well as in intracranial tumors, spinal cord compression and other degenerative or destructive processes. Available information on GFAP and S-100 proteins does not indicate that they can serve as markers of disease activity in MS (Massaro et al. 1985).

Immune System

Humoral Studies

The immunopathological uncertainty of the evolution of the tissue damage in MS is paralleled by the uncertainty of any direct or indirect immunological measure in CSF and blood as a monitor of disease activity. Many have been examined. The increase in CNS production of immunoglobulin and its restricted heterogeneity (oligoclonality) in MS are well known, but neither CSF immunoglobulin level nor the oligoclonal pattern varies with changes in disease activity (reviewed by Tourtellotte 1985). While the calculated rate of synthesis of IgG in the CNS may be reduced with treatment with ACTH and glucocorticoids, there is no change induced by such treatment on the oligoclonal band pattern nor is there a correlation with changes in clinical status (Tourtellotte et al. 1980). Serum immunoglobulins in MS are normal antibodies with specific reactivity to exogenous or endogenous antigens have shown no clear relationship with disease activity (Ivanainen 1981).

Cellular Studies

The number, subtype, markers and functions of blood and CSF lymphocytes from MS patients have been examined by a variety of methods (reviewed in Hafler and Weiner 1989). Since the late 1970s evidence has been gathered about an immunoregulatory T-cell defect in MS. The role of such cells in the formation of tissue lesions in MS is unresolved (Raine 1990). The CD8 cytotoxic/suppressor subset of T lymphocytes might participate in cytotoxicity or suppress immune events at sites of CNS inflammatory demyelination. Functional suppressor cell activity generated by the mitogen concanavalin A was shown to be reduced in acute phases of MS (Antel et al. 1978). Initial studies of lymphocyte subsets reported a reduction of T suppressor/cytotoxic cells during active phases of disease (Hauser et al. 1983b; Reinherz et al. 1980). While there may well be a defect in the function or generation of T suppressor cells in MS (Hafler and Weiner 1989; Morimoto et al. 1987), a number of studies have failed to confirm a consistent change in blood lymphocyte subsets temporally related to disease activity (Compston 1983; Paty et al. 1983; Zabriskie et al. 1985). CSF lymphocytes are activated in MS

(Hafler et al. 1985; Noronha et al. 1980) but are unlikely to provide a feasible biological measure.

Although the specific events remain ill-defined, the CNS tissue damage in MS is accompanied by the activation of infiltrating cells and resident glia (Raine et al. 1990a,b; Raine and Cross 1990). The activation of lymphocytes and macrophages results in the induction and release of certain membrane receptors and in the production of soluble mediators, referred to as cytokines. Cytokines and soluble receptors have been sought in CSF and blood as markers of disease activity. The cytokines interferon-gamma (Abbott et al. 1987), interleukin-1 beta (Hauser et al. 1990), interleukin-2 (Gallo et al. 1988), interleukin-6 (Hauser et al. 1990; Nishimoto et al. 1990), and tumor necrosis factor-alpha (Franciotta et al. 1989; Gallo et al. 1989a,b,c; Hauser et al. 1990) are either undetectable or not significantly different in CSF of MS patients and controls, or their levels in CSF or blood show no relationship to disease activity. The receptor for interleukin-2, IL-2R, is expressed on activated T cells from which it may be shed in a soluble form, sIL-2R (Rubin and Nelson 1990). A number of clinical immunologic studies have been performed on CSF and blood of MS patients (Adachi et al. 1990; Fesenmeier et al. 1990; Gallo et al. 1989a,b,c; Kittur et al. 1990). Available results are in disagreement as to whether 5IL-2R can be detected in CSF or correlates with disease activity. This may be a promising area for study.

Clinical Correlation of Biological Markers

Of the laboratory tests examined so far the measurement of MBP-like material has been the most thoroughly examined and useful in spite of technical demands on its performance. The clinical utility of the assay for MBP-like material in CSF is largely to document the presence, continuation, or resolution of CNS myelin damage. In individuals who have a disabling form of MS and in whom the degree of deficit is already marked, the presence of CSF MBP-like material may also provide documentation for another exacerbation when this is clinically uncertain. An elevated level of CSF MBP-like material may serve as an adjunct in the diagnosis of MS even though its presence is not disease-specific. In studies in which CSF MBP-like material, CSF immunoglobulins, and peripheral blood lymphocyte subsets have been examined in the same patients, only the CSF MBP-like material was shown to correlate with disease activity (Thompson et al. 1987). It has been noted that MS patients with high levels of MBP-like material in CSF have a higher incidence of late neurologic dysfunction (Matias-Guiu et al. 1986) while the absence of MBP-like material in CSF correlates with a benign course (Thompson et al. 1986). A longer follow-up and increased number of cases will make these correlations more persuasive. A fall in the level of MBP-like material in CSF of patients with MS who have been treated with either immunosuppressant drugs (Lamers et al. 1988) or glucocorticoids (Warren et al. 1986) correlates well with clinical improvement. Because of the known rapid changes in the MBP-like material in the CSF of untreated MS patients, proof of therapeutic efficacy with controlled studies of adequate duration is not yet available. No systematic study has been reported on the correlation of serial changes on cranial or spinal MRI or evoked potentials and the level of MBP-like material in CSF.

Overall Summary and Recommendations on Outcome Measures

The Kurtzke EDSS is the standard clinical outcome measure, and the functional scales (FS) should be done in parallel. Specific function measures should be used for symptomatic trials and for relapse therapy. However, the clinical measures do not measure the underlying extent (or burden) of the disease and much of the dynamic aspects of disease activity.

MRI and MRS hold the promise of not only being able to measure the extent and activity of disease, but also the type and severity of the damage. Biological markers of tissue damage or immunologic disturbances will provide insights into pathogenesis and severity of damage, but the precise methods to be used are not yet determined.

We suggest the following measures:

Clinical Outcome: The standard measure should be the EDSS. The Ambulation Index may be a useful addition if many of the trial patients are moderately disabled (EDSS 4.0–6.0). Selection of extra tests such as the ISS will depend on time and resources available and the special interests of the investigators. Restricted quantitative measures such as the Upper Extremity Index or a battery of such tests might be helpful as adjuncts. The tests of cognitive function most likely to prove valuable as a practical extra measure are intermediate-length tests such as the Neuro-psychological Screening Battery

Treatment of Acute Exacerbations: The EDSS should be the basic measure with consideration given to separate analysis of the functional systems most affected by the exacerbation

Treatment of Chronic Symptoms: An appropriate scale to grade the symptom of interest should be selected. If the symptom affects activities of daily living the ISS and/or the Ambulation Index should be considered for use

MRI and Evoked Potentials:

Quantitative: Entry and exit examinations using careful reproducibility controls

Serial for activity: Regularly spaced examinations, closely enough spaced to see the dynamic changes (example, every 6 weeks and at time of clinical relapse)

Biological Measures: Choose one as a research measure and carefully measure the changes to correlate with either the MRI, EP, or clinical changes.

Appendix. Suggested MRI Scanning Protocol for Clinical Studies

We would recommend that MRI be used carefully to study specific questions. As a final outcome measure of extent of disease one can do the following:

1. Quantitative measurements of the extent of the process at entry, midpoint, and exit from a clinical trial
2. Visual assessment of the outcome for individual lesions

If one wants to assess the dynamic aspect of the disease process over time one must do the following:

1. Frequent, evenly spaced scans with an assessment of individual lesion changes as well as the total extent of the process
2. Gd-enhancement, systematically done, will add additional information concerning BBB disruption as a marker of activity. However, since it is known that steroids probably reduce the degree of enhancement without changing the lesions themselves, one must evaluate morphological changes and enhancement separately. As in the clinical setting, with the use of steroids there may be a transient effect on one measure that is not reflected in a final reduction in the outcome measure

Frequency of Scanning

The optimum frequency of scanning, especially if gadolinium enhancement is used, would be every 2 weeks. One cannot get much dynamic information from a frequency of less than once every 6 weeks, at which point 50% of the activity data is lost.

Technical Aspects of Repeated Scanning

In order to have reproducible data, the results must be as consistent as possible both within sites and between sites. The procedure at the University of British Columbia is to identify the lesions on the films. We then use the image taken from the computer tape from the same machine, same examination, and quantitate the size, location, and total extent of the MS lesions for each examination. The standards and procedures given in this section are designed to minimize problems in clinical trials.

MRI centers may use instruments from one of several different manufacturers. Field strengths that are current used range from 0.15 to 1.5 Tesla. In order to maintain some sort of consistency, standardized pulse sequences must be adopted for scanning throughout the study. These standards must be selected to optimize the detection of MS lesions, delineate the limits of the ventricular system, and assure comparable entry and exit data despite anticipated equipment enhancement over the approximate 3-year interval of the study. The following imaging protocol is proposed:

1. Axial plane (coronal plane will add additional useful information, but will increase the time and cost of the procedure)

2. Minimum of 12 slices, 5–10 cm, preferably contiguous. Thinner slices may be used if done so consistently. Note that the gap between MRI slices varies between manufacturers. Some machines have a 50% gap between slices, though the MRI slices probably are thicker at the centre portion, filling in part of that gap. One must be aware of the extent of the gap in one's own machine and be careful that the gap does not create artifactual changes with repositioning.

It would be prudent to do several trials of repositioning and intentional displacement to see what effects these procedures have on one's own images

3. Consistency in studies is vital. The same parameters should be used on all examinations, including the same:
   a) Imaging machine
   b) Echo time (TE)
   c) Repeat time (TR)
   d) Number of views
   e) Acquisition matrix (frequency and phase encoding stops)
   f) Display matrix
   g) Number of excitations averaged
   h) Slice thickness
   i) Slice interval
   j) Slice gap
   k) Attenuation setting
   l) Reconstruction and filter
   m) Window and level for display
4. The suggested scanning parameters are as follows:
   a) Spin echo sequence
   b) Multiple echo studies should be used. At least one of the echo times should allow for the CSF to be dark or isodense with white matter and the lesions bright (TE 40–60, TR 2000). This sequence enables a distinction to be made between lesion and ventricle and optimizes contrast between lesion and white matter.
   Important. Because of problems involved with repositioning, follow-up studies may take about 20 min longer than the initial studies. This time factor should be considered in the planning stage and sufficient time be taken in order to produce optimum follow-up studies

First Examination

Position the patient comfortably in the head holder. Measure the angle of the radiographic baseline (RBL or canthomeatal line) as well as the angle between the tragus of the ear and the nasion with an anguliner. Record both of these external angles. On follow-up examinations the patient must be positioned so that these two angles are the same as on the first examination. The angle of the head is extremely important for repositioning as a slight difference (3°–4°) can make a dramatic difference in the scans. Remember that *patient comfort* is vital (see following).

Do a midline sagittal pilot or scout scan (short TR, approximately 300–500 ms, 128 matrix 1 excitation). Position the scan lines using a standard internal structure as a reference point. The top of the cerebellum can be used with scanners that use the middle slice of the series as a reference. Using the same structure on all patients makes the follow-up studies easier. It is very important that the patient be comfortable for the baseline scan. If comfortable, the patient is much easier to position for the follow-up scans.

From the pilot scan use the computer to measure an internal angle. The top of the cerebellum to the anterior superior portion of the sphenoid sinus works well. Photograph the pilot with the two points used on it as well as the angle measurement. On follow-up examinations, measure the same angle on the new pilot to check the patient position.

Follow-up Examinations

Position the patient so the RBL and tragus to nasion angles are the same as on the first examination. Do the midline sagittal pilot and check the internal angle used previously. If the internal angle varies more than 2° from the baseline scan then the patient's head should be adjusted accordingly and a second pilot scan done. Make sure that the patient is *comfortable*.

When the head position is satisfactory, position the scan lines as before. Position the lines seen on the pilot to match the lines on the original scan. If they do not match then the patient's head should be adjusted again until they match well. Only after they match are the actual evaluation scans obtained.

If a machine is available that scans in multiple oblique planes, patient position may not be as important. However, beware, because in some machines the oblique image is not the same as the standard one. Just match the scan lines on the pilots. As the scans come out compare each level with the corresponding level on the baseline scan. It is most efficient to do this procedure correctly the first time. If patients move during the scan that may mean they are not comfortable.

When the scans are photographed try to set the contrast and brightness levels so they look the same as on the first study, as this makes it easier to compare the two studies. If more than one follow-up study is being done, always use the first study as the reference scan.

This procedure can be quite time-consuming and frustrating, especially on patients who cannot stay perfectly still; however, it is important to the study for the imaging personnel to be patient.

Analysis of MRI Data

One way of assessing MRI activity is in terms of the rates of appearance of new lesions. Pilot studies indicate that, at least with scanning rates monthly or bi-weekly, scans with more than one new lesion are relatively frequent (1.7 lesions per active scan). Scans can be classified as either active or inactive. This method has the advantage of simplifying the analysis which can then be based upon the fraction of the scans for each patient exhibiting one or more new lesions.

Each patient has his/her own rate at which new lesions appear. The repeated scans on each patient permit rates to be calculated for individual patients and for the sample of patients. An assessment of how variable these rates are from patient to patient can be made. The within-patient estimation error component of variability and the patient-to-patient component of variability together determine the precision with which the underlying average rate for the collection of patients is determined. The estimation error component of variability can be controlled by including more patients in the sample. In such a setting, the relative allocation of effort to controlling the two different components of variability becomes a fundamental issue.

The results obtained in the pilot studies provide estimates of these components of variability for the groups of patients studied. These estimates have been employed in an evaluation of the adequacy of the sample sizes specified for ongoing multi-center beta-interferon clinical trials. However, this evaluation is at best an estimate because the relatively small number of patients involved in each of the pilot studies does not allow a precise estimation of the magnitude of the patient-to-patient component of variability. One of the objectives of future studies should be to obtain a more precise estimate of the components of variability for each group of patients studied, thereby allowing a more precise evaluation of necessary sample sizes for therapeutic trials. An assessment of the statistical power of doing repeated scans in the relapsing and remitting patients (UBC studies #1 and #2) showed that in a two-arm trial with monthly scanning over 24 months the chance that a two-sided statistical test carried out at 5% level will detect a 50% reduction in the average rate of appearance of new lesions would be 89% with a sample size of 35 in each of the two arms. The power with 25 in each arm would be 77%. If the number of patients in each arm is increased to 50 (or so) then the duration and follow-up necessary to detect statistical significance could be reduced to 1 year (John Petkau, unpublished calculations performed at UBC).

A variety of methods will be required to analyze the MRI data collected. Because many of the objectives concern the collection of additional information about disease activity, the primary emphasis will be on description. A basic scheme of scanning every 2 weeks should produce regularly-spaced data. Some of this data will be continuous (load) and can, perhaps after suitable transformation, be analyzed by repeated measures methods. Other of this data is of the presence/absence type (new lesions); a simple approach to the analysis of such data is through rates, as described above. These methods allow the description of a single group of patients, as well as the comparison of different groups.

Any scheme of serial MRI scanning involves a trade-off. Frequent scanning on a few individuals would provide detailed information on these individuals, but the information would not be applicable to all patients unless a large enough group could be studied. Less frequent scanning on a larger number of patients will provide a more broadly-based description of the nature of the disease activity.

Most schemes build on earlier studies and reflect the reality that patients will be reluctant, and in many cases unable, to present to scanning at frequencies greater than once every 2 weeks for extended periods of time. The basic scanning frequency proposed for use is once every 2 weeks and the feasibility of this frequency has been demonstrated in pilot studies.

Acknowledgements. We want to thank Lynne Hannay very much for her excellent work on putting this chapter together. We are also appreciative of the Multiple Sclerosis Society of Canada, the Medical Research Council of Canada, the British Columbia Health Care Research Foundation, and the

Jacob W. Cohen Fund for Research into Multiple Sclerosis all of which have contributed to the studies cited in this chapter.

References

Abbott RJ, Bolderson I, Bruer PJK, Peatfield RC (1987) Immunoreactive IFN-g in CSF in neurological disorders. J Neurol Neurosurg Psychiatry 50:882–885

Adachi K, Kumanoto T, Araki S (1990) Elevated soluble interleukin-2 receptor levels in patients with active multiple sclerosis. Ann Neurol 28:687–691

Alling C, Karlsson B, Vallfors B (1980) Increase in myelin basic protein in CSF after brain surgery. J Neurol 223:225–230

Alvord EC, Hruby S, Sires L (1979) Degradation of myelin basic protein by cerebrospinal fluid: preservation of antigenic determinants under physiological conditions. Ann Neurol 6:474–482

Amato MP, Fratiglioni L, Groppi C, Siracusa G, Amaducci L (1988) Interrater reliability in assessing functional systems and disability on the Kurtzke Scale in multiple sclerosis. Arch Neurol 45:746–748

Anderson DC, Slater GE, Sherman R, Ettinger MG (1987) Evoked potentials to test a treatment of chronic multiple sclerosis. Arch Neurol 44:1232

Antel JP, Richman DP, Medof ME, Arnason BGW (1978) Lymphocyte function and the role of regulator cells in multiple sclerosis. Neurology 28:106–110

Arnold DL, Matthews PW, Francis G, Antel J (1990) Proton magnetic resonance spectroscopy of human brain in-vivo in the evaluation of multiple sclerosis: Assessment of the load of disease. Magn Reson Med 14:154–159

Banik NL, Mauldin LB, Hogan EL (1979) Activity of 2′, 3′-cyclic nucleotide 3′-phosphohydrolase in human cerebrospinal fluid. Ann Neurol 5:539–541

Bashir RM, Whitaker JN (1980a) Molecular features of immunoreactive myelin basic protein in cerebrospinal fluid of persons with multiple sclerosis. Ann Neurol 7:50–57

Bashir RM, Whitaker JN (1980b) Metabolism of a peptide of human myelin basic protein in the rabbit. Neurology 30:1184–1192

Bastianello S, Pozzilli C et al. (1990) Serial study of gadolinium-DTPA MRI enhancement in multiple sclerosis. Neurology 40:591–595

Baumhefner RW, Tourtellotte W, Syndulko K et al. (1990) Quantitative multiple sclerosis plaque assessment with magnetic resonance imaging. Arch Neurol 47:19–26

Beatty WW, Goodkin DE (1990) Screening for cognitive impairment in multiple sclerosis: an evaluation of the Mini-mental State Examination. Arch Neurol 47:297–301

Becker WJ, Richards IM (1984) Serial pattern shift visual evoked potentials in multiple sclerosis. Can J Neurolog Sci 1:53–59

Bernard CC, Lamoureaux G (1975) Inhibition by serum of encephalitogenic activity of myelin basic protein. Intl Arch Allerg App Immunol 48:597–609

Bever CT, Whitaker JN (1985) Proteinases in inflammatory disease. Springer Sem Immunopath 8:235–250

Biber A, Englert D, Dommasch D, Hempel K (1981) Myelin basic protein in cerebrospinal fluid of patients with multiple sclerosis. J Neurol 225:231–236

Bornstein MB, Miller A, Slagle S et al. (1987) A pilot trial of COP 1 in exacerbating-remitting multiple sclerosis. N Engl J Med 317:408–414

Cammer W, Bloom BR, Norton WT, Gordon S (1978) Degradation of basic protein in myelin by neutral proteases secreted by stimulated microphages: a possible mechanism of inflammatory demyelination. Proc Natl Acad Sci USA 75:1544–1558

Cohen SR, McKhann GM, Guarnieri M (1975) A radioimmunoassay for myelin basic protein and its use for quantitative measurements. J Neurochem 25:371–376

Cohen SR, Herndon RM, McKhann GM (1976) Radioimmunoassay of myelin basic protein in spinal fluid: An index of active demyelination. N Engl J Med 295:1455–1457

Cohen SR, Brooks BR, Herndon RM, McKhann GM (1980) A diagnostic index of active demyelination: myelin basic protein in cerebrospinal fluid. Ann Neurol 8:25–31

Compston A (1983) Lymphocyte subpopulations in patients with multiple sclerosis. J Neurol Neruosurg Psychiatry 46:105–114

Cuzner ML, Davison AN, Rudge P (1978) Proteolytic activity blood leukocytes and cerebrospinal fluid in multiple sclerosis. Ann Neurol 4:337–344

de Weerd AW (1987) Variability of central conduction in the course of multiple sclerosis. Clin Neurol Neurosurg 9:89–91

Einstein ER, Csejtey J, Dalal KB, Adams CW, Bayliss OB, Hallpike JR (1972) Proteolytic activity and basic protein loss in and around multiple sclerosis plaques: combined biochemical and histochemical observations. J Neurochem

Eng LF (1980) The glial fibrillary acidic (GFA) protein. In: Bradshaw RA, Schneider DM (eds) Proteins of the nervous system. Raven Press, New York, pp 85–117

Fesenmeier JT, Herman PH, Walker DP, Whitaker JN (1990) Cerebrospinal fluid levels of myelin basic protein-like material and soluble interleukin-2 receptor in multiple sclerosis. Neurology 40:334

Folstein MF, Folstein SE, McHugh PR (1975) "Mini-Mental State": A practical method for grading the cognitive state of patients for the clinician. J Psychol Res 12:189–198

Franciotta DM, Grimaldi LME, Martino GV et al. (1989) Tumor necrosis factor in serum and cerebrospinal fluid of patients with multiple sclerosis. Ann Neurol 26:787–789

Franklin GM, Heaton RK, Nelson LM, Filley CM, Seibert C (1988) Correlation of neuropsychological and MRI findings in chronic/progressive multiple sclerosis. Neurology 38:1826–1829

Franklin GM, Nelson LM, Heaton RK, Filley CM (1990) Clinical perspectives in the identification of cognitive impairment. In: Rao SM (ed) Neurobehavioural aspects of multiple sclerosis. Oxford University Press, New York, pp 161–174

Gallo P, Piccinno, Pagni S, Tavolato B (1988) Interleukin-2 levels in serum and cerebrospinal fluid of multiple sclerosis patients. Ann Neurol 24:795–797

Gallo P, Cupic D, Bracco F, Krzalic L, Tavolato B, Battistin L (1989a) Experimental allergic encephalomyelitis in the monkey: humoral immunity and blood brain barrier function. Ital J Neurol Sci 10:561–565

Gallo P, Piccinno MG, Krzalic L, Tavolato B (1989b) Tumor necrosis factor alpha (TNFα) and neurological diseases: failure in detecting TNFα in the cerebrospinal fluid from patients with multiple sclerosis, AIDS dementia complex, and brain tumours. J Neuroimmunol 23:41–44

Gallo P, Piccinno MG, Pagni S et al. (1989c) Immune activation in multiple sclerosis: study of IL-2, sIL-2R, and g-IFN levels in serum and cerebrospinal fluid. J Neurol Sci 92:9–15

Gangji D, Reaman GH, Cohen SR, Bleyer WA, Poplack DG (1980) Leukoencephalopathy and elevated levels of myelin basic protein in the cerebrospinal fluid of patients with acute lymphoblastic leukemia. N Engl J Med 303:19–21

Goodkin DE, Hertsgaard D, Seminary J (1988) Upper extremity function in multiple sclerosis: improving assessement sensitivity with box-and-block and nine-hole peg tests. Arch Phys Med Rehabil 69:850–854

Goodkin DE et al. (1991) Inter- and intrarater variability for grades 1.0–3.5 of the Kurtzke Expanded Disability Sttatus Scale (EDSS). Neurology 41:145

Hafler DA, Weiner HL (1989) MS: A CNS and systemic autoimmune disease. Immunol Today 10:104–107

Hafler DA, Fox DA, Manning ME, Schlossman SF, Reinherz EL, Weiner HL (1985) In vivo activated T lymphocytes in the peripheral blood and cerebrospinal fluid of patients with multiple sclerosis. N Engl J Med 312:1405–1411

Hauser SL, Dawson DM, Lehrich JR et al. (1983a) Intensive immunosuppression in progressive multiple sclerosis. N Engl J Med 308:173–180

Hauser SL, Reinherz El, Hoban CJ, Schlossman SF, Weiner HL (1983b) Immunoregulatory T-cells and lymphocytotoxic antibodies in active multiple sclerosis: weekly analysis over a six-month period. Ann Neurol 13:418–425

Hauser SL, Doolittle TH, Lincoln R, Brown RH, Dinarello CA (1990) Cytokine accumulations in CSF of multiple sclerosis patients: Frequent detection of interleukin-1 and tumor necrosis factor but not interleukin-6. Neurology 40:1735–1739

Hawkins CP, Williams SCR, Barker GJ et al. (1990) Myelin breakdown products detected by magnetic resonance imaging in multiple sclerosis. Soc Magn Reson Med, p 149

Hayakawa T, Ushio Y, Mori T et al. (1979) Levels in stroke patients of CSF astroprotein and astrocyte-specific cerebroprotein. Stroke 10:685–689

Heaton RK, Thompson LL, Nelson LM, Filley CM, Franklin GM (1990) Brief and intermediate-length screening of neuropsychological impairment in multiple sclerosis. In: Rao SM (ed) Neurobehavioural aspects of multiple sclerosis. Oxford University Press, New York, pp 149–160

Hemphill M, Brooks B, Cohen S, Herndon R (1980) Cerebrospinal fluid myelin basic protein in children with multiple sclerosis. Ann Neurol 8:221

Honer WG, Hurwitz T, Li DKB, Palmer M, Paty DW (1987) Temporal lobe involvement in multiple sclerosis patients with psychiatric disorders. Arch Neurol 44:187–190

Huber SJ, Paulson GW, Shuttleworth EC et al. (1987) Magnetic resonance imaging correlates of dementia in multiple sclerosis. Arch Neurol 44:732–736

Huber SJ, Paulson GW, Chakeres D et al. (1988) Magnetic resonance imaging and clinical correlations in multiple sclerosis. J Neurol Sci 86:1–12

Iragui VJ, Wiederholt WC, Romine JS (1986) Serial recordings of multimodality evoked potentials in multiple sclerosis: a four year follow-up study. Can J Neurolog Sci 13:320-326

Isaac C, Li DKB, Genton M et al. (1988) Multiple sclerosis: a serial study using MRI in relapsing patients. Neurology 38:1511–1515

Itoyama Y, Sternberg NH, Webster HD, Quarles RH, Cohen SR, Richardson EP (1980) Immunocytochemical observations on the distribution of myelin-associated glyocprotein and myelin basic protein in multiple sclerosis lesions. Ann Neurol 7:167–177

Ivanainen MV (1981) The significance of abnormal immune responses in patients with multiple sclerosis. J Neuroimmunol 1:141–172

Jacobs JW, Bernhard MR, Delgado A, Strain JJ (1977) Screening for organic mental syndromes in the medically ill. Ann Int Med 86:40–46

Johnson MA, Li DKB, Bryant DJ, Payne JA (1984) Magnetic resonance imaging: Serial observations in multiple sclerosis. AJNR 5:495–499

Kappos L, Stadt D, Ratzka M et al. (1988) Magnetic resonance imaging in the evaluation of treatment in multiple sclerosis. Neuroradiology 30:299–302

Karlik SJ, Strejan G, Gilbert JJ, Noseworthy JH (1986) NMR studies in experimental allergic encephalomyelitis (EAE): Normalization of T1 and T2 with parenchymal cellular infiltration. Neurology 36:1112–1114

Karlsson B, Alling C (1984) Molecular size of myelin basic protein immunoactivity in spinal fluid. J Neuroimmunol 6:141–150

Kastrukoff LF, Oger JJ, Hashimoto SA et al. (1990) Systemic lymphoblastoid interferon therapy in chronic progressive multiple sclerosis. I. Clinical and MRI evaluation. Neurology 40:479–486

Katz D, Taubenberger J, Raine C, McFarlin D, McFarland H (1990) Gadolinium-enhancing lesions on magnetic resonance imaging: neuropathological findings. Ann Neurol 28:243

Kermode AG, Tofts PS, Thompson AJ et al. (1990) Heterogeneity of blood-brain barrier changes in multiple sclerosis: An MRI study with gadolinium-DPTA enhancement. Neurology 40:229–235

Kiel MK, Greenspun B, Grossman RI (1988) Magnetic resonance imaging and degree of disability in multiple sclerosis. Arch Phys Med Rehab 69:11–13

Kittur SD, Kittur DS, Soncrant TT et al. (1990) Soluble interleukin-2 receptors in cerebrospinal fluid from individuals with various neurological disorders. Ann Neurol 28:168–173

Kohlschutter A (1978) Myelin basic protein in cerebrospinal fluid from children. Eur J Pediatr 127:155–161

Koopmans RA, Li DKB, Grochowski E, Cutler PJ, Paty DW (1989a) Benign versus chronic progressive multiple sclerosis: magnetic resonance imaging features. Ann Neurol 25:74–81

Koopmans RA, Li DKB, Oger JJF et al. (1989b) Chronic progressive multiple sclerosis: serial magnetic resonance brain imaging over six months. Ann Neurol 26:248–256

Koopmans RA, Li DKB, Oger JJF, Mayo J, Paty DW (1989c) The lesion of multiple sclerosis: Imaging of acute and chronic stages. Neurology 39:959–963

Koopmans RA, Zhu G, Li DKB, Allen PS, Javidan M, Paty DW (1990) In vivo proton of the acute and chronic lesion of multiple sclerosis. Soc Magn Reson Med, abstracts, p 1205

Kurtzke JF (1955) A new scale for evaluating disability in multiple sclerosis. Neurology 5:580–583

Kurtzke JF (1961) On the evaluation of disability in multiple sclerosis. Neurology 11:686–694

Kurtzke JF (1983) Rating neurologic impairment in multiple sclerosis: an expanded disability status scale (EDSS). Neurology 33:1444–1452

Kurtzke JF (1986) Neuroepidemiology. Part II: Assessment of therapeutic trials. Ann Neurol 19:311–319

Kurtzke JF (1989) The disability status scale for multiple sclerosis: apologia pro DSS sua. Neurology 39:291

Lamers KJB, Uitdehaag BMJ, R. Ho, Doesburg W, Wevers RA, Geel WJA (1988) The short-term effect of an immunosuppressive treatment on CSF myelin basic protein in chronic progressive multiple sclerosis. J Neurol Neurosurg Psychiatry 51:1334–1337

Lees MB, Brostoff SW (1984) Proteins of myelin. In: Morell P (ed) Myelin. Plenum Press, New York, pp 197–224

Lennon V, Mackay IR (1972) Binding of 125-I myelin basic protein by serum and cerebrospinal fluid. Clin Exp Immunol 11:595–603

Li D, Mayo J, Fache S, Robertson WD, Paty D, Genton M (1984a) Early experience in nuclear magnetic resonance imaging of multiple sclerosis. Ann NY Acad Sci 436:483–486

Li D, Mayo J, Fache S, et al. (1984b) Lack of correlation between clinical manifestations and lesions of MS as seen by NMR. Neurology (Suppl 1) 34:136

Lowenthal A, Noppe M, Ghenens J, Karcher D (1978) α-albumin (glial fibrillary acidic protein) in normal and pathological human brain and cerebrospinal fluid. J Neurol 219:87–91

Ludwin SK (1979) An autoradiographic study of cellular proliferation in remyelination of the central nervous system. Am J Path 95:683–696

Massaro AR, Michetti F, Laudisio A, Bergonzi P (1985) Myelin basic protein and S-100 antigen in cerebrospinal fluid of patients with multiple sclerosis in the acute phase. Ital J Neurol Sci 6:53–56

Matias-Guiu J, Ruibal A, Martinez-Vazquez J-, Colomer R, Codina A (1986) Concentration of myelin basic protein in cerebrospinal fluid in prognosis of multiple sclerosis. Clin Chem 32:915–916

Matthews WB (1991) Treatment. In: Matthews WB (ed), McAlpine's multiple sclerosis, 2nd edn. Churchill Livingstone, Edinburgh

Matthews WB, Small DG (1979) Serial recording of visual and somatosensory evoked potentials in multiple sclerosis. J Neurol Sci 40:11–21

McPherson TA, Marchalonis JJ, Lennon V (1970) Binding of encephalitogenic basic protein by serum α-globulins. Immunology 19:929–933

Michetti F, Massaro A, Murazio M (1979) The nervous system-specific S-100 antigen in cerebrospinal fluid of multiple sclerosis patients. Neurosci Lett 11:171–175

Millar JHD et al. (1973) Double-blind trial of linokates supplementation of the diet in multiple sclerosis. Br Med J 3:765

Miller JP (1989) Statistical considerations for quantitative techniques in clinical neurology. In: Munsat TL (ed) Quantification of neurologic deficit. Butterworths, Boston, pp 69–84

Miller DH, Rudge P, Johnson G et al. (1988) Serial gadolinium-enhanced magnetic resonance imaging in multiple sclerosis. Brain 111:927–939

Morell P, Quarles RH, Norton WT (1989) Formation, structure, and biochemistry of myelin. In: Siegel GJ, Agranoff BW, Albers RW, Molinoff PB (eds) Basic neurochemistry. Raven Press, New York, pp 109–136

Morimoto C, Hafler DA, Weiner HL et al. (1987) Selective loss of the suppressor-inducer T-cell subset in progressive multiple sclerosis: analysis with anti-2H4 monoclonal antibody. N Engl J Med 316:67–72

Multiple Sclerosis Study Group (1990) Efficacy and toxicity of cyclosporine in chronic progressive multiple sclerosis: a randomized, double-blinded, placebo-controlled clinical trial. Ann Neurol 27:591–605

Narayana PA, Wolinsky JS, Fenstermacher MJ (1989) Proton magnetic resonance spectroscopy in multiple sclerosis. Soc Mag Reson Med p 457

National Multiple Sclerosis Society (1985) Minimal Record of Disability for Multiple Sclerosis. National Multiple Sclerois Society, New York

Newcombe J, Hawkins CP, Henderson CL et al. (1991) Histopathology of multiple sclerosis lesions detected by magnetic resonance imaging in unfixed post-mortem central nervous system tissue. Brain 114:1013–1023

Nishimoto N, Hoshizaki K, Eiraku N et al. (1990) Elevated levels of interleukin-6 in serum and cerebrospinal fluid of HTLV-I-associated myelopathy/tropical spastic paraparesis. J Neurol Sci 97:183–193

Noronha ABC, Richman DP, Arnason BGW (1980) Detection of in vivo stimulated cerebrospinal-fluid lymphocytes by flow cytometry in patients with multiple sclerosis. N Engl J Med 303:713–717

Noseworthy JH, Van de Voort MK, Wong CJ, Ebers JG (1988) Interrater variability with the Expanded Disability Status Scale (EDSS) and Functional Systems (FS) in a multiple sclerosis clinical trial. Arch Neurol 45:746–748

Nuwer MR, Packwood JW, Myers LW, Ellison GW (1987) Evoked potentials predict the clinical changes in a multiple sclerosis drug study. Neurology 37:1754–1761

Oger J, Kastrukoff LF, Li DKB, Paty D (1988) Multiple sclerosis: In relapsing patients, immune functions vary with disease activity as assessed by MRI. Neurology 38:1739–1744

Ohta M, Matsubara F, Konishi T, Nishitani H (1980) Radioimmunoassay of myelin basic protein in cerebrospinal fluid and its clinical application to patients with neurological diseases. Life Sciences 27:1069–1074

Ormerod IEC, Miller DH, McDonald WI et al. (1987) The role of NMR imaging in the assessment of multiple sclerosis and isolated neurological lesions. Brain 110:1579–1616

Palfreyman JW, Thomas DGT, Ratcliffe JG (1978) Radioimmunoassay of human myelin basic protein in tissue extract, cerebrospinal fluid and serum and its clinical application to patients with head injury. Clin Chim Acta 82:259–270

Palfreyman JW, Johnston RV, Ratcliffe JG, Thomas DGT, Forbes CD (1979) Radioimmunoassay of serum myelin basic protein and its application to patients with cerebrovascular accident. Clin Chim Acta 92:403–409

Paty DW (1988) Magnetic resonance imaging in the assessment of disease activity in multiple sclerosis. Can J Neurol Sci 15:266–272

Paty DW, Kastrukoff L, Morgan N, Hiob L (1983) Suppressor T-lymphocytes in multiple sclerosis: analysis of patients with acute relapsing and chronic progressive disease. Ann Neurol 14:445–449

Paty DW, Bergstrom M, Palmer M, MacFadyen J, Li D (1985) A quantitative magnetic resonance image of the multiple sclerosis brain. Neurology 35:137

Pedersen H (1974) Cerebrospinal fluid cholesterol and phospholipids in multiple sclerosis. Acta Neurol Scand 50:171–182

Pescovitz MD, Paterson PY, Kelly J, Lorand L (1978) Serum degradation of myelin basic protein with loss of encephalitogenic activity: evidence for an enzymatic process. Cell Immunol 39:355–365

Peyser JM, Edwards KR, Poser CM, Filskov SB (1980) Cognitive function in patients with multiple sclerosis. Arch Neurol 37:577–579

Poser S (1989) Disability Rating Scales for the Assessment of Multiple Sclerosis. In: Munsat TL (ed) Quantification of neurologic deficit. Butterworths, Boston, pp 163–169

Potvin AR, Tourtellotte WW (1975) The neurological examination: advancements in its quantification. Arch Phys Med Rehabil 56:427–437

Potvin AR, Tourtellotte WW, Syndulko K, Potvin J (1981) Quantitative methods in assessment of neurologic function. CRC Crit Review Bioeng 6:177–224

Price P, Cuzner ML (1979) Proteinase inhibitors in cerebrospinal fluid in multiple sclerosis. J Neurol Sci 42:251–259

Raes I, Weissbarth S, Maker HS, Lehrer GM (1981) 2,3′-cyclic nucleotide phosphodiesterase in cerebrospinal fluid. Neurology 31:1361–1363

Raine CS (1990) Multiple sclerosis: Immunopathologic mechanisms in the progression and resolution of inflammatory demyelination. In: Waksman BH (ed) Immunologic mechanisms in neurologic and psychiatric disease. Raven Press, New York, pp 37–54

Raine CS, Cross AH (1990) T-cell autoimmunity in the central nervous system: A new twist at an old rope. Lab Invest 62:133–134

Raine CS, Cannella B, Duijvestijn AM, Cross AH (1990a) Homing to central nervous system vasculature by antigen-specific lymphocytes. II. Lymphocyte/endothelial cell adhesion during the initial stages of autoimmune demyelination. Lab Invest 63:476–489

Raine CS, Lee SC, Scheinberg LC, Duijvestijn AM, Cross AH (1990b) Adhesion molecules on endothelial cells in the central nervous system: an emerging area in the neuroimmunology of multiple sclerosis. Clin Immunol Immunopathol 57:173–187

Rao SM (1986) Neuropsychology of multiple slcerosis: a critical review. J Clin Exp Neuropsychol 8:503–542

Reinherz EL, Weiner HL, Hauser SL, Cohen JA, Distaso JA, Schlossman SF (1980) Loss of suppressor T cells in active multiple sclerosis: analysis with monoclonal antibodies. N Engl J Med 303:125–129

Richards TL, Kenney JS, Rose LM et al. (1988) Detection of brain lipids in primates with experimental allergic encephalomyelitis by in vivo proton spectroscopy and in vitro histochemistry. Soc Mag Reson Med abstracts p 467

Rinne UK, Riekkinen P (1968) Esterase, peptidase and proteinase activities of human cerebrospinal fluid in multiple sclerosis. Acta Neurol Scand 44:156–167

Rosler N, Reuner C, Geiger J, Rissler K, Cramer H (1990) Cerebrospinal fluid levels of immunoreactive substance P and somatostatin in patients with multiple sclerosis and inflammatory CNS disease. Peptides 11:181–183

Rubin LA, Nelson DL (1990) The soluble interleukin-2 receptor: biology, function, and clinical application. Ann Int Med 113:619–627

Schumacher GA, Beebe G, Kibler RF et al. (1965) Problems of experimental trials of therapy in multiple sclerosis: report by the panel on the evaluation of experimental trials of therapy in multiple sclerosis. Ann NY Acad Sci 122:552–568

Simon JH, Fonte D (1988) Proton NMR spectroscopy of demyelination in experimental allergic encephalomyelitis. Soc Mag Reson Med abstracts p 69

Sipe JC, Knobler RL, Braheny SL, Rice GPA, Panitch HS, Oldstone MBA (1984) A Neurological Rating Scale (NRS) for use in multiple sclerosis. Neurology 34:1368–1372

Sprinkle TJ, McKhann GM (1978) Activity of 2′,3′-phosphodiesterase in cerebrospinal fluid of patients with demyelinating disorders. Neurosci Lett 7:203–206

Stewart WA, Hall LD, Berry K, Paty DW (1984) Correlation between NMR scan and brain slice data in multiple sclerosis. Lancet 2:412

Stewart WA, Hall LD, Berry K et al. (1986) Magnetic resonance imaging in multiple sclerosis: pathological correlation studies in eight cases. Neurology 36 (Suppl 1):320

Stewart WA, Alvord EC, Barwick SE, Hall LD, Paty DW (1988a) MRI of subclinical EAE: A model for relapsing-remitting MS. Ann Neur 24:475

Stewart WA, Barwick SE, Whittal K, Hall LD, Paty DW (1988b) In vitro multi-exponential relaxation in multiple sclerosis and experimental allergic encephalomyelitis. Soc Mag Reson Med p 36

Thompson AJ, Hutchinson M, Brazil J, Feighery C, Martin EA (1986) A clinical and laboratory study of benign multiple sclerosis. Q J Med 58:69–80

Thompson AJ, Brazil J, Hutchinson M, Feighery C (1987) Three possible laboratory indexes of disease activity in multiple sclerosis. Neurology 37:515–519

Thompson AJ, Kermode AG, MacManus DG et al. (1990) Patterns of disease activity in multiple sclerosis: clinical and magnetic resonance imaging study. Br Med J 300:631–634

Thompson AJ, Kermode AG, Wicks D et al. (1991) Major differences in the dynamics of primary and secondary progressive multiple sclerosis. Ann Neurol 29:53–62

Tourtellotte WW (1985) The cerebrospinal fluid in multiple sclerosis. In: Vinken PJ, Bruyn GW, Klawans HL, Koestsier JC (eds) Handbook of clinical neurology. Elsevier, Amsterdam, pp 79–130

Tourtellotte WW, Syndulko K (1989) Quantifying the neurologic examination: principles, constraints and opportunities. In: Munsat TL (ed) Quantification of neurologic deficit. Butterworths, Boston, pp 7–16

Tourtellotte WW, Baumhefner RW, Potvin AR et al. (1980) Multiple sclerosis de novo CNS IgG synthesis: effect of ACTH and corticosteroids. Neurology 30:1155–1162

Trotter JL, Wegescheide C, Lieberman L (1980) Myelin proteolipid protein (PLP) in sera and CSF after CNS damage. Trans Am Neurol Assoc 105:302–303

Warren KG, Catz I (1985) The relationship between levels of cerebrospinal fluid myelin basic protein and IgG measurements in patients with multiple sclerosis. Ann Neurol 17:475–480

Warren KG, Catz I (1987) A correlation between a cerebrospinal fluid myelin basic protein and anti-myelin basic protein in multiple sclerosis patients. Ann Neurol 21:183–189

Warren KG, Catz I, Jeffrey VM, Carroll DJ (1986) Effect of methylprednisolone on CSF IgG parameters, myelin basic protein and anti-myelin basic protein in multiple sclerosis exacerbations. Can J Neurolog Sci 13:25–30

Weiner HL, Ellison GW (1983) A working protocol to be used as a guideline for trials in multiple sclerosis. Arch Neurol 40:704–710

Weiner HL, Paty DW (1989) Diagnostic and therapeutic trials in multiple sclerosis: a new look. Neurology 39:972–976

Whitaker JN (1977) Myelin encephalitogenic protein fragments in cerebrospinal fluid of persons with multiple sclerosis. Neurology 27:911–920

Whitaker JN (1982) The antigenic reactivity of small fragments derived from human myelin basic protein peptide 43–88. J Immunol 129:2729–2733

Whitaker JN (1987) The presence of immunoreactive myelin basic protein peptide in urine of persons with multiple sclerosis. Ann Neurol 22:648–655

Whitaker JN, Heinemann MA (1983) The degradation of human myelin basic protein peptide 43–88 by human renal neutral proteinase. Neurology 33:744–749

Whitaker JN, Herman PK (1988) Human myelin basic protein peptide 69–89: immunochemical features and use in immunoassays of cerebrospinal fluid. J Neuroimmunol 19:47–57

Whitaker JN, Seyer JM (1979) The sequential limited degradation of bovine myelin basic protein by bovine brain cathepsin D. J Biol Chem 254:6956–6963

Whitaker JN, Chou CHJ, Chou FCH, Kibler RF (1977) Molecular internalization of a region of myelin basic protein. J Exp Med 146:317–331

Whitaker JN, Lisak RP, Bashir RM et al. (1980) Immunoreactive myelin basic protein in the cerebrospinal fluid in neurological disorders. Ann Neurol 7:58–64

Whitaker JN, Gupta M, Smith OF (1986) Epitopes of immunoreactive myelin basic protein in human cerebrospinal fluid. Ann Neurol 20:329–336

Whitaker JN, Sparks BE, Walker DP, Goodin R, Benveniste EN (1989) Monoclonal idiotypic and anti-idiotypic antibodies produced by immunization with peptides specified by a region of human myelin basic protein mRNA and its complement. J Neuroimmunol 22:157–166

Whitaker JN, Moscarello MA, Herman PK, Epand RM, Surewicz WK (1990) Conformational correlates of the epitopes of human myelin basic protein peptide 80–89. J Neurochem 55:568–576

Wiebe S, Karlik SJ, Lee DH et al. (1990) Serial cranial and spinal cord quantitative MRI in multiple sclerosis: clinical correlations. Neurology 40 (Suppl 1):377

Willoughby EW, Paty DW (1988) Scales for rating impairment in multiple sclerosis: a critique. Neurology 38:1793–1798

Willoughby EW, Grochowski E, Li DKB, Oger J, Kastrukoff LF, Paty D (1989) Serial magnetic resonance scanning in multiple sclerosis: A second prospective study in relapsing patients. Ann Neurol 25:43–49

World Health Organization (1980) International classification of impairments, disabilities and handicaps. WHO, Geneva

Yanagisawa K, Quarles RH, Johnson D, Brady RO, Whitaker JN (1985) A derivative of myelin-associated glycoprotein in cerebrospinal fluid of normal subjects and patients with neurological disease. Ann Neurol 18:464–469

Zabriskie JB, Mayer L, Fu SM, Yeadon C, Cam V, Plank C (1985) T cell subsets in multiple sclerosis: lack of correlation between helper and suppressor T cells and the clinical state. J Clin Immunol 5:7–12

Zomzely-Neurath CE, Walker WA (1980) Nervous system-specific proteins: 14-3-2 protein, neuron-specific enolase, and S-100 protein. In: Bradshaw RA, Schneider DM (eds) Proteins of the nervous system. Raven Press, New York, pp 1–57

Chapter 4

Design and Statistical Issues Related to Testing Experimental Therapy in Multiple Sclerosis

William Weiss and Emanuel M. Stadlan

Summary

The authors believe that neurologists planning a clinical trial of an experimental therapy for multiple sclerosis can select certain design elements that will enhance the sensitivity of the trial.

The typical trial will be multi-centered, double-blinded and randomized, with experimental therapy and placebo-treated patient groups.

The authors recommend that:

1. Admission to the trial should be restricted to those patients whose Extended Disability Status Scale (EDSS) scores do not exceed 3.5 at entry
2. Admission should be restricted to patients with relapsing forms of multiple sclerosis
3. One entry criterion should be evidence of disease activity: relapses during a pretrial period
4. There should be one primary response variable, based on the EDSS, and a restricted number of secondary response variables
5. An event should be defined as an increase in the EDSS score from baseline of at least one unit; it should be confirmed at a subsequent 3- or 6-month examination
6. The primary response variable should be defined as the "time to a confirmed event"
7. The clinical trial should include 3 years of treatment and follow-up for each patient
8. It should be estimated that 50% of the placebo patients will progress at least one confirmed EDSS unit during the trial
9. The minimum clinical effect of the experimental therapy to be demonstrated with high probability should fall in the range 30%–50% reduction in progression as compared to that in the placebo group
10. Interim analyses may be performed at 2 and $2\frac{1}{2}$ years to permit termination of the trial if a statistically significant difference between the therapy and placebo groups is observed

Introduction

Some of the major elements to be considered in the design of clinical trials of therapies for multiple sclerosis (MS) will be discussed in this chapter. The basic statistical methods employed in the experimental design and analysis of MS clinical trials are also applicable to the study of other chronic diseases. The characteristics of MS and of the patients with this disease, as well as the neurologists' objectives in undertaking the research, distinguish the MS clinical trial from trials for other chronic diseases. These distinctive features also provide the framework for the statisticians' contribution to the design of the MS clinical trial.

The readers will note, perhaps with surprise, numerous differences in the design elements among the individual clinical trials for MS that are described in this book. These trials also differ in their design from the one proposed in this chapter. This is so for a number of reasons. Treatments for MS began to proliferate only in the last two decades, so that experience in clinical trials for this disease is still somewhat limited. Some of the differences in approach, however, may be attributed to the knowledge gained from the earlier trials. There is also a considerable degree of patient variability in many of the characteristics of MS, so that patient cohorts (the populations from which patients are selected for the clinical trial) may vary from one trial to another, with consequent differences in design elements. For example, a clinical trial for chronic progressive MS patients may emphasize a comparison of changes in ambulation, whereas a trial involving patients with the relapsing/remitting type of MS may measure changes in the relapse rate.

Some recent and continuing epidemiological studies have the potential for providing insights that may influence clinical trial design (Weinshenker et al. 1987, 1989a,b, 1991a,b; Goodkin et al. 1989). They do so by providing a more precise characterization than now exists, of the various cohorts of MS patients available for participation in randomized clinical trials.

There is no unanimity of opinion among clinicians with clinical trial experience, nor among their statistical colleagues, regarding the specifics of certain important elements of these clinical trial designs. This is due, in part, to the fact that definitive data are rarely available. Also, committees of the National Institute of Neurological Disorders and Stroke that review clinical trial grant proposals modify their recommendations over time, due to an evolution in approach to critical design elements. Consequently they influence changes in the design of MS clinical trials. Similarly, the US Food and Drug Administration has had an impact on clinical trial design as it has refined its position regarding New Drug Applications (NDAs) for MS therapies.

The recommendations in this chapter are a consequence of the activities of the authors in clinical trials of MS. While these recommendations have been filtered through many conversations with statisticians and clinical trial neurologists, the reader can anticipate that the specifics of some of the design elements that are recommended will be met with spirited skepticism by some interested parties. Discussion of controversial issues can only be beneficial to the objectives of this book. The proposal that follows is not carved in stone, but is intended to be a waypoint toward a still evolving design for MS clinical trials.

This chapter is written for the practicing clinical neurologist interested in designing and participating in an MS clinical trial. It is not intended to be a primer on statistical methods. Rather, it is written to convey to the clinician with no considerable involvement in clinical trials, some of the design elements with statistical underpinnings which the neurologist must address. Only with an understanding of the role and contribution of the several disciplines involved, which will include that of biostatistics, can a lengthy, expensive, clinical trial of a chronic disease succeed.

The chapter is also not intended to cover all of the design elements for a clinical trial of MS. Those elements that are inherent in general clinical trial design for many disparate diseases are, to a great extent, not discussed, since this chapter would make no new contribution. Instead, the aspects of clinical trial design especially associated with MS are the major foci of attention. The statistician(s) collaborating with the clinical investigators will have ample resources upon which to rely for the statistical aspects of general application (Friedman et al. 1988; Matthews and Farewell 1988).

Even investigators whose clinical trial sophistication evolved from their own participation in trials, and for whom parts of this chapter will be redundant, may still gain some insights from reading it.

Initial Considerations

The general approach of this chapter will be to describe the salient features of an MS clinical trial by calling upon the reader to assume a participating role in the process of designing the trial. Let us assume that the reader is an investigator with an experimental therapy that is ready for testing in a clinical trial. While this experimental treatment may actually represent a complex therapeutic regimen, the therapy in this example will refer to an experimental drug. It will be necessary to develop portions of a protocol for a clinical trial that will test this drug for efficacy and for safety. If the drug is proven to have beneficial efficts, the investigator will compare its efficacy with its side effects, if any, and make a medical judgment about the value of the drug.

Since there is no generally accepted treatment for patients with MS, there is no ethical barrier to the inclusion in the trial of a group of patients who will be given a placebo while another group receives the experimental therapy. The changes in the characteristics of the disease in the placebo group of patients during the period of the trial will provide the basis for comparison with the experimental therapy group.

Comparison of the treatment group with an historical control group will not be an option, because in that case the differences found between the two groups of patients may be a function of other factors as well as that of the therapy being tested. These other factors, such as handedness, or history of allergic reactions, may be important but also may be unrecognized and therefore unrecorded, and thus are factors for which no adjustments can be made.

The application of statistical methods to this clinical trial requires that patients be randomly assigned to be in either the placebo group or the treatment group. This permits a statistical analysis to separate the effect of the treatment from that of the random changes found among patients within each of the two groups, to estimate the magnitude of the variability from each source, and to calculate the probability that the difference between treatment and placebo groups is due to the effect of the therapy rather than to chance.

Since the clinical trial will attempt to provide definitive answers regarding the usefulness of the therapy (in contrast to the goals of a small pilot study), the investigators should recruit several clinical centers to participate in the trial. Multiple centers will also permit a test of the consistency of any effect of therapy across centers, and provide a sufficient number of patients, which might exceed the patients available in any one of them.

Thus far the reader (investigator) has been asked to assume that a decision has been made to test an experimental drug for efficacy and safety, and to compare the response of the group of patients receiving the experimental therapy with the response of a placebo group in a multi-center trial.

Patient Eligibility

There are a number of early decisions that must be made, which can have a major effect on the potential for success or failure of the clinical trial. Some of these are critical although they may not be immediately recognized as such. The decision regarding the cohort from which patients will be eligible for inclusion in the trial is one of these, and one for which there is presently little consensus. For example, investigators usually employ the classification of MS patients as a means to identify the desired cohort of patients who will be eligible to enter the clinical trial. They may select for participation in the study, patients who have relapsing/remitting or chronic progressive disease. Some investigators have included patients with both types of MS (Milligan et al. 1987). A number of reasons are offered for restricting eligibility. One is that the specific objective of the clinical trial is to determine whether the treatment will reduce the number of relapses (Alter et al. 1987). This effectively restricts the eligible patients to those who have relapsing MS. Another reason, given to justify studying only those patients who are chronic progressive, is because of the impression that these patients will follow a regular pattern of worsening (Hauser et al. 1983). Still another is also the basis for entering only chronic progressive patients: the known toxicity of an experimental therapy justifies its use only in patients with advanced disease (Winter, 1989, personal communication) (see section *Testing for Efficacy*).

MS clinical trials have not yet been testing potential cures, or even therapy to halt the progress of the disease. Their more realistic objective has been to demonstrate an amelioration of the disease: a reduction in the number of relapses in patients, and/or a slowing of disease progression. If these are the objectives, the study will require patients who, without effective therapy, will continue to exhibit the characteristics of active disease, such as relapses, and/or progression. A patient who will remain stable during the period of trial, for example, will provide no opportunity to test an experimental therapy for slowing progression, since that patient will show no progression regardless of the therapy or lack thereof. By the same token, patients who are likely to show disease progression, but at a very slow rate during the period of the trial, may not progress sufficiently during the limited period of trial for a real difference to be demonstrated between those on the placebo and those on the therapy. Improved differentiation between these latter groups may be attained by lengthening the period of trial so that, over time, the advantage of therapy over placebo may become demonstrable. Increasing the number of patients in the trial may also serve the same purpose because larger numbers enable a smaller real effect of therapy to be demonstrated. However, increasing the number of patients will escalate the costs of the trial. This solution will also add more administrative complexity, for example, by adding more clinical centers in order to obtain the larger number of patients required within a reasonable time period.

There is an alternative approach to increasing the sample size which may improve the chances of demonstrating a real effect of the experimental therapy, if it exists, without substantially escalating the costs of the trial: choose patients with more active disease.

It is presently not possible to identify all patients who will demonstrate clinically active disease during a trial. However, over the years, the accumulating evidence has supported the impression that changes in the Kurtzke Extended Disability Status Scale (EDSS) occur more rapidly in less impaired patients with low scores on the EDSS than in those with high scores and greater impairment (Weinshenker et al. 1989a; Bornstein et al. 1987).

There are a number of reasons why this may be so. While the EDSS is an ordinal scale, it is not an interval scale. That is, while the scale shows an ordering from no disease involvement through degrees of increasing involvement to death, the amount of change is not equal between units of the scale. On the average, it may take a longer period of time for a patient to progress from an EDSS of 6 (walking with assistance) to 7 (wheelchair-bound), than from an EDSS of 2 (minimal disability in one Functional System) to 3 (moderate disability in one Functional System).

Another reason is that a patient at a stage early in the disease may actually progress more rapidly than a patient who has reached an advanced stage where progression has slowed substantially, even though the disease activity may not have changed. This may be so because pathological changes added at new levels to an already damaged fiber tract may cause little, if any, additional clinical impairment. Our inability to recognize a difference may also be related to insufficiently sensitive means for detecting changes.

For example, the nine-hole peg, and the box-and-block tests of upper extremity function have been reported to detect disease progression in 15% of MS patients in whom the EDSS was unchanged (Goodkin et al. 1988).

On the other hand, magnetic resonance imaging (MRI) studies of the brains of MS patients continue to disclose periodic changes that are unaccompanied by identifiable clinical manifestations. A recent study reveals MRI evidence of considerable disease activity in relapsing/remitting MS patients who have EDSS scores of 3.5 and under (Harris et al. 1991). The authors of that paper suggest that MRI is a sensitive procedure to detect disease activity and may be useful in clinical trials in patients with early relapsing/remitting MS.

It is reasonable to assume that patients with active disease will be better able to show a response to an effective treatment than patients who will show little clinical activity or remain stable during the trial period. The investigator should carefully attempt to regulate the entry into the trial of MS patients with active disease by defining the criteria for their admission. The authors recommend that this objective can be furthered by:

1. Entering only those patients whose EDSS scores at baseline do not exceed 3.5
2. Restricting accession of patients into the clinical trial to those who have relapsing MS

Support for these recommendations comes from data from a number of studies. As measured by the EDSS, one study of 50 relapsing/remitting patients showed sharp differences in disease progression in placebo patients in two baseline disability strata during the two years of the trial (Bornstein et al. 1987). Placebo patients who were less impaired upon admission (baseline Disability Status Scale [DSS] scores of 0–2), progressed an average of 1.2 units in the 2 years on trial. Those with more advanced disease (DSS 3–6), progressed only an average of 0.4 DSS units.

While 52% of the placebo-treated patients did not progress during the 2-year period of the trial, a breakdown by strata revealed that 30% of the patients with a DSS 0–2 at baseline did not progress. In contrast, 70% of the patients with DSS 3–6 at baseline did not progress. Subsequent analysis showed that baseline DSS 3 patients were similar to those in the baseline DSS 0–2 stratum in that 29% did not progress. During the 2 years of the trial the mean difference in disease progression between the therapy and placebo groups for the DSS 0–2 stratum was 1.7 DSS units in favor of the therapy, and only 0.1 DSS unit in the DSS 3–6 baseline stratum. It would appear that the patients with less severe disease progressed through the lower DSS scores at a more rapid rate, and were, therefore, more susceptible to the effect of therapy, as measured by changes in the DSS.

One negative aspect of restricting the cohort of patients who may participate in the trial to those who have relapsing MS and whose baseline EDSS scores are 3.5 or less is that it will reduce the number of MS patients eligible for admission into the trial. Nevertheless, the impact of this restriction may be small. In the study cited above of relapsing/remitting patients, entry was restricted to patients with baseline DSS scores of 6 or less. Of these, 71% of the patients had a DSS score of 3 or less. One study, which included 155 patients with stable relapsing/remitting MS, showed that over 80% of these had baseline EDSS scores of 3.0 or less (Goodkin et al. 1989). While restricting the cohort of patients to those with more active disease is important in clinical trial design, it need not jeopardize the successful acquisition of patients. The judicious selection of clinical centers with sufficient numbers of eligible patients, and, as specified in the protocol, sufficient time to enter them, can provide the necessary sample of patients.

The proportion of study patients who will progress during the clinical trial will, of course, depend in part on the magnitude of the change in the EDSS that will be required in order for a progression to be considered clinically meaningful. In another clinical trial of 106 chronic progressive patients, 50.9% of the placebo group had a confirmed progression defined as a change of ≥0.5 EDSS units after 2 years (Bornstein et al. 1991). When the change was defined to be ≥1 EDSS unit, only 24.5% of the placebo patients had a confirmed progression. In that trial, the mean EDSS score of the placebo group at baseline was 5.5 units. One of the possible inferences from these two studies is that, with less progression among the more disabled MS patients, as measured by the EDSS, it will be more difficult to demonstrate effects of therapy.

There is a logical reason for this to be so. The smaller the proportion of patients with active disease, the greater must be the effect of the experimental therapy on this latter subset of patients in order for statistically significant differences to be obtained between the placebo and therapy patient groups under study.

Assume, for example, that a trial is designed to have good power to detect a 50% increase in the rate of non-progressors in the experimental therapy group over that in the placebo group. That is, if the rate of non-progression in the placebo group is 30%, then the study will have adequate power to detect a rate of 45% or more in the experimental therapy group. For this to be accomplished, 21.4% of the potential progressors in the experimental therapy group would need to shift to the non-progressing column (see Appendix).

On the other hand, if the percent of the non-progressors in the placebo group is 50% rather than 30%, then 31.7% of the potential progressors in the experimental group would need to shift to the non-progressing column.

Thus, for a placebo rate of 30%, 21.4% of the actively progressing patients would need to respond to the drug by becoming non-progressors in order to demonstrate statistical significance. When the placebo rate is 50%, the effect of the drug on otherwise progressing patients would need to increase to 31.7% in order to demonstrate statistical significance.

In other words, the greater the proportion of non-progressors recruited into the trial, the greater the difficulty of detecting a pre-specified difference.

In previous clinical trials of MS, the percentage of patients who did not progress during the period of the trial has ranged from as low as 30%, for a stratum of placebo patients with early relapsing/remitting disease (DSS 0–3) (Bornstein et al. 1987), to 75% of all placebo patients in a study of chronic progressive patients (Bornstein et al. 1991).

Patient eligibility is frequently dependent on pre-trial disease activity, measured by the occurrence of relapses or progression. Consequently, investigators have a tendency to anticipate that during the period of trial the relative frequency of non-progression in the placebo group will be low. All too often, such speculation is faulty. Placebo rates for non-progressors have even been underestimated to be as low as 10% (Bornstein, 1988, personal communication).

That is yet another design element that has been used to increase the probability of admitting patients who will progress rapidly. To enter, a minimum number of relapses occurring in the recent past must have been reported. These relapses may have been determined either during a pretrial observation period, or from a review of the medical history of patients proposed for the trial. This requirement, of course, has been used in studies of patients with relapsing/remitting MS (British and Dutch MS Azathioprine Trial Group 1988). In some trials, the investigators required a total of at least two well-documented relapses during the prior 2 years (Bornstein et al. 1987; Camenga et al. 1986). In another, an average of at least 0.6 relapses per year was an inclusion criterion; actually the relapses averaged almost two per year in the pretrial period (Jacobs et al. 1987).

The occurrence of relapse during a pretrial observation period is no guarantee of commensurate relapse activity during the trial. While in one epidemiological study no significant change in the relapse rate was demonstrated over a period of 3 years (Goodkin et al. 1989), an opposite view was offered in another such study (Weinshenker and Ebers 1987). There is other evidence to suggest that the relapse rate, observed during a pretrial period, is likely to diminish during a period of trial (Camenga et al. 1986; Jacobs et al. 1987; Knobler et al. 1984). This was well illustrated in one study of relapsing/remitting MS: the placebo group, which averaged two relapses in each of the 2 prestudy years, showed a decrease of 55% in relapses over the 2-year period of the trial (Bornstein et al. 1987).

The drop in that relapse rate may be the consequence of a placebo effect. There are several additional possible reasons for the decrease in the number of relapses during that trial. The prestudy relapse rate was based on information obtained from the patients' private physicians and from MS clinics. These data may have been more variable and less reliable than information regarding relapse rate based upon in-trial observations. In addition, the study definition of a relapse was more rigorous in that objective changes had to be observed by the evaluating neurologist, and therefore differed from the prestudy definition.

The data might also have reflected a "regression to the mean", in that some of the patients may have been selected when they were having an unusually high relapse rate during the recruitment period, which later returned during the trial period to the earlier lower rate.

As discussed earlier regarding apparent slowing of disease progression with time, the change in relapse rate may also not be an accurate reflection of true change in disease activity; rather it may be due to cumulative lesions in the CNS. If a patient has normal strength in the legs, the occurrence of a lesion at any level in the corticospinal tract may present as an apparent weakness. On the other hand, if there is already leg paralysis from a lesion at T-4, for example, a new lesion at T-6 may not be reflected by a new clinical symptom, and a relapse could thus be missed.

Other potential artifacts include: a change in MS pattern from relapsing/remitting to chronic progressive, with a consequent reduction in relapse rate; loss of patient interest in reporting changes, especially mild ones, that would initiate a patient visit and examination; and a subtle change over the period of the trial in the examining neurologist's definition of a relapse.

In order to enhance the likelihood of clinical progression during the period of the trial, patients who have been clinically stable for an extended period should not be enrolled. Rather, it is reasonable to require that trial subjects show evidence of clinical disease activity during the months immediately preceding accession. Therefore, the authors offer another entry criterion: evidence of disease activity as measured by relapses during a pretrial period. The number of relapses, the length of the pretrial period, and whether or not monitoring is done during that period are considerations that need to be addressed and specified by the investigators. Because of the paucity of hard data, an ideal formula cannot be offered. It seems reasonable that the greater the activity and the more definite the determination of relapses, the better will the patient fill the needs of the study. Therefore a pretrial observation period of at least a year during which time a patient experiences at least one relapse, is recommended.

A recent extensive epidemiological investigation provides additional support for some of the observations reported in the relatively small-scale studies which have been cited. In a much-needed study of the natural history of MS, 1099 Canadian patients were followed. The investigators found that it took 7.7 years, on the average, for patients to reach a DSS of 3, 15 years to reach a DSS of 6, but 46.4 years to reach a DSS of 8 (Weinshenker et al. 1989a). It would appear from these data that clinical progression in less disabled patients is relatively rapid as measured by the Disability Status Scale (DSS), whereas progression is relatively slow in patients who have a DSS score of 6 or more.

There are other points of similarity among these investigations that support this observation. In one small trial of relapsing/remitting patients, there were relatively few patients with DSS of 4 or 5 (Bornstein et al. 1987). The most frequent DSS scores were 1, 2, 3 and 6. Another study also disclosed a bimodal distribution of all types of MS patients, with peaks at DSS 1 and DSS 6 (Weinshenker et al. 1989a). Again, relatively few patients with DSS 4 and 5 were found. Yet another study had similar findings (Goodkin et al. 1989). The recommendation made earlier that eligibility of patients be restricted to those whose baseline disability does not exceed 3.5 was, in part, predicated on these observations. The exclusion of patients with baseline EDSS scores of 4.0, 4.5, 5.0 and 5.5 would not significantly reduce the population of patients eligible for admission into a clinical trial. Moreover, it would narrow further the range of disability status, thus reducing variability, and favor inclusion of those most likely to have rapid progression through the DSS.

Nevertheless, future research may provide information to determine whether or not patients in the baseline EDSS range of 4.0–5.0 progress sufficiently rapidly to be considered for inclusion in relapsing/remitting MS clinical trials, in addition to those in the lower ranges of baseline EDSS.

Several current or proposed clinical trials of MS limit patients to those less disabled, as discussed here, or stratify the patients in order to highlight the *a priori* interest in the less disabled patients. These trials are limited to relapsing/remitting patients. One trial plans to limit the patients to a baseline EDSS score of 4.5 (Johnson, 1989, personal communication). Another study, recently funded, will limit the eligible patients to those whose baseline EDSS scores do not exceed 3.5 (Jacobs, 1990, personal communication). One constant objective of the investigators is to test the effect of therapy in patients they believe will be the most rapidly progressing.

There is, of course, an apparent negative aspect to the narrowing of the range of the eligibility of patients. It reduces the degree to which the patients in these clinical trials will represent the universe of patients with MS. As a matter of fact, most clinical trials of MS, or of any other disease, are not representative of the populations with the disease of interest. This is so for a number of reasons. The clinical centers involved in the trial are not randomly selected from all of the clinical centers that care for patients with MS. Some centers may be specializing in MS, and therefore may differ from some other centers in the types of MS patients seen; that is, the more serious, rapidly progressing patients with uncommon symptoms, may be referred to these tertiary care centers. Also, many MS patients may be seen only by their primary care physicians, and are not generally available to be entered into clinical trials. Patients with early symptoms of MS, who might have been diagnosed as having MS had they been seen by a neurologist, are excluded from consideration because the diagnosis is not established. Many patients, even those seen in clinics which provide patients for a clinical trial, are eliminated from consideration by other exclusion criteria: they are either too young or too old; they reside too far from the clinic; their family is not sufficiently supportive of their participation in the trial, or their primary physician does not support their participation in the trial; they are on medications which preclude their participation; they have other diseases; they are pregnant; their pre-trial disease activity does not meet the criteria set by the investigators; they are psychologically unprepared to participate in a clinical trial, and so on. It must be evident by this incomplete list that a very considerable proportion of the MS population is excluded from entering any clinical trial of the disorder.

This discussion raises two additional questions. If clinical trials offer so little representation of patients in the disease population, what purpose is served by the use of this expensive, difficult, and time-consuming procedure? And, what *can* a well-designed, well-run clinical trial demonstrate that may be useful? The answers to these questions are only partly satisfactory. The randomized, double-blind clinical trial is the generally accepted procedure for minimizing bias when testing the efficacy of an experimental therapy. Moreover, even if a beneficial effect of treatment is shown for only a subgroup of the MS population, it still is a critically important demonstration.

The proposal in this chapter is that clinical trials should test therapies in the potentially most rapidly progressing subgroup of MS patients, one in which an effect of therapy will most readily be demonstrated, if one exists. If the efficacy and safety of the therapy are demonstrated, there will be a very considerable incentive to proceed with the study of additional cohorts of the MS population. While there is, of course, the possibility that patient demand for treatment might preclude further research of a demonstrably efficacious therapy, an approach with wider-ranging eligibility criteria may be inefficient and unproductive.

There is nothing more discouraging of further investigation of an experimental therapy than a failed demonstration of efficacy following a long clinical trial. This is particularly unfortunate if the patients selected for study may not have been the most sensitive for testing efficacy, thereby masking an actual therapeutic effect.

Testing for Efficacy

In a clinical trial of MS there is no single measure of efficacy which will provide complete satisfaction. The DSS, now replaced by the EDSS, is frequently used in clinical trials of MS to measure the effect of therapy on the clinical course of the disease. Clinical trials restricted to relapsing/remitting patients on occasion have emphasized reduction in the frequency of relapses as the primary measure of efficacy. A variety of additional measures of response to therapy have also been studied in these clinical trials. They include lower extremity function, upper extremity function, neuropsychological changes, and activities of daily living (ADL). MRI is now emerging as a potentially powerful and sensitive objective measure of putative disease activity. Whether or not modulation of the MRI pattern by drug intervention will be reflected in the clinical course remains to be demonstrated. Until then, every clinical trial must, of course, include clinical neurological assessment.

The authors have thus far made two strong recommendations: EDSS scores at entry should not exceed 3.5, and only patients with relapsing disease should be admitted into a clinical trial of MS.

Thus, patients with chronic progressive MS would be excluded even though the authors suspect, without data to support their view, that patients with a chronic progressive type of MS from onset, in the same range of EDSS, may progress as rapidly as those who have relapsing disease. Such patients are relatively few in number. One study has shown that only approximately 3% of the MS patients in the DSS range 0–3 had chronic progressive disease (without accompanying relapsing/remitting components) (Goodkin et al. 1989).

An investigator who plans to test an experimental drug associated with known toxicity faces a more difficult ethical and scientific problem. The investigator may decide that the drug is too toxic for use in patients with early MS, and therefore proposes to test the drug in a cohort of patients with advanced MS. The investigator, before proceeding with the clinical trial, should resolve several issues:

1. Is it medically ethical to test a toxic drug in patients with advanced, chronic MS, who already suffer from the serious consequences of their disease?
2. Since the drug will, in all likelihood, be aimed at reducing the progression of the disease, to what degree will that drug advance the interests of patients who, on the average, may expect to remain in their chronic stage for many years?
3. Even if the drug slows the progression of the disease in those with chronic advanced MS, will the added side effects not reduce even more the patients' already compromised quality of life, and balance the positive effects of the therapy?
4. How will the investigator plan to demonstrate, even if the drug slows the progression of the disease in a trial lasting several years, that the added toxicity of the drug will not shorten the life span of the patients?
5. If the drug is found to slow progression in the patient with advanced disease, what are the likely consequences regarding the potential use of the drug in patients with early disease?
6. How will the investigator select the response variable(s) to test for efficacy in patients in a chronic stage of the disease, and whose progression is most likely proceeding at a very slow rate?
7. Finally, is it justifiable to provide potentially toxic drugs to patients in a clinical trial that has little likelihood for successful completion because large numbers of patients will probably drop out due to the extended length of time such a trial demands in order to demonstrate efficacy?

This concern is succinctly expressed: ". . . the central question regarding the use of patients with chronic progressive disease is whether it is ethical to test a toxic drug in patients who have the least chance of responding to the drug and therefore will have the highest likelihood of not providing an answer to the research question. From an ethical standpoint, it is difficult to justify doing an experiment if there is little potential for getting an answer." (McFarland, 1991, personal communication.)

Turning again to the selection of a response variable for testing efficacy, some investigators have preferred to use relapse frequency, since they considered it to be a more objective measure; it is an easier measure to define and observe, as compared to a measure of early disease progression (Bornstein, 1988, personal communication). Others prefer to count relapses because of their dissatisfaction with the recognized weaknesses of the EDSS. For investigators who prefer to use the frequency of relapses, rather than a measure of progression, as the response variable of interest, restricting entry to relapsing patients is, of course, obligatory.

The authors recommend that investigators focus on the EDSS, rather than on the frequency of relapses, in defining the primary response variable, for a number of reasons. One is based on an analysis of the baseline strata in one clinical trial (Bornstein, 1990, unpublished work). In that study, the investigators found that in demonstrating a statistically significant effect of the therapy on both relapse rate and progression, the level of significance attained was observed to be greater for the DSS response measure than that for relapse frequency. These data suggest that the DSS is at least as sensitive a measure for testing efficacy of therapy as is relapse frequency in the less disabled patient. A stronger statement regarding the sensitivity of these response variables is precluded until support is forthcoming from other studies demonstrating therapeutic efficacy.

Another reason for focusing on the EDSS is that the authors have noticed a change in the view of what should be the major objective of an experimental therapy for MS. There appears to be a general consensus that a diminution in progression of the disease is much more important than a decrease in relapse rate, and therefore should be the primary measure of efficacy of therapy for MS. The best means of measuring progression, however, is still being debated. A third reason for recommending the EDSS is that it would be a response variable applicable to all MS patients, whereas relapse frequency is meaningful only for one type of the disease.

Support for the belief that a slowing of progression should be the critical measure of efficacy stems as well from the observations and concerns of investigators and reviewers of current research efforts. In a review of a proposal for a clinical trial of relapsing/remitting patients, the NINDS grant review committee recommended to the investigators that they focus on progression rather than relapse frequency as the primary measure of efficacy. The investigators made that, and other, changes in a resubmission of the grant proposal, and the study was funded. An NINDS grant review committee also made a similar recommendation in reviewing another proposal for a multicenter clinical trial in relapsing/remitting MS patients.

Secondary Response Variables

The authors have proposed that the critical determinant of efficacy be the EDSS. Because of the wide variety of MS manifestations, other response variables of interest to the investigators may be assessed as well during the course of a clinical trial, and should be considered as secondary outcome measures. If a statistical demonstration of efficacy is made using the primary response variable, then these secondary outcome measures can provide additional important information about the impact of the experimental therapy on other clinical and laboratory expressions of the disease.

While the investigators should select the secondary response variables of interest to them, based on prior clinical trials of relapsing/remitting MS, it is likely that one or more secondary response variables would involve relapses.

Because of imperfections in the Kurztke EDSS and other assessment instruments, there is clearly a continuing need for alternative measures that will be sensitive to small changes in neurological function over the entire range of MS disability. A recently completed clinical trial of MS patients measured a large number of response variables and analyzed, *inter alia*, selected combinations of them (The MS Study Group 1990). One composite score based on activities of daily living (ADL) scales for dressing, grooming and feeding appeared to be useful in assessing chronic progressive patients falling within the EDSS range 3–7, but needs to be validated. Methodological investigations of the most sensitive measures remain to be accomplished.

Other specific secondary response measures that should be considered are the opinions of the patient and the blinded examining neurologist regarding whether the patient improved, remained stable, or progressed in disability during the course of the trial. These opinions should be recorded at the end of each patient's participation in the trial, and while still blinded. Also, the objective overall judgment of the examining neurologist performing the standardized neurological examination is particularly valued by many clinicians as the most important measure of the changing status of the patient.

The investigators should carefully consider whether magnetic resonance imaging should be part of the series of secondary response variables. MRI scans have the capability of providing a number of different response measures of interest. The relationships of MRI events, fundamental disease activity, and clinical manifestations of the disease have yet to be demonstrated. A reasonable schedule of MRI for each patient in a trial would add considerable cost to the clinical trial and, presently, is unlikely to provide a major pay-off in achieving the objectives of a clinical trial because of the poor correlation, as of this writing, between clinical manifestations and MRI activity. Nevertheless, ongoing research in MRI scans of MS patients is extensive, and the situation with regard to the use of MRI scans in these clinical trials may soon change. If, in fact, MRI events are demonstrated to be a sensitive measure of disease activity, as seems to be the case, and are early predictors of future clinical expression of the illness, MRI should provide a means to identify which interventions will be promising clinically, and thus worthy of investment of time and money. The critical decision regarding the use of MRI scans in these trials is predicated upon the conviction that they will further the specific objectives of the trial in the test of the experimental therapy; or that the investigators' special interests justify the added cost of response variables which would provide questionable support in meeting the primary objectives of the clinical trial.

Investigators should be wary of attempting an all-inclusive approach in selecting the secondary response variables to be employed in the trial. The aim should be for the minimum number of response variables that will provide a robust body of information should the therapy be demonstrated to be effective.

There are a number of disadvantages to the proliferation of response variables. They include: additional cost and effort on the part of the investigators and patients, increase in paperwork, data processing and quality control efforts, and a manifold increase in data analyses. Limiting the collection of clinical trial data to that which is critical to the objectives of the trial may also enhance the quality of the data, and may reduce the likelihood of reporting error.

Multiple Primary Response Variables

Thus far the authors have recommended that a primary response variable be related to the EDSS. Not infrequently, clinical trials include several primary response variables. A recently completed trial used three primary measures of progression (The MS Study Group 1990). The inclusion of more than one primary response variable stems from dissatisfaction with the weaknesses inherent in the EDSS; uncertainty as to which of the various ways a response variable, such as the EDSS, should best be measured; and/or a belief that no single measure is sufficient to measure the effect of an experimental therapy of a disease such as MS with its manifold manifestations. Perhaps more than one of these reasons apply.

Of course, there are few restrictions (except for reasonableness concerning the proliferation of response variables) to the use of any variables of interest as secondary response variables. As mentioned earlier, these secondary variables have the potential for providing a more robust picture of the effect of the experimental therapy, if the analysis of the primary response variable demonstrates efficacy. Several primary response variables, then, may be selected, not because they would all have to be shown to be beneficially affected by the experimental therapy before the therapy can be considered for general use, but because there is uncertainty as to the best measure of efficacy. A demonstrable, beneficial effect of therapy on any one of the variables would be considered salutary. The use of multiple primary response variables, on the other hand, creates some problems regarding the degree of statistical significance demonstrated by the trial results, and also problems of interpretation, if analysis of the primary response variables provides a mixture of significant and non-significant results.

One cannot infer, having achieved significance at the $p = 0.05$ level for only one of several primary response variables, that the experimental therapy had been demonstrated to be efficacious at that probability level.

These considerations can best be illustrated with an example. Assume that study investigators determined that an experimental therapy would be considered to be effective if the results showed statistical significance at a probability level of $p \leqslant 0.05$. (This means that the results, in a group of patients receiving an experimental therapy that is not effective may, just by a 1-in-20 chance, differ enough from results in a placebo group to show statistical significance. Since this is an unlikely event, if statistical significance is obtained at this level, it would be reasonable to conclude that the difference in results observed between the therapy group and the placebo group is due to the effect of the therapy.) If the clinical trial had included only 1 primary response variable, and if the results yielded a probability value of, say, $p = 0.04$, then it would be reasonable to conclude that the therapy was effective. However if, for example, there were 3 primary response variables, and only 1 of the 3 showed statistical significance, and that at the $p = 0.038$ level, it would be incorrect to conclude from this result alone that a demonstration of efficacy had been achieved. One may perhaps understand this intuitively since, if the therapy were ineffective, there would now be 3 chances (1 from each of the 3 primary response variables), rather than 1 chance, that a primary response variable should show significance at the $p = 0.05$ level.

A study of this problem, for a clinical trial with 3 primary response variables, revealed that for the results to be considered statistically significant, the significance level of any one of them would have to be as low as $p = 0.0167$, if the 3 variables were uncorrelated, to at least $p = 0.030$, if the 3 variables were highly correlated (Pocock et al. 1987). Only if the significance level appropriate to the degree of correlation of the variables were obtained would it be correct to conclude that statistical significance had been achieved at the $p = 0.05$ level. The reader may note that the level of significance to be obtained is $p = 0.0167$ if the 3 primary response variables are uncorrelated, that is, independent of each other. That level, multiplied by 3, would give an overall significance level of $p = 0.05$, which is intuitively reasonable.

There is an approximation frequently used to estimate the level of significance achieved, when there are multiple primary response variables, in order to determine whether or not statistical significance has been achieved at the $p = 0.05$ level. In the example just given, it is simply to multiply the highest level of significance that was calculated ($p = 0.038$) by the number of primary response variables (3), which would give a probability level of $p = 0.114$, which is not statistically significant. It would rectify the simplistic and false assumption that the calculated value $p = 0.038$ accurately represented the true level of statistical significance. For moderate degrees of correlation among the primary response variables, and for the presence of up to 5 variables, the estimate is conservative and closely approximates the true level.

There is an alternative procedure for calculating a single combined probability value for the 3 primary response variables, in order to avoid the approximation described above (O'Brien and Shampo 1988). A discussion of this procedure is beyond the scope of this chapter.

The investigators must decide which primary response variable(s) best meets the major objective of the clinical trial. If their judgment is that more than one primary response variable is necessary, then they must avoid a misinterpretation of the individual probability levels calculated from the group of primary response variables that have been chosen.

Alternative Primary Response Variables Based on a Single Measure

Once the EDSS has been selected as the measure of efficacy, the investigators must determine the specific way in which it will be used. For example, the response variable might be the difference between the final EDSS score and the baseline EDSS score for each patient in the trial. Another response variable might be a determination that the patients either progressed in their disability during the period of trial, that they remained stable, or that they improved in EDSS score from baseline. A closely associated response variable to the latter would be that a change of at least one full point on the EDSS during the period of trial would be necessary to measure progression of the disease or improvement of the patient. Otherwise the patient would be considered to be stable. Another measure would be to dichotomize the EDSS change from baseline as patients progressed, or did not progress, in disability.

The choice of a specific response variable can become complicated. A commonly-used measure is the time from baseline EDSS score to the occurrence of an EDSS event, where the event is an increase in EDSS score of a certain magnitude, and sustained for a specific length of time. The event might be an increase, from baseline, of a unit of EDSS score, or perhaps of a half unit. A clinical trial of therapy for chronic progressive MS, in which patients with a wide range of baseline EDSS scores were enrolled, considered an event to be a change of 1.5 EDSS units if the patient's baseline score were 5.5 or below, but only 1 unit if the patient's baseline score were 6 or above (Bornstein et al. 1991). This decision was made in an effort to achieve equivalence in the definition of progression at both ends of the scale.

In an effort to improve future trials, a post-trial analysis of this chronic progressive MS clinical trial was undertaken. The question was posed regarding the magnitude of EDSS changes in progression from baseline that would provide the greater sensitivity in testing the effect of the therapy, as compared to the placebo. Would the time to increase 1 or 1.5 EDSS units from baseline be a better discriminator of drug efficacy than, say, time to an increase of a 0.5 unit of EDSS? An analysis of these alternative response variables showed that the time to an increase of 1 or 1.5 units was the better discriminator than was the 0.5 unit change. Clinical neurologists are more likely to support the definition of an event to be the 1-unit change in EDSS as more meaningful than a change of a half unit, especially at the low end of the scale. While there is no evidence currently available to support a choice between the selection of 1-unit or 1.5-unit change in the EDSS to be considered an event, the authors opt for the 1-unit change since it will provide the greater number of events in the clinical trial. The demonstration of statistical significance will require a certain minimum number of events to occur.

Another potential response variable is the magnitude of change from baseline EDSS scores during the period of trial. For example, the improvement in patients may range anywhere from a reduction of 2 EDSS points over 2 years of trial, to a worsening of as much as 3 EDSS points. One could choose to compare the distributions of changes from baseline EDSS scores in the therapy and placebo groups.

Confirmation of an Event

Having selected a specific EDSS response variable, the investigators must now decide whether or not to require that the degree of progression to be considered an event should be confirmed by the next scheduled neurological examination(s) of the patient. Most MS clinical trials schedule a series of routine patient visits at which time the patients are examined and tested for the various primary and secondary response variables specified in the research protocol. These routine visits generally occur every 3 months, and in some trials, every 6 months. Most investigators believe that an EDSS progression, of any magnitude, should not be counted as an event if it does not persist for a predetermined period; that is, if the minimum progression to be considered an event is not found at the next routine examination. This is not necessarily a simple matter to ascertain.

Assume, for example, that the investigators have determined that an event will be defined as a confirmed increase of at least 1 unit from the baseline score. In this example, the patient's baseline EDSS score was found to be 1.0. At the neurological examination 6 months into the trial, the patient had a score of 2.5 EDSS units. At succeeding 6-month intervals the patient's scores were 1.5, 2, and, finally, another score of 2 at the 24-month examination. In this example, the event (the first score of 2) occurred at the 18-month examination, because it was confirmed at the next 24-month examination. The score of 2.5 EDSS units did not become an event because only a 0.5 unit increase from baseline (a score of 1.5) occurred at the next examination. The 18-month examination qualified as the time of an event because the EDSS score of 2 provided a unit increase over the baseline score, and the following score of 2, a 1-unit increase over the baseline score, was the confirming score. The time from the baseline examination to that in which the event was first identified becomes the "time to the confirmed event", and is a measure of the primary response variable.

One clinical trial protocol required confirmation of the event at two subsequent examinations (Cook et al. 1986). The authors consider this to be an excessive requirement.

The investigators in a trial of chronic progressive MS analyzed the effect of the requirement that progression of the disease be confirmed at the next routine 3-month neurological examination (Bornstein, 1989, unpublished work). With a total of 106 patients observed during the 2-year period of trial, the EDSS scores of 30 patients increased by 1 or 1.5 units, and these changes were confirmed at the next 3-month examination. The scores of an additional 19 patients progressed by the same magnitude, but the progression was not sustained and the patients could not be considered to have had a confirmed event. An analysis was performed on data from 48 patients who had a confirmed progression of 0.5 EDSS unit. A similar analysis was based on an additional 12 patients (added to the original 48) who had also progressed 0.5 EDSS unit but whose progression was not confirmed at the next examination. In both instances there was more variability and a lesser level of statistical significance in the data which included the unconfirmed progressions than in the confirmed progression data.

One may infer correctly from these results that excessive random variability is introduced into the trial by the use of unconfirmed events. A restriction of events to those which have been confirmed is advised.

The investigators must expect additional problems regarding the use of any primary response variable(s). It is important that these potential complications be anticipated in advance of the trial, and the manner in which they will be dealt with be described and incorporated into the trial protocol. Identifying the potential difficulties that may arise during the period of trial, and specifying in what manner the problems will be resolved, differentiates the experienced practitioner of clinical trials from the novitiate.

For example, if the protocol states that confirmation of the progression is required at the next routine examination of the patient, how will the problem of event definition be resolved if the progression is found at the patient's final formal visit in the trial? There are various alternative decisions that can be considered: the patient is considered not to have had an event; or, the progression is counted as an event even if no further examination is done; or, the patient is examined again in 3 months even though that would necessitate extending the patient's period in the trial by 3 months. This last alternative would serve to prolong the trial if the patient entered into the trial during the last 3 months of patient accession.

Another problem of a similar nature would occur if the patient showed the requisite progression at a scheduled examination, and then moved away and was subsequently unavailable for the follow-up examination. How would that situation be handled?

Selection of the Primary Response Variable

Of the various EDSS response variables available, the authors recommend that the primary response variable in MS clinical trials be the "time to the confirmed event": the measure of the time, from the baseline examination, to a 1-unit increase in the EDSS, confirmed at the next routine examination. If and when this confirmed event occurs, the usual procedure is to consider that the patient has completed the trial protocol, therapy may then be discontinued, and routine study examinations of that patient are stopped. Later in this chapter the authors suggest that this traditional approach is not the one recommended for MS clinical trials.

There are a number of reasons to support the selection of this primary response variable. The first relates to the problem of deciding how to evaluate the responses of those patients who do not complete the requirements of the protocol. These patients fall under the general category of "lost-to-study". They include patients whose treatment is terminated by the study physicians due to side effects, or for other reasons. Other patients are considered "dropouts". They stop treatment for one reason or another, and may or may not appear for their routine examinations. They may move, lose interest in participation in the trial, take medication not permitted by the protocol, be influenced by negative attitudes of their family, or drop out for other reasons. However, if the confirmed event has occurred before the patient leaves the study, then the patient has provided all of the information required by the protocol for that "time to the confirmed event" response variable. If the patient stopped all participation in the trial before the event occurred, the patient's data, up to that time, are also included in the analysis. In other words, the information provided by the patient up to the point of the event or dropout is utilizable in the analysis of the primary response variable, and reduces the number and impact of lost-to-study patients.

The Intent-To-Treat Analysis

Another reason to consider the use of a "time to the confirmed event" response variable is that it is in accord with an "intent-to-treat" approach in the analysis of the data. The statistical basis of clinical trials is that the randomization of patients into the study, into one treatment group or another, provides groups of patients whose departure from equivalence, if any, can be described in terms of probabilities. The loss of patients from the clinical trial tends to dissipate the effect of the randomization, which in turn can introduce bias into the analysis of the data. Assume that an important, but unknown, and therefore unrecorded, variable happens to be strongly correlated with the primary response variable. If the distributions of that variable in the two treatment groups differ, compensation for the resulting bias cannot be achieved in the analysis of the data (see earlier discussion of historical controls). Differences in the primary response variable between the treatment and placebo groups may then be partly, or even mostly, a function of the bias rather than of the effect of the experimental therapy. In order to minimize a potential bias, it is necessary to minimize the patient loss to the study.

An "intent-to-treat" approach to the data analysis is one which attempts to use the response variable data of every patient randomized into the trial. Statisticians differ regarding the degree to which an "intent-to-treat" analysis should be carried out. Assume, for example, that a patient who was randomized to the experimental therapy group, was given the placebo by mistake, and never received any of the experimental therapy. Some would insist that the data from that patient be analyzed as if that patient had received the experimental therapy in order to obtain the full benefit of randomization. The authors adopt a more moderate position. They recommend that several analyses be done, and that one of them be chosen in advance to be the primary analysis. In this particular example, they would probably include that patient in the placebo group in the primary analysis. In another analysis, an "intent-to-treat" analysis, that patient would be analyzed as an experimental therapy patient. In yet another analysis, the patient might be excluded from the analysis altogether. In the best of circumstances, the determination that the therapy was effective, or not effective, would be the same from all 3 analyses. If the result differed according to the analysis, then the investigators have a problem, suggesting that the demonstration of efficacy might, at best, be borderline.

An analysis of a "time to an event" response variable is called a survival analysis. For disorders, such as cancer, where the event might be death, neither treatment nor follow-up would be possible after the event. If the event were other than death, once the confirmed event had taken place and the protocol was completed, other options are possible. Typically, in such a clinical trial, treatment would then have been stopped and the patient no longer followed. In MS clinical trials, the event chosen is never death, but rather the development of further pathology such as progression, a relapse, or diminution in the activities of daily living. The authors recommend that the patients who have had an event should be continued on treatment and be subject to the routine examinations through the end of the trial. This would permit the recording of the secondary response variables for a more extended period. Thus, one of these secondary variables might be the change in EDSS from baseline until the end of the study period for each patient.

Duration of the Clinical Trial

The MS clinical trials in general have followed each patient for 2 or 3 years. While the advantage of a 2-year trial is the shorter time period for determining the efficacy of the experimental therapy, a number of recent trials have shown indications of therapeutic effect after 2 years of treatment and follow-up, but did not reach the desired level of statistical significance. If the period of trial had been 3 years, assuming that the experimental therapy were effective, statistical significance might have been achieved with the longer follow-up.

The authors recommend an approach which, to some extent, has advantages inherent in trial durations of both 2 and 3 years of patient follow-up. The protocol would provide for an in-trial period of 3 years. It would also call for two interim statistical analyses, as well as a third and final analysis at the end of the 3 years of trial. If the investigator chooses a similar approach, then the first interim statistical analysis should be accomplished when, on average, all patients had been in trial for 2 years; the second, at 2.5 years; and the final analysis, when all patients will have completed 3 years on study. The procedure can be designed so that, if the desired level of statistical significance is attained at any analysis, the trial may be terminated. Therefore, the trial has the potential for being completed at any of the interim periods.

Despite the two additional opportunities for trial termination, the overall risk of incorrectly finding statistical significance when the experimental therapy is ineffective can be designed to remain at, approximately, 0.05. If the statistical procedure of O'Brien and Fleming is used, then the first interim analysis would require a statistical significance level of 0.0005 to be achieved before the trial could be terminated (Geller and Pocock 1987). In other words, to consider stopping the trial at 2 years when efficacy of the experimental therapy has been demonstrated, a very large effect of the experimental therapy would need to be observed. If the first interim analysis did not demonstrate statistical significance, the clinical trial would continue. The second interim analysis, at 2.5 years, would have to demonstrate significance at the 0.014 level in order that there be consideration for stopping the trial. Finally, if neither interim analysis were to lead to termination of the study, then the final analysis would have to demonstrate statistical significance at the 0.045 level. The overall level of probability is not very different from the requirement of 0.05 had only one analysis been planned. Yet, this procedure permits an earlier termination of the study if a large effect of the experimental therapy were to be observed relatively early in the trial.

One additional, and not inconsequential, advantage of a trial that is carried out for 3 years is the increased credibility of the results, as compared to a trial of 2 years' duration.

Estimation of Sample Size

If the authors were to identify the statisticians' contribution of greatest import to the design of the clinical trial, they would consider it to be the estimation of the number of patients that must be admitted. This is so because the computation of the sample size assures that the investigators have made a number of decisions that will be critical to a successful trial. Some of these decisions are reached relatively easily, based on common practice among clinical trial investigators of MS. Others may be made with greater difficulty, since they should be based on prior information, which frequently is unavailable.

The investigators must decide on a minimally clinically important effect of the experimental therapy to be demonstrated with a high probability if the therapy, as measured by the primary response variable, were indeed effective in slowing progression.

Another is to decide what risk (alpha) to accept that the study results would, by chance, demonstrate statistical significance, if, in fact, the experimental therapy were ineffective. This decision is inextricably tied in with another choice: whether the risk should be considered one-tailed or two-tailed. That is, whether to exclude the possibility that the therapy may exacerbate the patients' disease progression (one-tailed), or to decide that the therapy may possibly affect the disease progression in either direction (two-tailed).

Another decision is to determine the acceptable power of the study (1-beta); that the results would demonstrate statistical significance if, in fact, the experimental therapy differed in efficacy from that of the placebo.

Finally, the investigators must estimate the proportion of the placebo patients in the trial who will remain event-free during the period of the trial.

In the past, but less frequently today, it was common practice among investigators to plan to enter as many patients as possible into a clinical trial within the constraints of their budget and their patient population. They might have selected the risk that they were willing to take of incorrectly demonstrating statistical significance, but might not have estimated the consequent power of the clinical trial. More frequently than not, these choices resulted in a smaller than optimal sample size, and a clinical trial of relatively low power. Thus, a major effort involving years of study might fail unless the effect of the experimental therapy was large.

Given the investigators' decisions regarding these design elements for a clinical trial, the sample size can be estimated.

Each of these decisions will be discussed in turn. The first decision is the choice of the minimal clinical effect of the primary response variable that the investigators want to demonstrate to be statistically significant, if there were a real effect. To do that, the investigators must estimate the proportion of placebo patients in the trial who will remain event-free during the period of trial. Reference has been made to a previous study, in which a group of placebo patients with baseline DSS scores ranging from 0 to 3 was compared, to determine what proportion progressed at least 1 DSS unit within the 2 years of trial. In the study, 30% of the placebo patients remained event-free (Bornstein et al. 1987). The authors are of the opinion, given the inclusion criteria recommended in this chapter, that a 50% non-progression rate is a conservative estimate, and can safely be used.

The authors have recommended that each patient remain in the trial for 3 years. The percentage of those not expected to progress at least 1 confirmed EDSS unit in 2 years would be further reduced over 3 years, which would provide an even more conservative estimate.

If the non-progression rate of the placebo group is less than 50%, the investigators will find that the power of their study is greater than estimated, other factors being equal.

In a study now under way, the investigators assume that 50% of the placebo patients will progress at least one EDSS unit during the 2-year trial period (Jacobs, 1990, personal communication). In that study, the progression needs to be confirmed at the next 6-month routine examination in order to be counted as an event. The investigators chose a one-third reduction in confirmed progressions (33% of the experimental therapy patients would progress) to be the minimal effect to be detected with high probability. Any larger effect obviously would be detected with even higher probability. The authors suggest that this is an achievable goal in terms of the number of patients that will be required. The authors believe that selection of the minimal effective reduction may reasonably range between a 30% reduction in confirmed progressions as a result of therapy, and a 50% reduction. If the minimal effect of interest is less than a 30% reduction, the number of patients required for admission into the trial will begin to escalate rapidly. On the other hand, if the trial design is aimed at measuring a minimal real effect of more than 50%, it may reasonably be assumed that smaller, though substantial, effects of therapy may be missed.

Readers will bear in mind that one of the critical factors recommended to maintain the percent of non-progression in the placebo group at no more than 50% is to restrict admission to relapsing patients with a baseline EDSS score of 3.5 or less.

Another decision that must be made is the selection of the alpha risk, that an ineffective therapy will incorrectly be judged to be effective. Investigators in MS clinical trials most often opt for an alpha risk of 0.05, a decision that a 1-in-20 risk of error is reasonable. In the study of other disorders, where the consequences of reaching a false conclusion of efficacy can be devastating to the patient who is given the ineffective therapy, investigators might choose a smaller alpha risk. This decision would increase the number of patients who must be admitted into the trial.

The decision concerning the choice of a one- or a two-tailed test of significance is more controversial among statisticians (Fleiss 1987; Peace 1989; Goodman 1988). The question refers to whether the experimental therapy may show a worse response, as well as a better response than the placebo. Generally speaking, in the case of clinical trials of MS, the prior animal research, pilot tests on patients, and/or dose–response studies on patients give sufficient indication that, while the experimental therapy may be effective or ineffective, it is unlikely to be deleterious when compared to the placebo group. Given this prior information, the authors might have recommended that a one-tailed test of significance be chosen. However, in a relatively recent clinical trial of gamma interferon, such background data was misleading (Panitch et al. 1987). Patients in the experimental therapy group rapidly showed clinical deterioration to the point that the trial was terminated early. Rather than assuming that the therapy will, at worst, be ineffective, it would be more prudent, in the opinion of the authors, to use a two-tailed test of significance.

The investigators must consider that making any of the above decisions more stringent will impact, perhaps heavily, on the number of patients required for admission into the trial. For example, other design elements being the same, and making certain choices (described later) regarding some of the above-mentioned design elements, a shift from an alpha risk of $p = 0.05$ to $p = 0.01$ would add more than 100 additional patients to the clinical trial. Additional protection against larger risks does not come cheaply in clinical trials. The choice of a two-tailed alpha risk will also increase the required number of patients needed to demonstrate efficacy.

The next decision is also relatively easy to make: the choice of the power of the clinical trial. To avoid an escalation in the number of patients to be admitted into the trial, a power of 0.80 is often chosen. It means that the investigator is willing to accept a 20% risk of missing the chosen minimal real effect. Again, an increase in the power of the trial requires a potentially substantial increase in the number of patients entered into the trial. For example, let us say that the investigators have assumed that 50% of the patients in the placebo group will have a confirmed progression during the period of trial. The investigators decide that it would be important to demonstrate that the progression rate in the experimental group will be 30% compared to 50% in the placebo group. Assume that the alpha risk is a two-tailed 0.05. If a decision is made to select a power of 0.90 rather than 0.80, approximately 80 additional patients would be required.

Given the choice of design elements specified above, the appropriate sample size can be estimated. Assume also that 50% of the patients entering the trial and randomized to the placebo group will have a confirmed progression of at least 1 full EDSS unit during the period of follow-up. The alpha risk is chosen to be a two-tailed 0.05, and the power is 0.80. The investigators, in our hypothetical example, have determined that the minimum real improvement to be detected with high probability is one of 40% below the rate in the placebo group (50% − 30% = 20%/50% = 40%). The appropriate sample size is approximately 200 patients, 100 in each treatment group.

There is, however, a need to account for patients lost-to-study. The primary response variable is "time to the event" so that the information collected before a patient may be lost-to-study is fully usable. If investigators focus in advance on procedures to keep patients in the study, and follow with routine examinations those who break the protocol, the patients lost-to-study should not exceed 10%. The size of the patient sample needs to be increased to adjust for this loss, but the consequences of the loss are greater than they appear to be. One can roughly estimate the percent by which the sample size must be increased, as 1 divided by $(1 - R)^2$, where R is the patient lost-to-study rate (Lachin 1981). For the example given above, if the loss rate were 10%, the sample size would have to be increased by 23%, for a corrected sample size of approximately 240 patients. It is evident that the penalty on sample size is severe as the anticipated loss rate increases.

All other design elements being equal, sample size escalates sharply the smaller the difference between the experimental and placebo rates. For example, if the experimental rate were 35%, that is, a reduction of 30% from the placebo rate, a sample size of 330 patients would be required to demonstrate statistical significance, including compensation for a 10% loss of patients from the trial. Given the design elements listed above, it would not appear that investigators have a great deal of leeway in reducing this selected minimum progression rate without an added penalty of substantially increased sample size.

Timely Patient Recruitment

Once the critical design elements are chosen, the investigators must examine their options for obtaining patients for the trial. These include, of course, the possibilities for collaborating with other centers, and the time frame for admitting patients. The advantage in having several collaborating centers is the greater patient representation inherent in the wider geographical areas, the more rapid admission of patients, and the ability to compare the consistency of the effect of the experimental therapy, if found, across clinical centers. The major disadvantage of increasing the number of collaborating centers is the added cost and complexity of administering the clinical trial, in order to maintain strict adherence to the protocol. The authors are of the opinion that a reasonable number of collaborating centers is 4–6. Four centers, randomizing 20 patients per year for 3 years, would provide 240 patients for the trial.

This sample size would permit patients to be randomized within centers, and within groups of 6, 3 to each treatment group. If the patients were randomized in pairs, one to the experimental therapy, and the other to placebo, once the first of the 2 patients is randomized, the second would be automatically allocated to the other treatment group. If, by chance, the treatment of one of the pairs of the patients were to be unblinded, and the pairing were known, it would automatically unblind the second patient of the pair. This unfortunate event is unlikely to occur if the randomized group were composed of 6 (or 4) patients rather than 2.

It is a matter of record that one of the most frequent breaches of protocol is in the inability of the investigators to enter the promised number of patients within the time frame specified, due to overly optimistic estimates of patient availability (Lee 1983). This extends the time span of the entire effort and can increase considerably the cost of the study. It is important that the prospective investigators provide solid data on their capacity to enter patients within the specified time frame. NINDS grant review committees have, in the past, concerned themselves with this issue when reviewing clinical trial protocols. It is not necessarily an easy matter to gather reliable data regarding potential patients. Investigators in one clinical trial, with a number of restrictive inclusion criteria, advertised for patients with relapsing/remitting disease (Bornstein et al. 1987). They obtained completed questionnaires from more than 900 patients; 15% of these were selected for examination for potential admission. Of the latter, 36% were eventually randomized into the trial. For centers without a registry, these data may indicate the potential difficulty that may be encountered in ascertaining the patient population in advance. Centers with computerized registries which include information about the characteristics of the patients and their disease are better able to predict the size of the pool of patients who will be eligible for entry into the trial.

Blinding

Acceptance by clinical neurologists of positive results from a clinical trial rests on the strength of the findings and the scientific integrity of the research, among other factors. One of the important aspects of the trial's scientific integrity is the requirement that neither the patient nor the examiner know the treatment the patient is receiving. The examiner may be the examining neurologist, or psychologist, or possibly a nurse obtaining responses to one of the test items. There is evidence to support the observation that a patient's participation in a clinical trial will affect the disease status in a positive way. Nevertheless, as long as the patient is unaware of the treatment received, in the absence of a therapeutic effect, it should not affect the difference in responses between the patients in both treatment groups.

The double-blinding (patient and examiner), or double-masking, according to some, may be thwarted to a degree through no fault of the investigators. Some of the side effects of the experimental therapy may reveal to the patient, and/or the examining neurologist, that the patient is likely to be receiving a treatment other than a placebo. The side effects, if not physically apparent, may be hidden from the examining neurologist if the protocol prohibits the patient from discussing apparent side effects with that clinician. Instead, the patients discuss their health status with a treating neurologist who assesses any untoward effect. In one clinical trial, hirsutism, which occurred in 66.5% of the experimental therapy patients, and in only 16.4% of the placebo patients, may have contributed to an unblinding of some of the patients and the examining neurologists (The MS Study Group). Questionnaires completed by patients at the end of their study period, in which they are asked to guess which treatment they received, and the reason for their guess, and similar questionnaires filled out by the examining neurologists after the last examination of each patient, can provide valuable evidence of the success or failure of the blinding.

The protocol should address the procedure for maintaining blindness of patient allocation to treatment group. During the trial, adherence to the blinding procedure should be vigorously monitored. As a matter of fact, only those study personnel who have a need to be unblinded should be so. They include the technicians who prepare the coded treatment medication for each patient, and the statisticians who will be examining the data quality and performing interim analyses during the course of the trial. The treating neurologist may need to become unblinded regarding a particular patient when dealing with serious side effects.

The authors recommend another area of blinding, in connection with interim data analyses. They have already suggested that the clinical trial of MS be planned for 3 years of patient follow-up, with interim analyses when all patients, on average, have had 2 and 2.5 years of follow-up. They recommend that all but a handful of participants in the trial be blinded to the results of the interim analyses regarding efficacy. This restriction would include the clinical trial director, members of the external advisory, monitoring, and steering committees, and all other personnel and patients except for the few with a need to know. The latter group is restricted to the statisticians and the computer and data processing personnel who produce the data for the interim analyses.

Monitoring and Advisory Committees

Multi-center clinical trial protocols include establishment of key committees that have responsibilities regarding the effective conduct of the trial. The steering committee is made up of investigators and is responsible for policy development, oversight and day-to-day conduct of the trial. An advisory committee, composed of other individuals within and/or external to the participating institution advises the principal investigator and steering committee on the conduct of the trial.

The ultimate responsibility for monitoring a multi-center clinical trial supported by the NINDS is assigned to a clinical trial monitoring committee or data and safety monitoring committee that is organized by the Institute. This committee is wholly independent of the investigators and has as its primary role the assurance of patient safety and well-being. It is composed of neurologists with expertise in MS and in clinical trials, and a statistician(s) having experience in clinical trial design, conduct and data analysis. Some clinical trials may require additional kinds of expertise, such as in pharmacology, depending on the nature of the therapy under study.

These committees serve important oversight and advisory functions. The role of each should be carefully defined in the protocol before the trial begins. Side effects, admission and lost-to-study data, data quality, trial management, and baseline equivalence data are monitored by these committees.

There is an ethical consideration that must be addressed, in advance, in the protocol. The clinical trial director and the members of those committees must routinely be kept informed about side effects, and be provided with information concerning the adherence to the specifications of the study protocol and the quality of the study data.

When the oversight of the data is directed toward side effects, regular monitoring is necessary, and the protocol should describe the procedures to be followed. At monitoring and other committee meetings, tables showing the distributions of the side effects should be presented, discussed and analyzed by treatment group, and by treatment group within centers.

The more serious side effects should be monitored daily, and their presence reported immediately by the principal investigator of a clinical center to the data center, and in turn to the statisticians and the clinical trial director. Should the clinical trial director consider the side effect(s) critical, the chairperson of the monitoring committee would be contacted to arrange for a special meeting of the committee. Further discussion would determine whether to revise the protocol, to continue the trial, or to terminate the study.

The authors have previously described a procedure for doing a limited number of interim analyses that may lead to consideration that the trial be stopped if a predetermined effect of the experimental therapy were demonstrated at an earlier stage of the trial. Monitoring and advisory committee meetings are generally held shortly after these interim analyses are completed. If the results of an interim analysis show that the data did not yet demonstrate statistical significance at the level of probability specified in the protocol, a statement would be made at a committee meeting only to that effect. None of the data in the efficacy analysis should be presented. On the other hand, if efficacy were demonstrated early, additional major statistical analyses should be accomplished, and presented to the committees and the principal investigators, in order to decide whether or not to continue the trial.

The monitoring committee's access to efficacy data, and consequent deliberations concerning the stopping of the trial for that reason, are a function of the interim data analyses. The committee has a full workload at each of its routine meetings. These should be held at least twice each year from the start-up of the trial to review of the final data analysis.

Reports concerning patient compliance procedures should also be reviewed. These procedures are designed to assure that patients' treatment is in accordance with the protocol of the trial. The best assurance of compliance is to assay blood or urine levels of an experimental drug or its metabolites. When this is not possible, and when the protocol directs that a supply of dosage vials is kept by the patients, an indirect method of assessing compliance is to count the accumulated empty vials of medication presented by patients when they return to receive a new supply of drug. Another compliance procedure might be to assay blood or urine for evidence of prohibited drugs. In general, these procedures attempt to limit ways in which the quality of the clinical trial may be degraded. The description and implementation of these procedures are indications of intent to manage the trial closely.

Reports concerning loss of patients to the trial must be closely monitored by the committee. These reports will compare the losses by treatment group and by center. The clinical trial director should be prepared to investigate those centers with unusually high loss rates, as compared to other centers, and to initiate action in their resolution.

During the period of admission of patients, routine reports of the effect of the randomization procedure must be provided to the committees. This is accomplished by comparing the baseline variables by treatment group, and by treatment group within centers, and by providing tests of significance of the differences. If unusual differences are found between treatment groups in certain baseline variables, for reasons which remain unknown, these differences can be compensated for by statistical methods in the analyses of the response variables.

Weaknesses in data collection, such as the proliferation of recording errors or data omissions, and inadequate data processing, will degrade the data flowing from the participating centers and contribute to substantial data errors. In order to minimize these errors, the data management center must devise operational quality control procedures that permit data checking at each stage of the data flow operation. Cross checks should be made of similar information on different data forms. Routine reports regarding the variety of such errors discovered, and their source, should be prepared for review by the clinical trial monitoring committee. In addition, the statisticians should identify certain of the key study variables, such as the primary response variable, and the baseline EDSS score for special attention. Apart from the routine data processing checks, the statisticians should hand review the computer printout of these variables, and compare them with data recorded on the original report forms which were forwarded to the data processing center, for every study patient.

Data Analysis

The clinical trial statisticians will accomplish a variety of analyses during the course of the trial. Routine data analyses of the differences in baseline variables between treatment groups will be presented at each monitoring

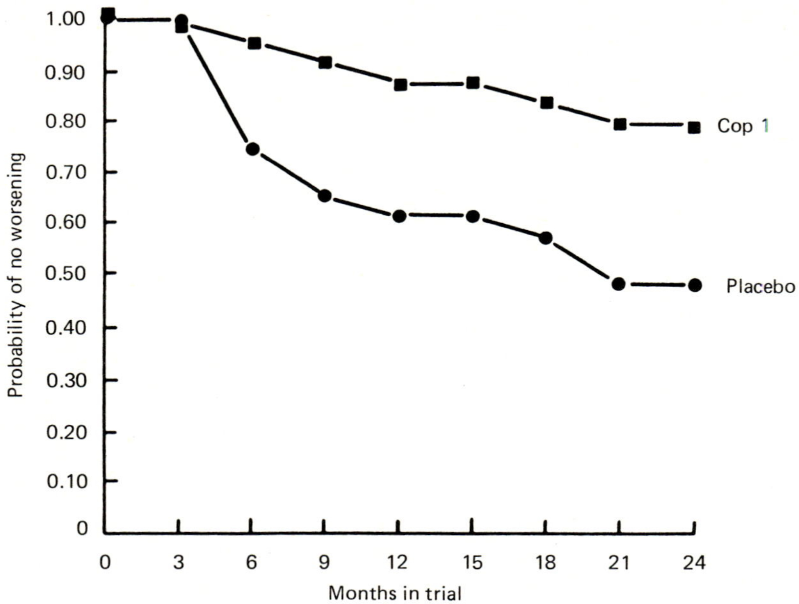

Fig. 4.1. Curves represent the probability of no worsening from the baseline DSS score (Bornstein et al. 1987).

committee meeting until all patients have been entered into the trial and the final baseline analyses have been accomplished. The primary purpose of these analyses is to determine if the randomization procedure has accomplished the objective of providing two treatment groups of patients with characteristics which are equivalent at entry into the trial.

At the end of the trial, a final baseline analysis will again be accomplished to test for equivalence of the treatment and control groups. This latter effort is especially important if the investigators decide that not all of the patients entered into the trial will be part of the major analysis; that is, if the "intent-to-treat" concept is modified. It would be important, in that case, to investigate the potential loss of equivalence at baseline between the two treatment groups of patients, due to the exclusion of some of the randomized patients. The investigators would hope to demonstrate that equivalence still existed between the two patient groups, if only based on those variables which were measured at baseline.

Statistically significant differences in baseline variables may also be found in analyses of all patients who are randomized. Randomization is no guarantor of equivalence; only that with observed differences of any given magnitude, the probabilities of their occurrence by chance can be calculated. All is not lost, nevertheless, if differences do appear in one or more of the baseline variables, since statistical procedures exist to adjust for these differences.

If the primary response variable is the "time to a confirmed EDSS unit increase", then a chart of the survival curves will be prepared, and a survival analysis made. Fig. 4.1 shows the survival curves of each treatment group in a study of relapsing/remitting patients (Bornstein et al. 1987). It shows, for each routine examination period, the probability of a patient not worsening. A statistical procedure exists for determining whether the two curves are the same, or different, in terms of probability calculations, over the entire period of the trial. The test of a difference is called a log rank test. Additional tests can be performed, seeking to determine whether the two curves differed at specific points in time, such as at 1, 2 and 3 years. The authors recommend that the primary analysis be of the comparison of the total survival curves, and that the analyses at specific time periods be considered secondary analyses. In addition to these analyses, which should be done at the end of the trial, survival analyses should also be accomplished as part of the interim analyses.

It may have become apparent from the discussions of the numbers of baseline variable analyses, analyses based on different numbers of patient subgroups, analyses of the primary as well as all of the secondary response variables, and analyses at interim periods during the trial, that a large number of statistical analyses are required. Additional analyses will certainly be needed, especially if there are losses of patients to the study, with consequent potential effects due to the loss of full randomization.

There are a number of patient characteristics or factors which have been of interest to clinical neurologists doing clinical trials of MS. These include the age of the patient at the time of admission into the trial, the length of time from first symptoms to time of admission, relapse rate and/or degree of EDSS change during a pretrial observation period, sex, EDSS score at admission, and the clinical center in which the patient was participating.

Some of the statistical analyses performed at the end of the trial will most likely include tests to determine whether these patient characteristics and factors are correlated with the primary and secondary response variables. Tests will also determine if observed differences in the primary and secondary response variables may, in part, be due to differences in the distributions of these characteristics or factors measured at baseline. If this is found to be so, an adjustment by statistical methods can eliminate their effect.

Some associations of factors with response variables can be troublesome. If, for example, the effect of the experimental therapy, as compared to that of the placebo, is demonstrably different from center to center, it is cause for concern, and further steps should be undertaken to understand the reasons for this anomaly.

Past studies suggest that the baseline EDSS score has been most frequently associated with EDSS response variables; that is, over a large range of EDSS scores, the more rapid changes in patient scores have occurred at the lower end of the scale. A statistical demonstration of this association is less likely to be obtained if the patients admitted to the trial are restricted to those whose baseline EDSS scores do not exceed 3.5.

The authors' experience is that, aside from the baseline EDSS variable, other baseline patient characteristics or factors are unlikely to be found to be important, given a proper randomization scheme.

Conclusions

This chapter has been devoted to some of the design and statistical issues that must be addressed by investigators planning to test experimental therapies in MS patients. Both statistical and neurological expertise are required in the planning stages to increase the likelihood of favorable assessment by grant reviewers, and in the execution phase to help assure patients' safety and interests and to derive interpretable results at the conclusion of the trial. By limiting the patient population in the clinical trial to MS patients who have more active disease, by careful definition and selection of response variables, estimating sample size, selecting a sufficiently long patient follow-up period and planning judicious interim analyses, the possibility of achieving the clinical trial objectives will be significantly enhanced.

Appendix. The Effectiveness of an Experimental Therapy Must Increase as the Percent of Non-progressing Patients in the Trial Increases, in Order to Achieve a Demonstration of Statistical Significance

Assume that, in a cohort of patients eligible for admission into a clinical trial, 30% of the patients treated with the placebo will not progress during the period of the trial.

Assume also that the trial has been designed so that statistical significance will be demonstrated if the experimental therapy group shows a 50% increase over the placebo group, in the percentage of patients who do not progress during the trial. That is, 45% (30% + 15%) of the patients in the experimental therapy group will not progress.

Assuming that certain other design parameters (not specified here) are held constant, the statistician projects that approximately 240 patients should be entered in the trial, with one half of these assigned at random to each of the experimental therapy and placebo groups.

If 30% of the patients entering the trial will not progress, then, because of randomization, the expectation is that 30% of the patients in each of the treatment groups will not progress. In the experimental therapy group, that will leave 84 patients (120 × 70%) to provide the base of potential progressors from which 18 patients (45% − 30% = 15% × 120 = 18) will have become non-progressors as a consequence of their receiving the experimental therapy.

In other words if, in the placebo group, there will be an estimated 36 patients (30% × 120) who will not progress during the trial, then 54 patients (36 + 18) must not progress in the experimental therapy group in order to provide the 50% increase in non-progressing patients that will be required in order for statistical significance to be attained.

Now, assume that the investigators have underestimated the percent of non-progressing patients entering the study, a common occurrence in MS trials, and consequently the placebo rate will not be 30%, but 50%.

The estimated number of non-progressing patients in each group is now 60 (120 × 50%), even if the experimental therapy is totally ineffective. An additional 19 non-progressing patients (60 × 15.8%) from among the potential progressors in the experimental therapy group would now be required in order to achieve a demonstration of statistical significance. That is, 31.7% (19/60) of the experimental therapy patients expected to progress during the trial must become non-progressors.

To sum, if the percent of non-progressors entering the trial were to be 30%, then 21.4% of the actively progressing patients would need to respond to the experimental therapy for statistical significance to be achieved. When the percent of non-progressors entering the trial is 50%, the effect of the experimental therapy would need to increase to 31.7% of the actively progressing patients in order to achieve statistical significance.

References

Alter M, Greenstein J, Camenga D, LaRue L (1987) Alpha interferon clinical trial for multiple sclerosis: design considerations. Neuroepidemiology 6:85–92

Bornstein MB, Miller A, Slagle S et al. (1987) A pilot trial of COP 1 in exacerbating-remitting multiple sclerosis. N Engl J Med 317:408–414

Bornstein MB, Miller A, Slagle S et al. (1991) A placebo-controlled, double-blind, randomized two-center, pilot trial of COP 1 in chronic progressive multiple sclerosis. Neurol 41:533–539

British and Dutch Multiple Sclerosis Azathioprine Trial Group (1988) Double-masked trial of azathioprine in multiple sclerosis. Lancet 2:179–183

Camenga DL, Johnson KP, Alter M et al. (1986) Systemic recombinant alpha-2 interferon therapy in relapsing multiple sclerosis. Arch Neurol 43:1239–1246

Cook SD, Devereux C, Troiano R et al. (1986) Effect of total lymphoid irradiation in chronic progressive multiple sclerosis. Lancet 1:1405–1409

Fleiss JL (1987) Some thoughts on two-sided tests. J Controlled Clin Trials 8:394

Friedman LM, Furberg CD, DeMets DL (1988) Fundamentals of clinical trials, 2nd ed. PSG, Littletown, New York

Geller NL, Pocock SJ (1987) Interim analyses in randomized clinical trials: ramifications and guidelines for practitioners. Biometrics 43:213–223

Goodkin DE, Hertsgaard D, Seminary J (1988) Upper extremity function in multiple sclerosis: improving assessment sensitivity with box-and-block and nine-hole peg tests. Arch Phys Med Rehabil 69:850–854

Goodkin DE, Hertsgaard D, Rudick RA (1989) Exacerbation rates and adherence to disease type in a prospectively followed-up population with multiple sclerosis. Arch Neurol 46:1107–1112

Goodman S (1988) One-sided or two-sided p values? J Controlled Clin Trials 9:387–388

Harris JO, Frank JA, Patronas N, McFarlin DE, McFarland HF (1991) Serial gadolinium enhanced magnetic resonance imaging scans in patients with early relapsing-remitting multiple sclerosis: implications for clinical trials and natural history. Ann Neurol 29:548–555

Hauser DL, Dawson DM, Lehrich JR, Beal MF, Kevy SV, Weiner HL (1983) Immunosuppression and plasmapheresis in chronic progressive multiple sclerosis. Arch Neurol 40:687–690

Jacobs L, Salazar AM, Herndon R et al. (1987) Intrathecally administered natural human fibroblast interferon reduces exacerbations of multiple sclerosis. Arch Neurol 44:589–595

Knobler RL, Panitch HS, Braheny SL et al. (1984) Clinical trial of natural alpha interferon in multiple sclerosis. Ann NY Acad Sci 436:382–388

Lachin JM (1981) Introduction to sample size determination and power analysis for clinical trials. J Controlled Clin Trials 2:93–113

Lee YJ (1983) Interim recruitment goals in clinical trials. J Chron Dis 36:379–389
Matthews DE, Farewell VT (1988) Using and understanding medical statistics 2nd edn. Karger, Basel
Milligan NM, Newcombe R, Compston DAS (1987) A double-blind controlled trial of high dose methylprednisolone in patients with multiple sclerosis: 1. Clinical effects. J Neurol Neurosurg Psychiatry 50:511–516
O'Brien PC, Shampo MA (1988) Statistical considerations for performing multiple tests in a single experiment. 5. Comparing two therapies with respect to several endpoints. Mayo Clin Proc 63:1140–1143
Panitch HS, Hirsch RL, Haley AS, Johnson KP (1987) Exacerbations of multiple sclerosis in patients treated with gamma interferon. Lancet 1:893–895
Peace KE (1989) Second thoughts: the alternative hypothesis: one-sided or two-sided? J Clin Epidemiol 42:473–476
Pocock SJ, Geller NL, Tsiatis AA (1987) The analysis of multiple endpoints in clinical trials. Biometrics 43:487–498
Rudick RA (1990) Helping patients live with MS. What primary care physicians can do. Postgrad Med 88:197–207
The Multiple Sclerosis Study Group (1990) Efficacy and toxicity of cyclosporine in chronic progressive multiple sclerosis: a randomized, double-blinded placebo-controlled clinical trial. Ann Neurol 27:591–605
Weinshenker BG, Ebers GC (1987) The natural history of multiple sclerosis. Can J Neurol Sci 14:255–261
Weinshenker BG, Bass B, Rice GPA et al. (1989a) The natural history of multiple sclerosis: a geographically based study. 1. Clinical course and disability. Brain 112:133–146
Weinshenker BG, Bass B, Rice GPA et al. (1989b) The natural history of multiple sclerosis: a geographically based study. 2. Predictive value of the early clinical course. Brain 112:1419–1428
Weinshenker BG, Rice GPA, Noseworthy JH, Carriere W, Baskerville J, Ebers GC (1991a) The natural history of multiple sclerosis: a geographically based study. 3. Multivariate analysis of predictive factors and models of outcome. Brain 114:1045–1056
Weinshenker BG, Rice GPA, Noseworthy JH, Carriere W, Baskerville J, Ebers GC (1991b) The natural history of multiple sclerosis: a geographically based study. 4. Applications to planning and interpretation of clinical therapeutic trials. Brain 114:1057–1068

Chapter 5

Pathogenesis of Multiple Sclerosis: Relationship to Therapeutic Strategies

Richard M. Ransohoff

Introduction

Ten chapters of this book are devoted to specific therapeutic strategies for multiple sclerosis (MS). It will be immediately noted that all of these strategies involve manipulation of the patient's immune system. These immune-modulatory strategies comprise a broad spectrum. At one end are the global immunosuppressives, both anti-inflammatory (corticosteroids), cytotoxic (azathioprine, cyclophosphamide), and total lymphoid irradiation and plasmapheresis. Slightly more specific immune modulators include cyclosporine A and anti-T cell antibodies. The rationale for using interferons to treat MS relies primarily on their immunoregulatory potential although antiviral effects may also be desirable. Finally, several elegant strategies for specific immunotherapy directed against small numbers of presumed pathogenic immunocompetent cells are also described. If the majority of effort in studying experimental therapies for MS is directed at manipulating the immune system, then the task of explaining the rationale for this approach reduces to explaining why MS is thought to be an immune-mediated disorder. In this chapter, the concept of MS immunopathogenesis will be reviewed, with concentration primarily on the epidemiologic data and derivative clinical investigations. Where possible, references are to reviews, to facilitate further reading.

Historical Background

The gross pathology of MS was described approximately 150 years ago, and 30 years later Charcot described the histopathology and clinical characteristics of MS (Adams 1983). Until the early 1950s, despite intensive investigation, there was very little agreement about the pathogenesis of the demyelinating disorders (Wolf 1952). Investigations carried out since then have served to focus attention progressively on immune-mediated tissue injury. It is important, however, to remember that a variety of other possibilities have been considered and extensively pursued. The essential characteristics of the MS pathologic lesion are not in doubt. They include: perivascular inflammation, segmental demyelination and reactive gliosis (Adams 1983; Lampert 1983; Lassmann 1983). Interpretation of the preferential destruction of myelin in these lesions has been difficult in that myelin is the most sensitive component of the CNS to injurious influences of all sorts. Therefore, the selective destruction of myelin in MS invited two possible explanations: either the pathologic process was directed specifically at myelin, or a low-intensity pathologic process could damage myelin while leaving other elements of the CNS unharmed. A variety of exogenous toxins, all capable of producing demyelinating lesions, have been considered as potential causes of MS. These include carbon monoxide, lead and arsenic poisoning, and a variety of biologically-derived exotoxins (Merritt 1970; Scheinberg and Korey 1962; Wolf 1952). There has never been evidence implicating these toxic substances or processes related to them (such as anoxia) in the human demyelinating disorders. A recent observation of an occupational cluster of MS may in the future provide some further insight into this issue (Stein et al. 1987).

As an alternative to exogenous toxins, it was proposed that endogenous toxins might activate myelinolytic enzymes within CNS white matter. A suggestion that subclinical hepatic insufficiency might lead to accumulation of endogenous toxins which could activate myelinotoxic processes was extensively investigated in both human and animal material in the 1930s and 1940s (Wolf 1952). No circulating substances specific to MS and capable of inducing demyelination could be demonstrated. It remains possible that inflammatory cells produce or induce myelinolysis, as part of the final common pathway of immune-mediated demyelination (Lampert 1983).

The occurrence of demyelination in association with pernicious anemia led to the suggestion that other demyelinations might similarly be a consequence of nutritional deficiency. However, dietary manipulation in MS patients has been generally unrewarding. Furthermore, it has not been possible to produce experimental animal models of nutritional deficiency which closely mimic the spontaneous human demyelinating disorders.

Early pathologic descriptions of MS lesions remarked on the similarity of their distribution to the consequences of embolic showers. Indeed, in the late 1930s vascular thrombosis was advocated as a prominent component of MS pathogenesis. However, multiple negative investigations for occlusive vascular phenomena cast doubt on this hypothesis, and disappointing results were obtained in clinical studies of anticoagulation as an MS treatment (Wolf 1952).

The occurrence of a clinico-pathologically distinct demyelination in association with metabolic disturbance (central pontine myelinolysis (CPM)) provoked interest in altered homeostasis as a causative factor for spontaneous inflammatory demyelination. However, CPM was subsequently attributed to rapid correction of hyponatremia, without any evidence that similar metabolic aberrancy underlies MS.

Epidemiology

The genetic and environmental components of MS pathogenesis appear to underlie the complex epidemiology of the disease (Acheson 1985; Kurtzke

1983). MS epidemiology has provided highly suggestive data despite extraordinary difficulties imposed by the absence of a sensitive and specific laboratory diagnostic test (Acheson 1985). MS is accordingly a clinical diagnosis. Further, because the prevalence of MS is low, the diagnostic data for epidemiologic studies are generated by local practitioners. The effect of this circumstance is to bias prevalence data to distribute an excess of MS diagnoses to regions of more accessible medical care and cases are included and excluded with variable accuracy. Therefore, prevalence data are reliable only insofar as they are obtained from regions with comparable levels of access and quality of neurologic care. Bearing these limitations in mind, the following observations have consistently emerged in carefully-performed epidemiologic studies:

1. MS occurs in women more frequently than in men with a relative risk of approximately 1.8
2. Onset of MS symptoms shows a world-wide unimodal peak beginning in mid-adolescence, with maximal rates in the late twenties or early thirties and a drastic decline after age 60
3. In both northern and southern hemispheres, the occurrence of MS increases with increasing distance from the equator. This MS risk gradient has been carefully documented in the USA, Australia, and in comparisons of genetically-similar populations in South Africa and the British Isles
4. Migration from a high-risk to a low-risk area in early life confers a significant reduction in risk. The most convincing evidence in support of this notion comes from the US Veterans study; compatible data have been derived in studies of Israeli immigrants, South African immigrants, and others
5. Different racial groups are differentially susceptible to MS. For groups of low susceptibility, prevalence rates are low regardless of geographical location. For groups of high susceptibility, rates are significantly affected by geography
6. MS clusters in families. Sibs of patients with MS carry a greater-than-tenfold excess of MS relative to the population at large
7. Other clusters of MS occur. The best-documented of these occurred in the Faroe Islands after World War II (Acheson 1985; Kurtzke 1983).

These observations may be considered useful insofar as they provide testable hypotheses about the etiology of MS. The universal excess in women and globally-uniform age of onset provide some reassurance that MS in differing locales is a single disease, but have not otherwise been informative. The predilection for MS to occur in some racial backgrounds while sparing others suggests that MS, as practically every disease of humans, expresses itself differentially according to innate differences in susceptibility. The distinctive geographic distribution of MS cases has been a focus of intense speculation and study. The relationship to latitude implies a relationship to climate and thus to two major factors affected by climate: diet and social conditions affecting transmission of infection. As is noted above, the world-wide relationship to latitude in the face of variable geology, soil and water supply makes it extremely unlikely that a single trace constituent of diet is causally related to MS. Similar comments may be made about the influence upon diet of climate, namely that diets in high-risk and low-risk zones for MS are so extraordinarily variable that a single protective or deleterious component is unlikely to be identified.

Efforts to understand further the clues provided by these epidemiologic studies have focused, therefore, on the attempt to understand the virology and genetics of MS.

Virology

For many years, speculation has centered upon the role of infectious agents in MS (Johnson 1982, 1983; ter Meulen and Stephenson 1983). Several hypotheses have been considered: that MS could be associated with a slow virus infection; that MS could be a rare sequela of a common human infection or family of infections; that MS could be a common sequela of exposure to a pathogen for which humans are an accidental host. With the accumulation of epidemiologic data about geographical case distribution these speculations have been extended to postulate either that early exposure to a common enteric pathogen in regions of low prevalence is protective against MS or that late-childhood exposure to a respiratory pathogen in high prevalence areas is an inciting event, followed after a latent period by emergence of neurologic disease. The enterovirus hypothesis is made somewhat less likely by the failure of late-childhood migration from high-risk zones to low-risk zones to confer increased risk of MS for those migrants.

The notion that a unique virus infection could be causally implicated in MS is supported by the occurrence of viral demyelinating disorders of several mammalian species including humans (Johnson 1983; Johnson and McArthur 1987). Both progressive multifocal leukoencephalopathy (PML) and subacute sclerosing panencephalitis (SSPE) were investigated in parallel with MS as cryptogenic demyelinating disorders for many years. PML has been attributed to papovavirus infection of immunocompromised individuals, while SSPE is caused by a persistent measles virus infection (Johnson 1982).

Very recently, a demyelinating leukoencephalomyelitis variously described as HTLV-I-associated myelopathy (HAM) or tropical spastic paraparesis (TSP) has been firmly linked to infection with the lymphotropic retrovirus HTLV-I (Brew and Price 1988; Jacobsen et al. 1988; Johnson and McArthur 1987).

Demyelination is also associated with post-infectious sequelae of human viral infections, most prominently observed with measles (Johnson 1982). Several viral demyelinating diseases also occur in other mammalian species. These include visna virus infection of sheep, canine distemper virus of dogs, Theiler's virus infection of mice, and rodent infection with variant strains of mouse hepatitis virus (Johnson 1983; Knobler and Oldstone 1983; Narayan et al. 1983).

Two major hypotheses about the pathogenesis of virus-induced demyelination have been entertained. In one case direct viral impairment of oligodendrocyte function is proposed, while in the second case virus-induced immune-mediated tissue injury is proposed. Of the mammalian viral demyelinations, Theiler's virus murine encephalomyelitis (TME) and mouse hepatitis virus (MHV) infection of rats have been studied most intensively. In the case of TME, persistent virus infection of oligodendroglia appears likely, and demyelination may be mediated by immune mechanisms directed against viral determinants expressed on infected cells (Rodriguez et al. 1987). In the case of MHV-induced demyelination in rats, it has been demonstrated that T-cell recognition of myelin antigens occurs during the course of disease, which can be passaged to syngeneic uninfected rats with lymphocyte transfer (Knobler and Oldstone 1983). Therefore, virus-induced demyelination in these model systems utilizes a variety of mechanisms including direct viral tissue injury and immunologic attack upon viral and host antigens.

Virologic studies of MS patients have focused on evaluation of viral antibodies, attempts to isolate viruses, and morphologic studies. Both intrathecal and circulating antiviral antibodies are significantly elevated in MS material. The most significant elevations, both in terms of absolute titres and frequency, are against measles virus, but intrathecal antibodies directed against numerous paramyxoviruses, poxviruses, herpes viruses, orthomyxoviruses and others can be detected. It is not clear whether the elevated viral antibodies are of pathogenic significance or reflect non-specific polyclonal B cell recall responses, in the context of intrathecal immune dysregulation (Salmi et al. 1983).

Viral (and spirochetal) isolates from MS tissue have a venerable and uniformly disappointing history. More than 20 viruses have been "isolated" from MS tissue, using a variety of methods including coculture with tissue culture cells; intrathecal or intravenous inoculation of pathogenic tissue in recipient animals which are screened for viral antibodies or pathology; and molecular cloning experiments. To date, none of these isolates has been reproducibly obtained by a majority of investigators (Johnson 1982). Recently, molecular cloning experiments which initially suggested the presence of an HTLV-I-like retrovirus in MS lymphocytes could not be reproduced, and the potential involvement of a pathogenic retrovirus in MS remains indeterminate (Bangham et al. 1989; Reddy 1989; Richardson et al. 1989; Waksman 1989). These studies are important, since lymphotropic retroviruses have a distinct capacity to cause peripheral immune dysregulation (as in HIV infection) and inflammatory demyelination (as in HAM). The failure to isolate a virus from MS tissues is consistent with the possiblity that the virus–host interaction results in virus clearance, but elicits pathogenic autoimmunity. According to this notion, virus infection could induce autoreactivity to myelin antigens in the appropriate susceptible host (Waksman 1983). The feasibility of this concept was demonstrated by Johnson and co-workers who documented lymphocyte proliferative responses to myelin basic protein in post-measles encephalomyelitis patients (Johnson 1982).

Genetics

Evidence favoring a genetic component to MS susceptibility came early in assessment of the epidemiology of the disease. Racial groups exhibiting distinct disparity in MS prevalence were described by numerous epidemiologic studies in the 1950s, 1960s and 1970s. The disparate occurrence of MS cases in different racial groups appeared particularly striking in high-risk geographic locales, as noted above (Acheson 1985; Johnson and McArthur 1987). Familial clustering of MS cases has also been a focus of epidemiologic study and is consistent with the postulate of genetic susceptibility to MS (Batchelor 1985). More recently, population-based studies of MS concordance in monozygotic and dizygotic twins were reported (Ebers et al. 1986; Kinnunen et al. 1987). Significantly, MS concordance in dizygotic twins approached expected rates for siblings, while monozygotic concordance rates were at least ten-fold higher (Ebers 1986). Such studies strongly support the hypothesis of a genetic component to MS susceptibility, since both monozygotic and dizygotic twins tend to share a common environment. These studies also imply a contribution of environment to occurrence of MS since monozygotic concordance rates were far short of 100%.

Over 20 years ago, Fog and co-workers reported an association of MS with certain HLA antigens (Jersild et al. 1972). Numerous studies have subsequently confirmed these associations and it has been clarified that allelic variation in the D/DR locus accounts for the increased susceptibility (Stewart and Kirk 1983). In Caucasian populations, HLA-DR2/Dw2 is very significantly over-represented in MS patients compared with relevant control populations. It is most important to note that different racial groups possess different MS-susceptible HLA-D haplotypes (McFarlin and Lachman 1989). Recent studies on the function of the gene products of the HLA-D locus (in the human major histocompatibility complex class II region) in determining specificity of immune responses (see R.B. Bell and L. Steinman in this volume) have excited great interest in these associations. The finding that different HLA haplotypes confer increased MS risk in different genetic backgrounds has several potential explanations. One possibility is that the different HLA-DR alleles are in linkage disequilibrium with another polymorphic susceptibility gene. In this regard, suggestive evidence was provided by Vartdal and colleagues that HLA-DQβ-chain alleles common to a number of susceptible HLA-DR haplotypes shared structural features in the predicted antigen binding cleft (Vartdal 1989). This intriguing report requires wider confirmation. An alternative explanation for different HLA-linked susceptibility genes in different racial groups could be that a number of different pathogens can each elicit autoimmunity to myelin in the appropriate susceptible host, determined in part by HLA haplotype. Reports of myelin basic protein (MBP) peptides which are differentially encephalitogenic in mice, as determined in part by Class II MHC haplotype, are consistent with this concept (Weller 1985).

To date, investigations of various polymorphic MHC loci have failed to disclose MS associations tighter than those with HLA-DR. Indeed associations tend to become less significant as one evaluates markers either centromeric or telomeric of HLA-D/DR suggesting that HLA-D antigen genes may indeed encode susceptibility factors.

Epidemiologic studies of populations using HLA antigens as genetic markers can establish association, but cannot address linkage to disease. Two studies of HLA haplotype-sharing in affected sibling pairs from multiplex MS families have demonstrated linkage between inheritance of the HLA-bearing chromosome and susceptibility to MS (Batchelor 1985).

With advancing suspicion that MS could be a reflection of cell-mediated immunopathology, attention has turned to genetic analysis of T-cell receptor (TCR)-associated MS susceptibility. As indicated by Bell and Steinman, the

TCR is a critical component of antigen-specific immune recognition. Molecular characterization of the T-cell receptor germ-line repertoire has allowed both association and linkage studies to be performed. Unrelated patients were screened for biased inheritance of TCR variable region genes by Beall and co-workers (Beall et al. 1989). Significant biases were demonstrated in MS patients' germ-line TCR β-chain repertoire. Hauser and co-workers performed elegant TCR β-chain polymorphism linkage analysis in affected sibling pairs of MS multiplex families, analogous to earlier studies of HLA haplotype-sharing. A highly-significant increase in haplotype-sharing among affected sibs was demonstrated, linking inheritance of chromosomes containing the TCR β-chain with MS susceptibility (Seboun et al. 1989). In the aggregate, results described in this section are consistent with the linkage of inheritance of immune-recognition molecules with MS susceptibility. As described by Bell and Steinman, analogous observations have been made in regard to murine and rat susceptibility to autoimmune demyelination.

The third component of immune recognition of myelin, in addition to the HLA antigens and T-cell receptors, is the antigenic myelin peptide. To date, polymorphisms in the coding sequence of the important myelin antigens (myelin basic protein, myelin proteolipid protein, myelin-associated glycoprotein) have not been described. Therefore, genetic susceptibility in MS appears to be determined in part by the genes encoding immune-recognition molecules. It should be noted that the best estimate of the contribution of these genes to genetic susceptibility of MS is approximately 30% indicating that other inherited traits must also be implicated in MS susceptibility (Seboun et al. 1989).

Immunology and Immunopathology

Immunologic abnormalities have been described in a wide variety of studies of MS peripheral blood, cerebrospinal fluid (CSF), and brain tissue. None of the individual observations is uniquely observed in MS and it has not been possible to define the detailed mechanism of immune-mediated tissue injury through such studies. Furthermore, immune activation clearly could be secondary to the host response to a pathogenic orgainsm. Thus immunologic aberrations observed in MS are important only in that they indicate the presence of potential targets of therapeutic intervention, monitoring or etiologic insight. In this regard, the bulk of evidence strongly suggests the presence of an activated T-lymphocyte-directed immune response in patients with MS.

The immune aberration most characteristic of MS is elevated immunoglobulin protein of restricted heterogeneity within the CSF (Walsh and Tourtellotte 1983). This elevated immunoglobulin is directed in part against multiple viral antigens, although antibody reactivity to myelin antigens has also been described. The majority of intrathecal immunoglobulin is of unknown specificity. While it has not been directly proven, there is strong evidence to support the assertion that this oligoclonal immunoglobulin is synthesized within the central nervous system.

An "immunologic profile" of circulating components in MS patients consists of: normal serum immunoglobulin levels; detectable circulating immune complexes; normal T-lymphocyte numbers with normal reactivity to mitogen and recall antigens; intermittent moderate distortion of T-lymphocyte subsets with decreased numbers of CD8+ and CD45R+ T-cells; decreased functional in vitro T-cell suppressor activity (Leibowitz 1983; Batchelor 1985). These studies have provided an impression of disturbed immune regulation and are in many respects consistent with studies of patients with other proposed immunopathologic conditions such as rheumatoid arthritis and systemic lupus erythematosus.

Studies of CSF T-lymphocytes have been difficult due to limited availability of cells. Recent advances in techniques for T-cell culture and analysis have permitted studies of T-cells in CSF. In regard to subset representation, these T-cells reflect the composition of peripheral blood. Activated T-lymphocytes in CSF from patients with MS have been described by several techniques including flow cytometric quantitation of DNA content and expression of activation antigens. Recently, analysis by Hafler and co-workers of TCR gene rearrangements in T-cell clones derived from CSF provided evidence in favor of the "oligoclonality" of the intrathecal T-cell population (Hafler et al. 1988). This observation would be consistent with the postulate of an antigen-specific immune response occurring within the CNS compartment.

Clearly, the demonstration of T-cell recognition of myelin antigens in MS patients would be of tremendous importance in supporting an immunopathologic mechanism of disease. Several elegant and powerful studies have recently addressed this issue. Allegretta and co-workers documented the presence of increased numbers of MBP-reactive activated T-cells in MS patients (Allegretta et al. 1990). More recently, Hafler and co-workers described responses to an immunodominant epitope of MBP in MS patients. The further evaluation of the human response to the important myelin encephalitogens MBP and PLP is a very active focus of on-going research. The implications of such work for specific immunotherapy are described in the chapters by Bell and Steinman and by Hafler, Brod, and Weiner.

The pathologic characteristics of the MS lesion have suggested the presence of pathogenic inflammation to observers since Dawson's seminal work of 85 years ago. With the advent of specific reagents for defining components of the immune system within these inflammatory lesions has come delineation of the composition of the cellular infiltrate, demonstration of the presence of immunologically functional secretory products and definition of cell membrane expression of the molecules of immune recognition. The cellular infiltrate in MS is mononuclear and is composed primarily of T-cells and macrophages (Traugott et al. 1983; Hayashi et al. 1988). The T-cells may express either CD8 or CD4 phenotypes, without a clear-cut predilection for either. The CD45R+ T-cell subset appears to be depleted in MS brain, in comparison with control inflammatory lesions (Sobel et al. 1988). Unambiguous delineation of the cellular composition of the MS inflammatory infiltrate has been hampered by variable tissue preservation in autopsy material available to different investigators (Sobel 1989).

Several studies have addressed the presence of secretory immune mediators within MS tissue. Hofman and co-workers documented the presence of interleukins and tumor necrosis factor in easily-detectable amounts in the MS lesion (Hofman et al. 1986; Hofman et al. 1989). Traugott and co-workers have carefully delineated the presence and distribution of interferons in MS lesions (Traugott and Lebon 1988a). These investigators have also underscored the elevated expression of MHC Class I and II antigens on parenchymal brain cells, endothelial cells and infiltrating leukocytes within MS lesions; the expression of intercellular adhesion molecule (ICAM-1), a significant accessory molecule for immune recognition events, was also demonstrated (Traugott 1987; Traugott and Lebon 1988a,b). In summary, the requisite components for a cell-mediated immune response have been demonstrated in MS plaques.

Conclusion

Convergent lines of evidence suggest that tissue injury in MS results from aberrant immune reactivity to one or more myelin antigens. These suggestive data are summarized above, and include the fruits of epidemiologic, genetic, pathologic and immunologic investigations. The effects of intervention with immunomodulatory agents are also consistent with this concept, since treatments which augment immune function (from intrathecal tuberculin to interferon-gamma) have tended to exacerbate disease activity, while immunosuppressive treatments have produced neutral or beneficial consequences.

Lately, the great bulk of attention has focused on T-lymphocyte-directed immunopathologic mechanisms. This development has been hastened by rapid progress in understanding the role of T-cells in EAE, a highly-informative animal model of myelin-specific autoimmunity. Studies in MS patients have produced suggestive data about the potential parallels between EAE and MS. Virtually every element in the intricate and complex cascade of the immune response can now be considered a potential target for therapeutic intervention. Candidates include: the T-cell antigen recognition event, as described by Hafler and Steinman and their colleagues; a different approach is represented by copolymer 1, described by Bornstein. T-lymphocyte activation, proliferation and effector functions can be affected by corticosteroids, azathioprine, cyclophosphamide, total lymphoid irradiation or cyclosporine A, as described by Myers, Hughes, Weiner, Cook and Wolinsky. In some cases these agents affect laboratory indices of disturbed immunoregulation, such as antigen-nonspecific T-cell suppressor function or intrathecal immunoglobulin synthesis. Our current level of knowledge about the pathophysiology of MS does not allow any firm conclusion about whether these latter effects are relevant for clinical response. Following T-cell antigen recognition, a multitude of secreted polypeptides, collectively termed cytokines, serves locally to amplify the number and activation state of immunocompetent cells within tissue sites of inflammation. The first attempt to manipulate the cytokine environment in MS is represented by clinical trials of interferons, as described by Jacobs. It is possible that plasmapheresis, described by Noseworthy, may also have the effect of modifying cytokine levels. The explosive growth in understanding immunobiology should promote the detection of progressively more effective means of downregulating pathogenic autoimmunity in the near future. With these techniques will come the critical test of the immunopathogenesis hypothesis for MS: ability to temper the course of the disease by modulating function of the immune system.

References

Acheson E (1985) The epidemiology of multiple sclerosis. In: Matthews W, Batchelor J, Acheson E, Weller R (eds) McAlpine's multiple sclerosis. Churchill Livingstone, Edinburgh, pp 3–46

Adams C (1983) The general pathology of multiple sclerosis: morphological and chemical aspects of the lesions. In: Hallpike J, Adams C, Tourtellotte W (eds) Multiple sclerosis: pathology, diagnosis and management. Chapman and Hall, London, pp 203–240

Allegretta M, Nicklas JA, Siram S, Albertini RJ (1990) T cells responsive to myelin basic protein in patients with multiple sclerosis. Science 247:718–721

Bangham C, Nightingale S, Cruickshank J, Daenke S (1989) PCR analysis of DNA from multiple sclerosis patients for the presence of HTLV-I. Science 246:821

Batchelor J (1985) The immunological and genetic aspects of multiple sclerosis. In: Matthews W, Batchelor J, Acheson E, Weller R (eds) McAlpine's multiple sclerosis. Churchill Livingstone, Edinburgh, pp 479–513

Beall S, Concannon P, Charmely P, McFarland H, Gatti R, Hood L, McFarlin D, Biddison W (1989) The germline repertoire of T-cell receptor β-chain genes in patients with chronic progressive multiple sclerosis. J Neuroimmunol 21:59–66

Brew B, Price R (1988) Another retroviral disease of the nervous system: chronic progressive myelopathy due to HTLV-I. N Engl J Med 318:1195–1197

Ebers G, Bulman D, Sadovnick A (1986) A population based study of multiple sclerosis in twins. N Engl J Med 315:1638–1642

Hafler DA, Duby AD, Lee SJ, Benjamin D, Seidman JG, Weiner HL (1988) Oligoclonal T lymphocytes in the cerebrospinal fluid of patients with multiple sclerosis. J Exp Med 167:1313–1322

Hayashi T, Morimoto C, Burks J, Kerr C, Hauser SL (1988) Dual-label immunocytochemistry of the active multiple sclerosis lesion: major histocompatibility complex and activation antigens. Ann Neurol 24:523–531

Hofman FM, von Hanwehr RI, Dinarello CA, Mizel SB, Hinton D, Merrill JE (1986) Immunoregulatory molecules and IL-2 receptors identified in multiple sclerosis brain. J Immunol 136:3239–3247

Hofman FM, Hinton DR, Johnson K, Merrill JE (1989) Tumor necrosis factor identified in multiple sclerosis brain. J Exp Med 170:607–612

Jacobsen S, Raine C, Mingioloi E, McFarlin D (1988) Isolation of an HTLV-1-like retrovirus from patients with tropical spastic paraparesis. Nature 331:540–543

Jersild C, Svejgard A, Fog T (1972) HLA antigens and multiple sclerosis. Lancet 1:1240–1241

Johnson R (1982) Viral infections of the nervous system. Raven, New York

Johnson R (1983) Persistent viral infections and demyelinating diseases: an overview. In: Mims C, Cuzner M, Kelly R (eds) Viruses and demyelinating diseases. Academic Press, London, pp 7–20

Johnson R, McArthur J (1987) Myelopathies and retroviral infections. Ann Neurol 21:113–116

Kinnunen E, Koskenvuo M, Kaprio J, Aho K (1987) Multiple sclerosis in a nationwide series of twins. Neurology 37:1627–1629

Knobler R, Oldstone M (1983) The role of host genes and virus-cell tropism in coronavirus-induced demyelination: a unique murine experimental model for understanding human demyelinating disease. In: Mims C, Cuzner M, Kelly R (eds) Viruses and demyelinating diseases. Academic Press, London, pp 53–66

Kurtzke J (1983) Fine structure of the demyelinating process. In: Hallpike J, Adams C, Tourtellotte W (eds) Multiple sclerosis: pathology, diagnosis and management. Chapman and Hall, London, pp 47–96

Lampert P (1983) Fine structure of the demyelinating process. In: Hallpike J, Adams C, Tourtellotte W (eds) Multiple sclerosis: pathology, diagnosis and management. Chapman and Hall, London, pp 29–46

Lassmann H (1983) Comparative neuropathology of chronic experimental allergic encephalomyelitis and multiple sclerosis. Springer Verlag, Berlin

Leibowitz S (1983) The immunology of multiple sclerosis. In: Hallpike J, Adams C, Tourtellotte W (eds) Multiple sclerosis: pathology, diagnosis and management. Chapman and Hall, London, pp 379–412

McFarlin D, Lachman P (1989) Hopeful genes and immunology. Nature 341:693–694

Merritt H (1970) Multiple sclerosis: a clinical science review. Med World News, July 24

Narayan O, Strandberg J, Griffin D, Clements J, Adams R (1983) Aspects of the pathogenesis of Visna in sheep. In: Mims C, Cuzner M, Kelly R (eds) Viruses and demyelinating diseases. Academic Press, London, pp 125–140
Reddy E (1989) PCR analysis of DNA from multiple sclerosis patients for the presence of HTLV-I. Science 246:823–824
Richardson J, Wucherpfennig K, Endo N, Rudge P, Dalgleish A, Hafler D (1989) PCR analysis of DNA from multiple sclerosis patients for presence of HTLV-I. Science 246:821–823
Rodriguez M, Oleszak E, Leibowitz J (1987) Theiler's murine encephalomyelitis: a model of demyelination and persistence of virus. CRC Crit Rev Immunol 7:325–365
Salmi A, Arnadottir T, Reunanen M, Ilonen J (1983) The significance of viral antibody synthesis in the central nervous system of multiple sclerosis patients. In: Mims C, Cuzner M, Kelly R (eds) Viruses and demyelinating diseases. Academic Press, London, pp 141–152
Scheinberg L, Korey S (1962) Multiple sclerosis. Annu Rev Med 13:411–430
Seboun E, Robinson M, Doolittle T, Ciulla T, Kindt T, Hauser S (1989) A susceptibility locus for multiple sclerosis is linked to the T cell β chain complex. Cell 57:1095–1100
Sobel RA (1989) T-lymphocyte subsets in the multiple sclerosis lesion. Res Immunol 140:208–211
Sobel RA, Hafler DA, Castro EE, Morimoto C, Weiner HL (1988) The 2H4 (CD45R) antigen is selectively decreased in multiple sclerosis lesions. J Immunol 140:2210–2214
Stein EC, Schiffer RB, Hall WJ, Young N (1987) Multiple sclerosis and the workplace: Report of an industry-based cluster. Neurology 37:1672–1677
Stewart, G, Kirk R (1983) The genetics of multiple sclerosis: the HLA system and other demyelinating diseases. In: Hallpike J, Adams C, Tourtellotte W (eds) Multiple sclerosis: pathology, diagnosis and management. Chapman and Hall, London, pp 241–274
ter Meulen V, Stephenson J (1983) The possible role of viral infections in multiple sclerosis and other genetic markers. In: Hallpike J, Adams C, Tourtellotte W (eds) Multiple sclerosis: pathology, diagnosis and management. Chapman and Hall, London, pp 241–274
Traugott U (1987) Multiple sclerosis: relevance of class I and class II MHC-expressing cells to lesion development. J Neuroimmunol 16:283–302
Traugott U, Lebon P (1988a) Demonstration of alpha, beta, and gamma interferon in active chronic multiple sclerosis lesions. Ann NY Acad Sci 540:309–311
Traugott U, Lebon P (1988b) Interferon-gamma and Ia antigen are present on astrocytes in active chronic multiple sclerosis lesions. J Neurol Sci 84:257–264
Traugott U, Reinherz E, Raine C (1983) Multiple sclerosis: distribution of T-cell subsets within active chronic lesions. Science 219:308–310
Vartdal F (1989) HLA association in multiple sclerosis: implications for immunopathogenesis. Res Immunol 140:192–196
Waksman B (1983) Viruses and immune events in the pathogenesis of multiple sclerosis. In: Mims C, Cuzner M, Kelly R (eds) Viruses and demyelinating diseases. Academic Press, London, pp 155–166
Waksman B (1989) Multiple sclerosis: relationship to a retrovirus? Nature 337:599
Walsh M, Tourtellotte W (1983) The cerebrospinal fluid in multiple sclerosis. In: Hallpike J, Adams C, Tourtellotte W (eds) Multiple sclerosis: pathology, diagnosis and management. Chapman and Hall, London, pp 275–358
Weller R (1985) Experimental demyelinating diseases and their relevance to multiple sclerosis. In: Matthews W, Batchelor J, Acheson E, Weller R (eds) McAlpine's multiple sclerosis. Churchill Livingstone, Edinburgh, pp 344–348
Wolf A (1952) A review of experimental studies on the etiology of the human demyelinating diseases. In: The First International Congress of Neuropathology. Tipografia G. Dommini, Rome, pp 1–60

Chapter 6

Treatment of Multiple Sclerosis with ACTH and Corticosteroids

Lawrence W. Myers

Introduction

Adrenocorticotrophic hormone (ACTH) and glucocorticosteroids (GCS) have potent anti-inflammatory and immunosuppressive effects. They were introduced as therapeutic agents in the late 1940s and in spite of their limitations and adverse effects GCS remain the mainstay of treatment for allograft protection and for autoimmune diseases including multiple sclerosis (MS). In this chapter I will discuss the physiology and pharmacology of these agents as it relates to their use in MS. For more detailed discussion of the pharmacology of these hormones the interested reader is referred elsewhere (AHFS 1990; Haynes 1990). I will review the literature which provides the rationale for why, when, and how we use these agents in MS. I will also present my current recommendations for their use and suggest future studies.

ACTH

Normal Physiology

ACTH is a 39-amino-acid polypeptide with a molecular weight of 4500, which is secreted by the anterior pituitary and stimulates the adrenal cortex to secrete a number of different hormones with a variety of physiological effects. Normally there is a diurnal fluctuation in the secretion of ACTH, with maximum release in the early morning and a nadir around midnight. Superimposed upon this process are intermittent small bursts throughout the day. The plasma half-life of ACTH is 15 min. Physiological stress from trauma, burns, cold, infection, surgery, parturition, physical exertion, or emotional reactions leads to increased release of corticotrophin-releasing factor by the hypothalamus, increased secretion of ACTH by the pituitary and increased synthesis and release of adrenal cortical hormones.

Based on their biological activity, these steroids are divided into glucocorticoids (GCS) if their primary activity is to increase the body's stores of glucose and glycogen, and minerocorticoids if their primary action is to increase the body's stores of sodium and water. In actuality the adrenal cortical steroids have both effects but for each steroid one effect predominates over the other. ACTH also stimulates the secretion of a number of weakly androgenic substances from the adrenal glands but these are not of physiological importance.

Physiologically, cortisol is the most important glucocorticoid in humans and is secreted by the zona fasciculata of the adrenal cortex. Aldosterone, secreted from the zona glomerulosa, is the body's principal minerocorticoid. The glucocorticoid potency is quantitated in a bioassay which measures the stimulation of glycogen deposition in the liver of rats. Cortisol is 3–4 times as potent as aldosterone in this assay. Minerocorticoid activity is quantitated in a bioassay which measures the reduction of sodium excretion by the kidney in adrenalectomized rats. Aldosterone has 300 times the minerocorticoid potency of cortisol. The anti-inflammatory potency may be quantitated in a bioassay that measures the suppression of swelling of rat paw or rabbit ear induced by an irritant such as caregeenan or turpentine. The anti-inflammatory potency parallels the glucocorticoid potency.

Mechanism of Action

The primary physiological and pharmacological effect of ACTH results from the secretion of adrenal cortical steroids (Haynes 1990). In-vitro studies show that ACTH can directly suppress antibody production (Johnson et al. 1982) but it is unclear how important this is therapeutically.

Preparations

Currently there are 3 different preparations of ACTH available for therapeutic use in the United States (AHFS 1990). Natural ACTH is generally extracted from the pituitary glands of pigs. Corticotropin for injection is a lyophilized powder which is reconstituted as an aqueous solution which may be administered subcutaneously, intramuscularly, or intravenously. For therapy in MS it is usually administered in a dose of 25–40 units dissolved in 500 ml 5% dextrose in water and infused intravenously (IV) over 8 h.

Cosyntropin is a synthetic polypeptide identical with the first 24 amino acids of natural ACTH and is also administered as an aqueous solution. A dose of 0.25–0.5 mg dissolved in 500 ml 5% dextrose in water and administered intravenously over 8 h is generally used for MS.

Corticotropin repository is ACTH in a solution of partially hydrolyzed gelatin. It is generally administered intramuscularly in a dose of 40–80 units once or twice daily. A gel form of the synthetic ACTH is available in some countries but not in the USA. The only clear advantage of the synthetic ACTH over the natural preparation is a slightly lower risk of allergic reactions with the former although allergic reactions to synthetic ACTH have also been reported. Some investigators feel that the synthetic preparation is more stable and gives a more consistent response although that has not been clearly demonstrated. Some physicians use higher than ordinary doses e.g., 100 units bid of ACTH gel, because of concerns with the stability and potency of the natural preparation.

Clinical Trials (Table 6.1)

Detailed reviews of the various clinical trials of ACTH and GCS have recently been published (Ellison 1990; Myers and Ellison 1990; Troiano et al. 1990) and will only be summarized here.

ACTH has been shown to hasten recovery from exacerbations of MS (Miller et al. 1966; Rinne et al. 1968; Rose et al. 1970) but it is not effective in preventing relapses or progression (Millar et al. 1967). Based upon the claims by Alexander and Cass (1963) and subsequent experience with the use of GCS for treating autoimmune diseases one could argue that a suboptimal regimen was used in Millar's study and that an induction phase using higher doses and increased dosing during relapses should have been used. However, it is clear that a hyperadrenal state was produced with the regimen used and in spite of significant toxicity from this treatment there was no hint of efficacy. In a follow-up study the same investigators found no evidence that withdrawal of ACTH had any effect on the frequency or severity of relapses or rate of deterioration in 156 of the patients who had received ACTH injections for 18 months compared to 150 of the controls (Millar et al. 1970).

Glucocorticosteroids

Normal Physiology

Although 28 different steroids have been extracted from the adrenal cortex only 5 are biologically active (Haynes 1990). Cortisol is the principal GCS secreted by the adrenals. The normal rate of secretion of cortisol is about 20 mg/day. The plasma half-life is approximately 1.5 h but the biological half-life is 8–12 h.

Mechanism of Action

GCS alter the immune network at a number of different levels (Kurki 1984; Haynes 1990). GCS cause a rapid lysis of lymphocytes in some species, such as mice and rats, but not in other species, including man (Clamen 1972). There is a 70% decrease in lymphocytes and a 90% decrease in monocytes in the peripheral blood within 4–6 h of exogenous GCS administration but this is due to redistribution rather than lysis (Cupps and Fauci 1982). T cells are affected more than B cells and helper cells more than suppressor cells (Haynes and Fauci 1978). GCS cause a rise in blood neutrophils by increasing their release from the bone marrow and vascular endothelium and decreasing their removal from the blood. The gradual decrease in lymphoid tissue with the hypercorticoid state in humans in thought to be due to the protein catabolism caused by GCS and not lympholysis (Haynes 1990).

GCS suppress antibody-mediated allergic reactions such as urticaria, eczema, and asthma through anti-inflammatory effects and by suppressing the release of histamine, bradykinin and anaphylactin by basophils. Cell-mediated immunity

Table 6.1. Clinical trials with adrenal cortical trophic hormone (ACTH)

Protocol	Phase	Number treated				Comments	Reference
		Total	Better	Same	Worse		
50–100 mg IM tid × 5 d–4 mo.	NS	8	4	4	0	Open, uncontrolled. No definite evidence of efficacy	Glaser et al. (1950)
25 mg IM initially & 5 mg q3 h up to 300 mg	NS	4	3	1	0	Open, uncontrolled. ACTH can be tried & should be started quickly after relapse	Jonsson et al. (1951)
20–25 mg IM q6 h × 5–14 d repeat × 1 or cortisone 200 mg IM × 1 then 100 mg IM qd × 2–4 wks	NS	33	12	NS	NS	Open, uncontrolled. ACTH and/or cortisone not recommended	Glaser and Merritt (1952)
60 U IM bid × 7 d then 40 U IM bid × 7 d then taper over 7 d	Relapse	22	11	8	3	Double-blind, randomized. ACTH significantly better than saline placebo at 3 wks	Miller et al. (1961b)
Saline placebo	Relapse	18	4	7	7		
40 U IV × 10 d or 60 U IM bid × 10 d then 60 U IM bid × 11 d then taper to 20 U IM 3 × /wk up to 3 mo.	NS	94	78	NS	NS	Open, nonrandomized. High dose most effective, low dose less effective but better than no treatment	Alexander and Cass (1963)
40 U IM qd × 3 wks then taper to 20 U IM 3 × /wk up to 3 mo.	NS	19	9	NS	NS		
No treatment	NS	18	5	NS	NS		
40 U IV or 60 U IM bid × 10 d then 60 U IM bid × 11 d then taper to 20 U IM 3 × /wks × 1–6 yr	NS	37	30	NS	NS	Open, nonrandomized. Prolonged benefit especially after high dose, increased doses required for worsening	Alexander and Cass (1963)
40 U IM qd × 2 d then taper to 20 U IM 3 × /wk for 1–4 yr	NS	12	4	NS	NS		

40 U IM qd × 6–14 d then taper to 30 U qd × 1, 20 U qd × 1, 10 U qd × 6 wks	NS	14	NS	NS	NS	Open, nonrandomized. Rapid improvement with ACTH and slow improvement with PT. PT should be used and ACTH reserved for relapse	Blomberg (1965)
Or 10 U IM qd × 6 mo.	NS	4	NS	NS	NS		
Physical therapy (PT)	NS	10	NS	NS	NS		
15–25 U IM qd × 18 mo. plus thiamine 100 mg IM q mo. × 18 mo.	NS	181	45	76	60	Open, randomized. Relapse rate also identical, ACTH does not prevent worsening	Millar et al. (1967)
Thiamine 100 mg IM q mo. × 18 mo.	NS	169	37	76	56		
90 U IM qd × 35 d then taper 1 wk	Relapse	13	NS	NS	NS	Double-blind, randomized. ACTH significantly better than placebo, low dose better than high dose	Rinne et al. (1968)
30 U IM qd × 35 d then taper 1 wk	Relapse	10	NS	NS	NS		
Saline placebo	Relapse	13	NS	NS	NS		
90 U IM qd × 35 d then taper 1 wk	Mixed	14	NS	NS	NS	Double-blind, randomized. All 3 groups improved significantly, but no significant difference between groups	Rinne et al. (1968)
30 U IM qd × 35 d then taper 1 wk	Mixed	9	NS	NS	NS		
Saline placebo	Mixed	14	NS	NS	NS		
40 U IM bid × 7 d then 20 U bid × 4 d then 20 U qd × 3 d	Relapse	103	84	14	5	Double-blind, randomized. ACTH significantly better than placebo at 1, 2, & 3 wks but not at 4 wks, little justification for ACTH	Rose et al. (1970)
Inert placebo	Relapse	94	65	18	11		

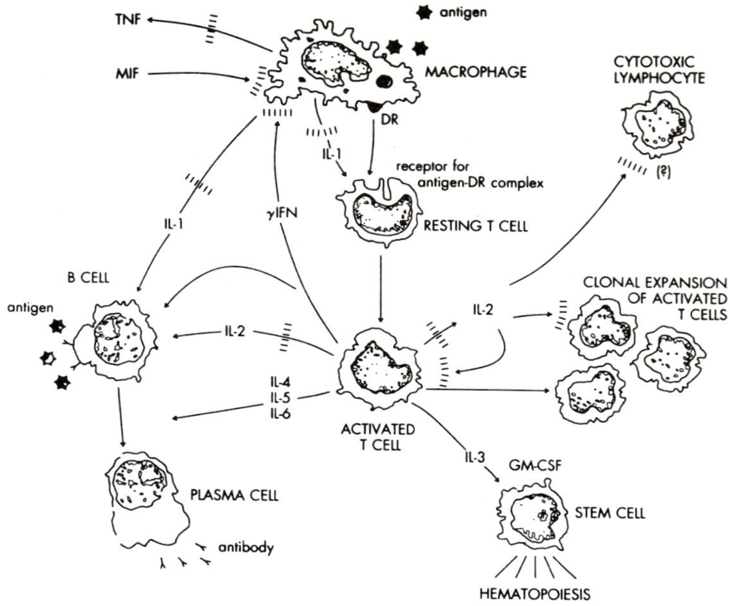

Fig. 6.1. Sites of action of glucocorticoids in the immune network. (From Haynes (1990), reprinted with permission of Pergamon Press, New York.)

implicated in allograft rejection and autoimmune diseases is also suppressed. Although there is a gradual decrease in lymphoid tissue and blood immunoglobulin levels from chronic hypercorticism, it is not the blocking of antigen–antibody or antigen–lymphocyte interactions that accounts for the immunosuppressive effect of GCS (Haynes 1990). Rather, GCS block the cascade of events following these interactions (Fig. 6.1). GCS block clonal expansion of T cells and B cells by blocking the release of IL1 from macrophages and the release of IL2 from lymphocytes. The clonal expansion of B cells is also reduced by the blocking of IL4, IL5, and IL6. Large doses of GCS decrease serum IgG concentrations but the ability to produce a normal antibody response to antigen is retained (Butler 1975). Complement levels (Atkinson and Frank 1973) and circulating immune complexes (Liebling et al. 1982) are reduced. By blocking release of gamma interferon, the activation of macrophages and expression of MHC molecules is decreased.

Secretion of migration-inhibition factor (MIF) is not affected but the macrophage response to MIF is inhibited thereby allowing egress of macrophages from the target tissue (Balow and Rosenthal 1973). GCS cause an increase in synthesis of lipocortin in lymphocytes and monocytes which inhibits phospholipase A. This leads to decreased availability of arachidonic acid and therefore decreased synthesis and release of prostaglandins and leukotrienes (DiRosa et al. 1985). By blocking release of tumor necrosis factor, prostaglandins, and leukotriene, inflammation is suppressed. GCS decrease Fc receptor expression on K cells and macrophages and thereby decrease antibody-dependent cellular cytotoxicity mediated by these cells.

At inflammatory sites, GCS decrease capillary dilatation, edema, fibrin deposition, and migration of leukocytes into the area. GCS stabilize leukocyte lysosomal membranes and decrease the release of destructive acid hydrolases. Animal studies show a suppression of experimental allergic encephalomyelitis (Kibler 1965) and lysolecithin-induced demyelination (Herndon 1987).

The potent immunosuppressive and anti-inflammatory effects of GCS are thus the result of suppression of a large number of important pathways. However, because these reactions are rapidly reversible and require high levels of GCS the immunosuppressive and anti-inflammatory effects can be overcome by sustained potent immunological reactions.

Most investigators suggest that the rapid onset of improvement following intravenous methylprednisone (MP) is probably related to a reduction in inflammation and tissue edema (Dowling et al. 1980; Buckley et al. 1982; Abbruzzese et al. 1983; Barnes et al. 1985; Durelli et al. 1986). Troiano et al. (1984) reported that contrast enhancement of MS plaques seen on brain computer-assisted tomography was reduced or eliminated within 8 h of the first infusion of MP.

Intravenous mannitol may produce a rapid improvement in neurological signs in patients with MS due to its anti-edema effect (Stefoski et al. 1985). The beneficial effect of the mannitol is transient and phase-locked to the treatment, whereas the beneficial effects of GCS administration may persist for months (Abbruzzese et al. 1983; Barnes et al. 1985). Presumably the GCS are suppressing events in the inflammatory cascade that cause the fluid accumulation in the MS plaques.

Effects on Intra Blood–Brain Barrier (IBBB) Synthesis of Immunoglobulin G (IgG)

In the early phase of the disease or in patients with minimal central nervous system (CNS) involvement, aproximately 65% of patients show an increase in IgG content in the cerebrospinal fluid (CSF). This figure rises to 90% in the later stages of the disease or in patients with extensive involvement (Yahr and Kabat 1957). Using newer techniques these figures may be increased to 90% and 100% respectively (Tourtellotte et al. 1985). Once elevated, the IgG tends to remain so with only minor variations. The IgG levels do not fluctuate with clinical fluctuations. Whether the IgG is directly involved in the pathogenesis of the disease or is an epiphenomenon is unclear. Regardless, the increased IBBB IgG synthesis may be considered a marker for the disease and eradication of this activity may be an indication of an effective therapy. To date no treatment has been found capable of eradicating the IBBB synthesis of IgG in MS. How close a treatment comes to achieving that goal might be considered a measure of the relative efficacy of the treatment.

Several investigators have studied the effect of ACTH and/or GCS administration on CSF IgG synthesis in MS (Yahr and Kabat 1957; Goldstein et al. 1962; Torbergsen 1972; Massaro 1978; Brooks et al. 1979; Trotter and Garvey 1980; Tourtellotte et al. 1980; Naess and Nyland 1981; Durelli et al. 1986; Warren et al. 1986; Compston et al. 1987; Milanese et al. 1989; Baumhefner et al. 1989). In general, there is a correlation between the frequency and degree

Table 6.2. Biological activity of commonly used glucocorticosteroids

	Glucocorticoid activity	Minerocorticoid activity	Biological half-life (h)
Cortisol	1	1	8–12
Prednisone	4	0.8	24–36
Prednisolone	4	0.8	24–36
Methylprednisolone	5	0.5	24–36
Dexamethasone	25	0	56–96

of reduction in IBBB IgG synthesis and the dosage of ACTH or GCS but there is no correlation between the reduction in IBBB IgG synthesis and the clinical response. It is still unclear what is the optimum regimen for reducing the IBBB IgG synthesis.

Warren et al. (1986) have reported that "high" (160 mg/day) or "mega" (2 g/day) doses of IV MP for 10 days produce a significant reduction in antibody to myelin basic protein in CSF of patients with MS. No such reduction occurred in patients treated with bedrest alone or in patients treated with ACTH 60 units IV daily for 10 days. The IgG index was also significantly decreased with both the "high" and "mega" doses of MP but not with bedrest or ACTH.

Future studies need to look at the correlation between the reduction in IBBB IgG synthesis and duration of remission or stabilization. Milanese et al. (1989) reported that normalization of CSF pleocytosis correlated with clinical outcome following ACTH or GCS treatment. This has not been noted by others.

Presumably, alterations in the inflammatory response account for the rapid and reversible improvements, and alterations in the immune response account for the more persistent benefits following ACTH or GCS treatment in MS. Against this hypothesis is the lack of evidence for any correlations between the immunological measurements and the clinical measurements. Furthermore it is clear that there are receptors for GCS in the brain and GCS can alter a number of brain functions (McEwen et al. 1986; Funder and Shephard 1987).

Preparations

Although cortisol and cortisone have anti-inflammatory effects they are generally not used for this purpose. Synthetic analogs with stronger glucocorticoid and weaker minerocorticoid properties, such as prednisone, prednisolone, methylprednisolone, and dexamethasone are most commonly used (Table 6.2). The fluoride-containing GCS such as triamcinolone have fallen out of favor because of increased risk of myopathy associated with their systemic use. GCS may be administered orally, intramuscularly, intravenously, intrathecally, directly into site of inflammation (intrasynovially, periarticularly, retroorbitally) or topically. For MS the oral and intravenous route are generally used. GCS are said to be readily absorbed after oral administration (AHFS 1990). However a comparison of intravenous and oral absorption efficacy using 1000-mg doses suggests individual variability with the oral absorption ranging from 70% to 80% of the levels from IV administration (Narang et al. 1983).

Clinical Trials (Table 6.3)

Jonsson et al. (1951) were the first to report the use of cortisone in MS.

The earliest studies of GCS in MS in the USA were conducted by Glaser, Merritt et al. (Glaser and Merritt 1952; Merritt et al. 1954). They concluded that ACTH and cortisone are not suitable therapeutic agents for multiple sclerosis.

Although oral GCS are commonly used to treat acute exacerbation of MS, I am not aware of any controlled study demonstrating their efficacy for this indication.

Miller et al. (1961) conducted the first placebo-controlled double-blind randomized clinical trial in multiple sclerosis. They concluded that daily oral prednisone in a dose of 15 mg/day for 8 months followed by 10 mg/day for 10 months was ineffective. Tourtellotte and Haerer (1965) obtained essentially the same results in a double-blind randomized clinical trial using oral methylprednisolone 8–12 mg/day for 18 months. Retrospective analyses by several investigators have also reached the conclusion that the chronic use of oral GCS does not significantly alter the course of the disease (Fog 1965; Cendrowski 1975).

Because the above-cited studies used relatively low doses of GCS, there was nagging doubt in some people's minds as to whether or not GCS had been used in adequate doses for a sufficient period of time. To address these questions, Brooks et al. (1979) treated 11 patients with relapsing/progressive (RP) MS and 11 patients with progressive (P) MS with oral prednisone 170 ± 40 (X ± SD) mg every other day for 12–15 months. The relapse rate was 1.6 ± 0.8 relapses per patient per year for the RP group and 0.5 ± 0.5 for the P group. These rates are comparable to those experienced by 11 patients with RP MS 1.5 ± 1.2 and 14 patients with P MS 0.4 ± 0.5 not on prolonged therapy. Mean disability status scale (DSS) scores (Kurtzke 1965) and functional scores did not change significantly but quantitative assessment of lower extremity function worsened in both groups and was not statistically different. The treatment caused a significant ($p < 0.01$) decrease in serum IgG (937 ± 159 mg/dl before, 575 ± 136 mg/dl during) but not serum IgA or IgM, nor in CSF IgG/protein ratios or incidence of CSF oligoclonal bands. Elevations in CSF myelin basic protein (MBP) occurred in association with relapses in the prednisone-treated patients and elevations persisting up to 6 months were seen in 6 of the RP patients. In 2 patients with accelerated progression, increasing elevations (18–40 ng/ml) occurred over 4–8 months. The progressive MS patients also had intermittently low (5–10 ng/ml) elevations in CSF-MBP. Thus, even with prolonged high-dose oral GCS administration, there was clinical and laboratory evidence of disease progression. We are forced to conclude that chronic daily or every-other-day oral GCS administration alone is not effective in preventing disease progression in MS. Nevertheless, physicians and patients continue to be seduced into the chronic use of oral GCS by the sometimes dramatic improvements seen with their initial use and the increasing disability associated with their withdrawal.

In the early 1970s the use of "pulses" of high doses (1000 mg/day) of IV MP were introduced for the treatment of allograft rejections (Bell et al. 1971). Shortly thereafter, this approach was being used for suppressing autoimmune diseases such as lupus nephritis (Cathcart et al. 1976) and rheumatoid arthritis

Table 6.3. Clinical trials with glucocorticosteroids

Protocol	Phase	Number treated: Total	Better	Same	Worse	Comments	Reference
Cortisone 900 mg–2000 mg po total dose, protocol otherwise NS	NS	7	7	0	0	Nonrandomized, improvement not as pronounced as with ACTH	Jonsson et al. (1951)
ACTH 20–25 mg IM qd × 5–14 d or cortisone 25–50 mg po tid–qid × 2 wks	NS	19	14	NS	NS	Open, nonrandomized, not a suitable treatment	Merritt et al. (1954)
Or × 3.5–27 mo.	NS	19	4	10	5		
Prednisone 15 mg po qd × 8 mo. then 10 mg qd × 10 mo.	Mixed	26	3	10	13	Double-blind, randomized, relapse rate also the same, disease activity not influenced	Miller et al. (1961a)
Calcium aspirin 3.5 g po qd × 18 mo.	Mixed	24	5	11	8		
Placebo	Mixed	29	3	13	13		
Methylprednisolone (MP) 8–12 mg po qd × 18 mo.	Mixed	38	5	23	10	Double-blind, randomized, trends in favor of MP but few stastistically significant differences	Tourtellotte and Haerer (1965)
Cyanocobalamin 1–1.5 μg po qd × 18 mo.	Mixed	38	3	16	19		
Prednisone or equivalent po initially high dose tapered to 15 mg/d for 1–3 mo. (12), 4–12 mo. (36), 1–2 yr (16) or >2 yr (12)	NS	77	10	29	38	Open, uncontrolled, course of disease not influenced in spite of side effects	Fog (1965)
Prednisone 50 mg po q 6 h × 7–10 d then taper over 3–4 wks	Relapse	12	12	0	0	Open, 9 patients, 12 relapses, all but 1 returned to prerelapse by 10 wks. 6 subsequent relapses >5 mo. after treatment. Large controlled trial needed	Kibler (1965)
Dexamethasone 4–8 mg po qd × 4–5 wks repeated 1–4 × over 14 mo.	Mixed	21	NS	NS	NS	Open, uncontrolled, did not affect overall rate of deterioration	Cendrowski (1975)
Prednisone 170 ± 40 mg po qd × 12–15 mo.	Mixed	22	NS	NS	NS	Open, uncontrolled, clinical & laboratory evidence of disease progression	Brooks et al. (1979)
MP 125, 250, or 300 mg IV initially then 125–250 mg IV q 6 h × 14–60 h then prednisone 100 mg po & tapered over 10–18 wks	Relapse	7	5	2	0	Open, uncontrolled, well tolerated, controlled study recommended	Dowling et al. (1980)

MP 250 mg IV qd × 5 d or 500 mg IV qd × 2 d then 250 mg IV qd × 3 d or 1000 mg IV qd × 3–5 d	Relapse	6	6	0	0	Open, uncontrolled, controlled trial recommended	Buckley et al. (1982)
MP 1 g IV qd × 5–7 d with oral prednisone taper over 1 wk	Relapse	98	32	47	19	Open, uncontrolled, 98 courses in 61 patients. Rapid responses. Does not prevent subsequent worsening	Newman et al. (1982)
MP 1 g IV qd × 5 d	Relapse	13	13	0	0	Open, uncontrolled, larger trial recommended	Goas et al. (1983)
MP IV 20 mg/kg/d × 3 d then 10 mg/kg/d × 4 d, then 5 mg/kg/d × 3 d then 1 mg/kg/d × 5 d	Relapse	30	21	9	0	Open, randomized. No significant differences at end of treatment or 18 mo. later. MP regarded as useful	Abbruzzese et al. (1983)
ACTH synthetic 0.5 mg IV bid × 15 d	Relapse	30	22	8	0		
MP 1 g IV qd × 7 d	Relapse	14	NS	NS	NS	Blind observer, randomized. MP group better than ACTH group at 3, 7, & 28 d but not at 3 mo.	Barnes et al. (1985)
ACTH IM 60 U, 40 U, 20 U each × 7 d	Relapse	11	NS	NS	NS		
MP IV 15/mg/kg/d × 3 d then 10 mg/kg/d × 3 d, then 5 mg/kg/d × 3 d, then 2.5 mg/kg/d × 3 d, then 1 mg/kg/d × 3 d	Relapse	11	10	1	0	Double blind, randomized. MP significantly better than placebo at end of treatment	Durelli et al. (1986)
Placebo	Relapse	10	4	6	0		
MP 500 mg IV qd × 5 d	Relapse	12	11	1	0	Randomized, double blind. MP significantly better than placebo, no long term benefit	Milligan et al. (1987)
Placebo	Relapse	9	2	6	1		Milligan et al. (1988)
MP 500 mg IV qd × 5 d	Progressive	13	6	7	0		
Placebo	Progressive	15	0	13	2		
MP IV 20 mg/kg/d × 3 d then 10 mg/kg/d × 3 d then 5 mg/kg/d × 3 d	Stationary	10	9	1	0	Open, uncontrolled. Beneficial and may persist up to 6 mo.	Citterio et al. (1987)
Followed 3 mo.		8	7	1	0		
Followed 6 mo.		3	3	0	0		
MP 1 gm IV qd × 5 d	Relapse	15	12	3	0	Open, randomized, 5 days effective, 1 day not effective	Bindoff (1988)
MP 1 gm IV qd × 1 d	Relapse	17	0	14	3		
MP 1 gm IV qd × 3 d	Relapse	29	NS	NS	NS	Double-blind, randomized, no significant differences at 3, 7, 14, 18, or 84 days except fewer adverse effects with MP	Thompson et al. (1989)
ACTH 40 U IM bid × 7 d, then 20 U bid × 4 d then 20 U qd × 3 d	Relapse	32	NS	NS	NS		

(Fan et al. 1978). In 1980 the first reports of the use of this approach in multiple sclerosis appeared (Dowling et al. 1980; Trotter and Garvey 1980).

Several uncontrolled trials as well as two placebo-controlled double-blind randomized clinical trials have demonstrated the efficacy of high-dose IV "pulse" MP for treatment of acute exacerbations (Table 6.3). Milligan et al. (1987, 1988) also found transient improvement in patients with chronic/progressive MS.

Comparison of ACTH and Glucocorticosteroids

Debate over the relative merits of ACTH versus GCS has existed since their introduction into clinical medicine 40 years ago. In 1951, Jonsson et al. commented that improvement with cortisone treatment was not as pronounced as with ACTH. This comment was based upon an experience in which 7 patients had been treated with cortisone and 4 patients treated with ACTH. Details of the cases and of the treatment are not given. The authors felt the difference might be related to the fact that the cases treated with cortisone were more "inveterate". Alexander was one of the strongest proponents of ACTH over GCS (Alexander and Cass 1963). However, he was much more aggressive with the ACTH treatment than with the GCS. Of the 38 patients treated with cortisone, 23 received 25 mg qd (slightly above a physiological dose), 1 received 25 mg every other day and 14 received up to 75 mg qd (Alexander et al. 1961). Of the 25 patients treated with prednisone, only 7 received more than 40 mg daily, a relatively low dose by today's standards.

Alexander noted that ACTH caused an elevation of excretion of 17 ketosteroids in the urine and suggested that perhaps the beneficial effect of ACTH was related to release of androgens as well as GCS from the adrenals induced by ACTH. Although androgenic steroids may help counteract the negative nitrogen balance caused by GCS, they have no significant effect on the neurological status or course of MS (Cendrowski and Curan 1972).

Proponents for ACTH also argue that there are receptors for ACTH within the CNS and ACTH may exert direct beneficial effects on the CNS in MS (Davis and Stefoski 1988; Poser 1989). However, the role of ACTH as a neurotransmitter and the effects within CNS remain speculative.

There are also receptors for GCS in the CNS and activation of these receptors causes numerous physiological changes (McEwen et al. 1986). However, it is unclear how these changes relate to the therapeutic benefit of GCS in MS. They may be more important in explaining the adverse effects.

There are 3 reports in which direct comparative trials of ACTH and high-dose IV MP for treating relapses of MS have been conducted (Abbruzzese et al. 1983; Barnes et al. 1985; Thompson et al. 1989) (Table 6.3). Thompson et al. found 3 days of IV MP was equivalent in efficacy to IM ACTH given for 14 days. Barnes et al. reported that 7 days of IV MP produced more rapid and greater improvement than 4 weeks of IM ACTH. Abbruzzese et al. found no difference between 15 days of IV MP and 15 days of IV synthetic ACTH. All 3 reports suggest that IV MP is preferable to ACTH because of the rapid onset of improvement with fewer adverse effects.

Several studies have shown that the adrenal secretion of GCS in response to pharmacologic stimulation with ACTH is highly variable from patient to patient or even within the same patient from day to day (Alexander and Cass 1963; Alexander et al. 1971; Ketelaer and Delmotte 1972; Maida and Summer 1979; Snyder et al. 1981). Also the potency of various ACTH preparations as measured by the 24-h urinary excretion of 17-hydroxysteroids and 17-ketosteroids is highly variable (Rinne et al. 1968). Therefore, for maximal and dependable dosing the use of high-dose intravenous MP is recommended.

I have previously recommended an initial course of 500 mg IV daily for 5 days with an increase in dose to 1000 mg daily for an additional 3–5 days if no response (Myers 1990a). This recommendation was based upon the results reported by Milligan et al. (1987) using 500 mg daily for 5 days. I am now of the opinion that the 500 mg daily dose gives less consistent and less impressive results than 1000 mg daily doses. I now give 1000 mg IV daily for 7 days but stop after 5 days if the neurological improvement is striking or continue up to 10 days for an unsatisfactory response. Some neurologists very experienced in treating MS tell me they give 500 mg IV q 8 h for 5 days and others routinely give 1000 mg/day for 10 days. Clearly the optimum regimen is unknown.

Uncertainty regarding the need for an oral taper also exists. Troiano et al. (1987) recommend a routine taper of 8–14 weeks with oral prednisone. I also favor a taper with oral prednisone. I currently start the taper at a dose of 1 mg/kg every other day for 2 doses and reduce the dose by 20-mg increments every 2 doses. Randomized clinical trials are needed to clarify the need for a taper and, if needed, to determine the optimum regimen.

Intrathecal Glucocorticosteroids (Table 6.4)

The use of intrathecal (IT) GCS to treat multiple sclerosis has had a long and controversial history. Until recently the studies had been open and uncontrolled with varying indications and protocols and with conflicting claims of efficacy and safety. In the 1960s most reports indicated a beneficial effect from IT-GCS. In the 1970s reports of the adverse effects from IT depot methylprednisolone acetate (DMPA) appeared. Studies implicated the polyethylene glycol in the DMPA as the cause of the meningeal irritation (CSF pleocytosis, aseptic meningitis) and adhesive arachnoiditis. By the 1980s, with a few notable exceptions (Rivera 1989) the neurological community had abandoned the use of IT-DMPA for MS. However, in 1988 Rohrbach et al. reported that 3–4 IT injections of a crystalline suspension of triamcinolone acetonide had been found to be superior to an unspecified regimen of oral triamcinolone for improving lower extremity function in a double-blind study in patients with chronic progressive MS (Rohrbach et al. 1988). Further double-blind studies comparing the safety and efficacy of IT-GCS and high-dose IV-GCS are in order.

Table 6.4. Clinical trials with intrathecal glucocorticosteroids

Protocol	Indication	Number treated				Comments	Reference
		Total	Better	Same	Worse		
HC 10, 20, 10, 40, 40, 20 mg consecutive d & 20 mg on d 17 & ACTH 10–45 mg IM qd d 4–20	NS	3	3	0	0	Open, no adverse effects	Kamen and Erdman (1953)
HC, protocol NS	NS	7	7	0	0	Open, no adverse effects	Boudin et al. (1953)
MPA 20–80 mg q 2–3 wks × 6 plus PT & OT	NS	12	12	0	0	Open, heachaches occasional, staggering – 1 pt × 2	Boines (1961)
MPA 40 mg, p 2 wks 60 mg, p 4 wks 80 mg then 120 mg q 6 wks × 3 & booster q 3–12 mo. prn & PT, OT, special diet	NS	30	29	0	1	Open, remission 3–12 mo., headache – 3 pts, vertigo – 1 pt, sciatic pain – 1 pt	Boines (1963)
MPA 40 mg q 2 wks × 3–6	Relapse	8	5	NS	NS	Open, variable decrease CSF IgG	Goldstein et al. (1962)
MPA 40–80 mg q 1–2 wks × 4–8	Relapse	38	30	NS	NS	Open, follow up 2–8 yr, adhesive arachnoiditis – 1 pt, aseptic meningitis – 1 pt, marked increase CSF protein – 4 pts. Weight gain, increased appetite and fluid retention – 9 pts. Severe headache – 3 pts, bloody CSF – 1 pt, urinary retention – 1 pt, decreased CSF IgG if elevated. Treatment not recommended	Goldstein et al. (1970)
MP 20, 40, 60, 80 mg at weekly intervals, & 80–100 mg monthly up to 16 mo.	NS	20	13	NS	NS	Open, duration 1 wk–16 mo., relapses – 6 pts (11 relapses), transient decreased spasticity & improved bladder control. Urinary retention – 2 pts. No long term benefit	Van Buskirk et al. (1964)
MPA 20–40 mg q 1–2 d × 3	Spastic paraparesis	10	3	NS	NS	Open, CSF pleocytosis – 2 pts, no serious side effects, no consistent change in CSF IgG, further testing warranted	Kane (1964)

MPA 80 mg q 2–3 d × 3 then q 2–4 wks up to 2.5 yr	NS	30	25	NS	NS	Open, duration 2 mo. to 2.5 yr, no serious side effects, headaches – occasional, fluid retention – 2 pts, increased appetite – 7 pts	Baker (1967)
MPA 40 mg, p 2 wks 60 mg, p 4 wks 80 mg, p 6 wks 100 mg, then 100 mg q 8 wks or prn plus PT	NS	8	7	0	1	Open, duration 7–22 mo., weight gain – 5 pts, duodenitis – 1 pt, headache – 1 pt	Ringer (1968)
MPA 40, 60, 80, 100 mg at 1, 2, 4 & 4 wk intervals plus PT	Spastic paraparesis	17	13	4	0	Open, 8/13 subsequently worsened, urinary retention & leg pain – 1 pt	Lance (1969)
MPA 40 mg	Relapse	16	3	8	5	Open, adhesive arachnoiditis – 2 pts, aseptic meningitis – 1 pt, not recommended	Nelson et al. (1973)
MPA 40 mg	Spastic paraparesis	7	1	4	2		
MPA, protocol NS	NS	NS	NS	NS	NS	Reported 3 more cases of adhesive arachnoiditis	Nelson (1976)
MPA 80 mg × 8 over 1 yr	NS	1	1	0	0	Case report – pachymeningitis	Bernat et al. (1976)
MPA 80 mg q 3–6 mo. × 24 mo.	Spastic paraparesis	100	100	0	0	Open, no adverse effects, not a replacement for systemic steroids	Rivera (1981)
MPA 40 mg q 4 d × 3–5	Relapse	31	14	17	0	Open, 28 patients, 3 treated twice, no difference from historical controls, no advantage over systemic routes	Mazzarello et al. (1983)
MPA – repeated courses over 4 yr	NS	1	1	0	0	Case report, adhesive arachnoiditis	Carta et al. (1987)
Triamcinolone 80 mg × 3–4	Relapse	22	NS	NS	NS	Double-blind, randomized, no serious complications, systemic side effects equal, intrathecal better than oral	Rohrbach et al. (1988)
Triamcinolone PO, protocols NS	Relapse	20	NS	NS	NS		
MPA 80 mg 2 × /wk × 5 wks (washed with Elliott's B solution)	Stationary	9	0	9	0	Open, aseptic meningitis – 1 pt, weakness – 1 pt, decreased CSF IgG, dangerous, should not be used	Baumhefner et al. (1989)

Adverse Effects

The adverse effects of ACTH and GCS administration are generally well-known (AHFS 1990). Patients and their significant others need to be aware of these possibilities so they can make an informed decision whether or not to accept the treatment and also to be prepared to deal with the adverse effects if they do occur. I find it helpful to relate the adverse effects to the physiological effects of steroids.

The binding of ACTH and GCS to receptors in the brain probably explains the most common adverse effects, namely, euphoria, insomnia, restlessness, hallucination, paranoid ideation, psychoses, or seizures. Patients with a history of depression, or a family history of mental disturbances or alcoholism are reported to be at increased risk for hypomanic reactions (Minden et al. 1988).

The minerocorticoid effects may cause sodium and water retention which may result in pedal edema, a bloated feeling, hypertension, and even congestive heart failure.

The androgenic effects may cause acneform rashes, hirsutism, loss of scalp hair, and menstrual irregularities.

The glucocorticoid effects may lead to hyperglycemia, glucosuria, redistribution of body fat accounting for the well-known "moon facies" and "Buffalo hump". The catabolism of proteins underlies many of the adverse effects of prolonged GCS administration such as thinning of the skin and mucosal lining of the gastrointestinal tract, myopathy, neuropathy, cataracts, and osteoporosis.

GCS also alter calcium (Ca) metabolism which contributes to osteoporosis (Bockman and Weinerman 1990). GCS decrease Ca absorption from the gastrointestinal tract and increase renal excretion of Ca. There is an increase in parathormone secretion which stimulates osteoclast activity with resultant increase in bone resorption. Trabecular bones of the vertebral bodies and ribs are particularly affected. The use of oral hydroxyvitamin D and calcium may retard the process (Di Munno et al. 1989).

Osteonecrosis or aseptic necrosis of bone is a serious complication of GCS. An incidence of 1% has been reported (Zizic and Marcoux 1985). The pathophysiology is poorly undertstood. The proximal head of the femur and humerus are most commonly affected. MRI may be used to verify the diagnosis (Kalurian et al. 1989). It is non-reversible and prosthetic replacement of the joint may be required.

Ulceration of the gastrointestinal tract is another relatively rare complication of GCS treatment. Messer et al. (1983) pooled data from 71 clinical trials in which patients were randomized to GCS or non-GCS treatment for a variety of conditions. They found that 2% of patients treated with GCS developed peptic ulcers and 1% of non-GCS treated patients developed peptic ulcers. The routine prescribing of a histamine H_2-receptor antagonist prophylactically adds to the complexity and cost of GCS treatment and increases the risk of adverse effects to the antagonist for a relatively low risk problem (Spiro 1983).

The risk of ulceration, hemorrhage, and perforation of the lower gastrointestinal tract is as great a risk as peptic ulcer disease from GCS use (Fadul et al. 1988). Constipation, which is a common problem in MS, should be treated aggressively when GCS are administered to minimize this risk.

Allergic reactions may occur with administration of any medication including natural hormones such as ACTH and GCS. Fatal anaphylaxis has been reported following IV MP (Prysee-Phillips et al. 1984). Sudden cardiovascular collapse on a non-allergic basis has also been reported following high-dose IV MP (McDougal et al. 1976). For these reasons we dilute the 1000 mg of MP in 100 ml 5% dextrose in water and drip it in slowly over 30–60 min rather than giving it in the 16 ml diluent as an IV push. We commonly administer the high-dose IV MP to outpatients, in which case the first dose is given in our outpatient facility where a nurse, physician, and medical supplies for treating anaphylaxis or cardiovascular collapse are immediately available. Subsequent treatments are generally administered at the patient's home by a home nurse.

With the administration of high-dose IV MP a facial flush may suddenly appear and a facial erythema may persist throughout the period of treatment (5–7 days). It is important that this be distinguished from an allergic reaction and that patients be aware that this will probably occur. This very common reaction may break the code in double-blind studies. We found that the addition of 1 mg nicotinic acid to each IV dose induced a transient facial flush to help maintain blinding (Ellison 1989a,b). A metallic taste during the IV administration is also common and this can be masked by having the blinded recipient dissolve a fruit-flavored candy in the mouth.

The frequency and severity of adverse effects of GCS treatment increases with the dose and especially the duration of treatment. The introduction of "pulse" administration appears to have not only increased the efficacy but decreased the risk of GCS treatment in MS (Lyons et al. 1988).

Conclusions

GCS and ACTH, acting primarily through stimulation of the synthesis and release of GCS from the adrenal glands, have potent anti-inflammatory and immunosuppressive effects. Numerous studies and 40 years of clinical experience clearly indicate that these agents hasten the rate of recovery from acute exacerbation of MS. Studies to date have not been properly designed to determine whether or not the use of these agents for treatment of acute exacerbations reduces the risk of persistent deficits caused by the exacerbation. The studies do indicate that a short course of treatment (days to weeks) does not have any long-term effect ($\geq$12 months) after treatment. Future studies should compare not only the rate and extent of recovery from exacerbations but also the duration of the improvement e.g., mean time to subsequent worsenings (acute exacerbation or slow progression).

Comparative studies to date indicate that the risk/benefit ratio is better with high-dose intravenous "pulse" MP than with ACTH or oral GCS for treating exacerbations of MS. However, studies comparing comparable high doses administered orally and intravenously have not yet been reported. There are no studies comparing the use of "pulses" with and without a tapering regimen of oral GCS. The optimum dosing regimen for "pulse" treatment needs to be established using double-blind randomized clinical trials.

Anecdotal experience and limited clinical studies indicate that "pulse" GCS also produce improvement in a substantial percentage of patients in the chronic/progressive phase of their disease. Again, studies are needed to determine the extent and duration of improvement and also to determine the optimum dosing regimen for treating such patients. Clearly there are sufficient studies demonstrating that the chronic use of ACTH of GCS is not effective in preventing acute exacerbations or chronic progression. Because of the adverse effects caused by the chronic use of these agents and their lack of efficacy such regimens should not be used. However, the possible use of intermittent "pulses" to prevent worsening of MS (exacerbations and progression) should be studied in placebo-controlled, double-blind, randomized clinical trials. Careful evaluation of the risks as well as benefits of such an approach is essential.

While it is clear that GCS are not the optimal treatment for MS and that studies to find the cause and a better treatment are essential, it is also clear that GCS will remain important agents in the care of patients with MS for the foreseeable future. Therefore, carefully designed clinical studies should be conducted to determine the optimum route, dose, and regimen for their use.

Acknowledgements. Thanks to Richard Burger for manuscript preparation; Pamela Latham for administrative assistance; Sharon Craig, RN, for nursing care; George W. Ellison, MD, for encouragement; the People of the State of California; the Conrad N. Hilton Foundation, the Southern California Chapter of the National Multiple Sclerosis Society, the Joe Gheen Fund and Various Donors to the UCLA Multiple Sclerosis Research and Treatment Program for financial support.

References

Abbruzzese G, Gandolfo C, Loeb C (1983) Bolus methylprednisolone versus ACTH in the treatment of multiple sclerosis. Ital J Neurol Sci 4:169–172

AHFS (1990) Pituitary and adrenal hormones and synthetic substitutes. In: McEvoy GK (ed), AHFS Drug Information 90. American Society of Hospital Pharmacists, Bethesda, pp 1722–1745, 1820–1824

Alexander L, Cass LJ (1963) The present status of ACTH therapy in multiple sclerosis. Ann Int Med 58:454–71

Alexander L, Cass LJ (1971) ACTH-induced adrenocortical response patterns in multiple sclerosis and their relation to the clinical effectiveness of ACTH therapy. Confinia Neurologica 33:1–24

Alexander L, Berkeley AW, Alexander AM (1961) Multiple sclerosis prognosis and treatment. Charles C Thomas, Springfield, ILL

Atkinson JP, Frank MM (1973) Effect of cortisone therapy on serum complement components. J Immunol 111:1061–1066

Baker (1967) Intrathecal methylprednisolone for multiple sclerosis: evaluation by a standard neurological rating. Ann Aller 25:665–672

Balow JE, Rosenthal AS (1973) Glucocortical suppression of macrophage inhibition factor. J Exp Med 137:1031–1039

Barnes MP, Bateman DE, Cleland PG et al. (1985) Intravenous methylprednisolone for multiple sclerosis in relapse. J Neurol Neurosurg Psychiatry 48:157–159

Baumhefner RW, Tourtellotte WW, Syndulko K, Staugaitis A, Shapshak P (1989) Multiple sclerosis intra-blood-brain-barrier IgG synthesis: effect of pulse intravenous and intrathecal corticosteroids. Ital J Neurol Sci 10:19–32

Bell PRF, Briggs JD, Calman KC, Paton AM, Wood RFM, MacPherson SG (1971) Reversal of acute clinical and experimental organ rejection using large doses of intravenous prednisolone. Lancet 1:876–880

Bernat JL, Sadowsky CH, Vincent FM, Nordgren RE, Margolis G (1976) Sclerosing spinal pachymeningitis. J Neurol Neurosurg Psychiatry 39:1124–1128

Bindoff L (1988) Methylprednisolone in multiple sclerosis: a comparative dose study. J Neurol Neurosurg Psychiatry 51:1108–1109

Blomberg LH (1965) Comments on treatment of multiple sclerosis with ACTH. Acta Neurol Scand 41 (suppl 13):485–486

Boines GJ (1961) Remissions in multiple sclerosis. Delaware Med J 33:230–235

Boines GJ (1963) Predictable remissions in multiple sclerosis. Delaware Med J 35:200–202

Bockman RS, Weinerman SA (1990) Steroid-induced osteoporosis. Orthop Clin North Am 21:97–107

Boudin G, Barbizet J, Guihard J, Clop H (1953) Intraspinal hydrocortisone. Clinical applications, particularly in the treatment of tuberculous meningitis. Presse Medicale 63:1072

Brooks BR, Jubelt B, Cohen S, O'Donnelly P, Johnson RT, McKhann G (1979) Cerebrospinal fluid (CSF) myelin basic protein (MBP) in multiple sclerosis (MS): effect of prolonged high single-dose alternate-day prednisone therapy. Neurology 29:548

Buckley C, Kennard C, Swash M (1982) Treatment of acute exacerbations of multiple sclerosis with intravenous methylprednisolone. J Neurol Neurosurg Psychiatry 45:179–180

Butler WT (1975) Corticosteroids and immunoglobulin synthesis. Transplant Proc 7:49–53

Carta F, Canu C, Datti R, Guiducci G, Pisani R, Silvestro C (1987) Calcification and ossification of the spinal arachnoid after intrathecal administration of Depo-Medrol. Zentralbl Neurochir 48: 256–261

Cathcart ES, Idelson BA, Scheinberg MA, Counser WG (1976) Beneficial effects of methylprednisolone "pulse" therapy in diffuse proliferative lupus nephritis. Lancet 1:163–166

Cendrowski WS (1975) Pilot-study on large-dose alternate-day steroid therapy in multiple sclerosis. Schweiz Arch Neurol Psychiatr 117:197–203

Cendrowski W, Kuran W (1972) Results of combined administration of anabolic steroids in patients with multiple sclerosis. Neurol Neurochir Pol 6:573–576

Citterio A, Bergamaschi R, Vercesi S, Cosi V (1987) High-dose methylprednisolone infusion in multiple sclerosis. Riv Neurol 57:105–106

Clamen HN (1972) Corticosteroids and lymphoid cells. N Engl J Med 287:388–397

Compston DA, Milligan NM, Hughes PJ et al. (1987) A double-blind controlled trial of high dose methylprednisolone in patients with multiple sclerosis. 2. Laboratory results. J Neurol Neurosurg Psychiatry 50:517–522

Cupps TR, Fauci AS (1982) Corticosteroid-mediated immunoregulation in man. Immunol Rev 65:133–155

Davis FA, Stefoski D (1988) Is steroid therapy in multiple sclerosis superior to corticotropin therapy? Arch Neurol 45:1180

Di Munno O, Beghe F, Favini P et al. (1989) Prevention of glucocorticoid-induced osteopenia: effect of oral 25-hyroxyvitamin D and calcium. Clin Rheumatol 8:202–207

DiRosa M, Calignano A, Carnuccio R, Lalenti A, Sautebin L (1985) Multiple control of inflammation by glucocorticoids. Agents Actions 17:284–289

Dowling PC, Bosch VV, Cook SD (1980) Possible beneficial effect of high-dose intravenous steroid therapy in acute demyelinating disease and transverse myelitis. Neurology 30:33–36

Durelli L, Cocito D, Riccio A et al. (1986) High-dose intravenous methylprednisolone in the treatment of multiple sclerosis: clinical-immunologic correlations. Neurology 36:238–243

Ellison GW (1990) Chronic progressive multiple sclerosis: steroids and immunosuppressive drugs. In: Cook SD (ed) Handbook of multiple sclerosis. Marcel Dekker Inc, New York, pp 371–402

Ellison GW, Myers LW, Mickey MR et al. (1989a) Clinical experience with azathioprine: the pros. Neurology 38 (suppl 2):20–23

Ellison GW, Myers LW, Mickey MR (1989b) A placebo-controlled, randomized, double-masked, variable dosage, clinical trial of azathioprine with and without methylprednisolone in multiple sclerosis. Neurology 39:1018–1026

Fadul CE, Lemann W, Thaler HT, Poser JB (1988) Perforation of the gastrointestinal tract in patients receiving steroids for neurologic disease. Neurology 38:348–352

Fan PT, Yu DTY, Clements PJ, Eisman J, Bluestone R (1978) Effect of corticosteroids on the human immune response: comparison of one and three daily 1 gm intravenous pulses of methylprednisolone. J Lab Clin Med 91:625–634

Fog T (1965) The long-term treatment of multiple sclerosis with corticoids. Acta Neurol Scand Suppl 13:473–484

Funder JW, Sheppard K (1987) Adrenocortical steroids and the brain. Annu Rev Physiol 49:397–411

Glaser GH, Merritt HH (1952) Effects of corticotropin (ACTH) and cortisone on disorders of the nervous system. JAMA 148:898–904

Glaser GH, Randt CT, Hoefer PFA, Merritt HH, Traeger CH (1950) The influence of adrenocorticotropic hormone (ACTH) on central nervous system and neuromuscular functions. Trans Am Neurol Assoc 75:98–104

Goas JY, Marion JL, Missoum A (1983) High dose intravenous methylprednisolone in acute exacerbations of multiple sclerosis. J Neurol Neurosurg Psychiatry 46:99

Goldstein NP, McKenzie BF, McGuckin WF (1962) Changes in cerebrospinal fluid of patients with multiple sclerosis: A preliminary report. Proc Mayo Clin 37:657

Goldstein NP, McKenzie BF, McGuckin WF, Mattox VR (1970) Experimental intrathecal administration of methylprednisolone acetate in multiple sclerosis. Tran Am Neurol Assoc 95:243–244

Haynes RC Jr (1990) Adrenocorticotropic hormone: adrenocortical steroids and their synthetic analogs: inhibitors of the synthesis and actions of adrenocortical hormones. In: Gilman AG, Rall TW, Nies AS, Taylor P (eds), Goodman and Gilman's pharmacological basis of therapeutics, 8th edn. Pergamon Press, New York, pp 1440–1462

Haynes BF, Fauci AS (1978) The differential effect of in vitro hydrocortisone on the kinetics of subpopulations of human peripheral blood thymus-derived lymphocytes. J Clin Invest 61:703–707

Herndon RM (1987) The effect of drugs on oligodendrocyte proliferation and myelin regeneration. Prog Brain Res 71:485–491

Johnson HM, Smith EM, Torres BA et al. (1982) Regulation of the in vitro antibody response by neuroendocrine hormones. Proc Natl Acad Sci US 79:4171–4174

Jonsson B, von Reis G, Sahlgren E (1951) Experience of ACTH and cortisone treatment in some organic neurological cases. Acta Psychiatr Neurol Scand (Suppl 74) 60–63

Kalurian KC, Hahn BH, Bassett L (1989) Magnetic resonance imaging identifies early femoral head ischemic necrosis in patients receiving glucocorticoid therapy. J Rheumatol 16:959–963

Kamen GF, Erdman GL (1953) Subdural administration of hydrocortisone in multiple sclerosis: effect of ACTH. J Am Geriatr Soc 1:794–804

Kane CA (1964) Skeletal muscle spasms and spasticity: clinical considerations. Clin Pharmacol Ther 5:852–858

Ketelaer CJ, Delmotte P (1972) Results of adrenal and pituitary stimulation tests in patients with multiple sclerosis. Acta Neurol Scand 48:467–478

Kibler RF (1965) Large dose corticosteroid therapy of experimental and human demyelinating diseases. Ann NY Acad Sci 122:469–479

Kurki P (1984) The effects of "pulse" corticosteroid therapy on the immune system. Scand J Rheumatol 154 (Suppl):13–15

Kurtzke JF (1965) Further notes on disability evaluation in multiple sclerosis with scale modifications. Neurology 15:654–661

Lance JW (1969) Intrathecal "Depo-Medrol" for spasticity. Med J Aust 2:1030

Liebling MR, McLaughlin K, Boonsue S, Kasdin J, Barnett EW (1982) Monthly pulses of methylprednisolone in SLE nephritis. J Rheumatol 9:543–548

Lyons PR, Newman PK, Saunders M (1988) Methylprednisolone therapy in multiple sclerosis: a profile of adverse effects. J Neurol Neurosurg Psychiatry 51:285–287

Maida E, Summer K (1979) Serum cortisol levels of multiple sclerosis patients during ACTH treatment. J Neurol 220:143–149

Massaro AR (1978) Modifications of the cerebrospinal fluid IgG concentrations in patients with multiple sclerosis treated with intrathecal steroids. Neurology 219:221–226

Mazzarello P, Poloni M, Piccolo G, Cosi V, Pinelli P (1983) Intrathecal methylprednisolone acetate in multiple sclerosis treatment. Acta Neurol Belg 83:190–196

McDougal BA, Whittier FC, Cross DE (1976) Sudden death after bolus steroid therapy for acute rejection. Transplant Proc 8:493

McEwen BS, DeKloet ER, Rostene W (1986) Adrenal steroid receptors and actions in the nervous system. Physiol Rev 66:1121–1188

Merritt HH, Glaser GH, Herrmann C (1954) Study of short- and long-term effects of adrenal steroids on clinical patterns of multiple sclerosis. Ann NY Acad Sci 58:625–632

Messer J, Reitman D, Sacks HS, Smith H Jr, Chalmers TC (1983) Association of adrenocorticosteroid theapy and peptic-ulcer disease. N Engl J Med 309:21–24

Milanese C, LaMantia L, Salmaggi A et al. (1989) Double-blind randomized trial of ACTH versus dexamethasone verus methylprednisolone in multiple sclerosis bouts. Eur Neurol 29:10–14

Millar JHD, Vas CJ, Noronha MJ, Liversedge LA, Rawson MD (1967) Long-term treatment of multiple sclerosis with corticotrophin. Lancet 2:429–431

Millar JHD, Rahman R, Vas CJ, Noronha MJ, Liversedge LA, Swinburn WR (1970) Effect of withdrawal of corticotrophin in patients on long-term treatment for multiple sclerosis. Lancet 1:700–702

Miller H, Newell DJ, Ridley A (1961a) Multiple sclerosis trials of maintenance treatment with prednisolone and soluble aspirin. Lancet 1:127–129

Miller H, Newell DJ, Ridley A (1961b) Multiple sclerosis. Treatment of acute exacerbations with corticotrophin (ACTH). Lancet 2:1120–1122

Milligan NM, Necombe R, Compston DA (1987) A double-blind controlled trial of high dose methylprednisolone in patients with multiple sclerosis: 1. Clinical effects. J Neurol Neurosurg Psychiatry 50:511–516

Milligan NM, Newcombe R, Compston DAS (1988) A double-blind controlled trial of high dose methylprednisolone in patients with multiple sclerosis. J Neurol Neurosurg Psychiatry 51:597–598

Minden SL, Orav J, Schildkraut JJ (1988) Hypomanic reactions to ACTH and prednisone treatment for multiple sclerosis. Neurology 38:1631–1634

Myers LW (1990) Management of multiple sclerosis. Autoimmunity Forum Neurology 2:3–5

Myers LW, Ellison GW (1990) The peculiar difficulties of therapeutic trials for multiple sclerosis. Clin Neuropharmacol 8:119–141

Naess A, Nyland H (1981) Effect of ACTH treatment on CSF and blood lymphocyte subpopulations in patients with multiple sclerosis. Acta Neurol Scand 63:57–66

Narang PK, Wilder R, Chatterji DC, Yeager RL, Gallelli JF (1983) Systemic bioavailability and pharmacokinetics of methylprednisolone in patients with rheumatoid arthritis following high-dose pulse administration. Biopharm Drug Dispos 4:233–248

Nelson D (1976) Arachnoiditis from intrathecally given corticosteroids in the treatment of multiple sclerosis. Arch Neurol 33:373

Nelson DA, Yates TS Jr, Thomas RB Jr (1973) Complications from intrathecal steroid therapy in patients with multiple sclerosis. Acta Neurol Scand 49:166–188

Newman PK, Saunders M, Tilley PJB (1982) Methylprednisolone therapy in multiple sclerosis. J Neurol Neurosurg Psychiatry 45:941–942

Poser S (1989) Corticotropin is superior to corticosteroids in the treatment of MS. Arch Neurol 46:946

Prysee-Phillips WEM, Chandra RK, Rose B (1984) Anaphylactoid reaction to methylprednisolone pulsed therapy for multiple sclerosis. Neurology 34:1119–1121

Ringer WA (1968) The treatment of multiple sclerosis with intrathecally administered methylprednisolone acetate. J Indiana St Med Assoc 61:1213–1215

Rinne JK, Sonninen V, Tuovinen T (1968) Corticotrophin treatment in multiple sclerosis. Acta Neurol Scand 44:207–218

Rivera VM (1981) Intraspinal steroid therapy. Neurology 31:1060

Rivera VM (1989) Safety of intrathecal steroids in multiple sclerosis. Arch Neurol 46:718

Rohrbach E, Kappos L, Stadt D et al. (1988) Intrathecal versus oral corticosteroid therapy of spinal symptoms in multiple sclerosis: A double-blind controlled trial. Neurology 38 (suppl 1):256

Rose AS, Kuzma JW, Kurtzke JF, Namerow NS, Sibley WA, Tourtellotte WW (1970) Cooperative study in the evaluation of therapy in multiple sclerosis: ACTH vs. placebo. Final report. Neurology 20:1–59

Snyder BD, Lakatua DJ, Doe RP (1981) ACTH-induced cortisol production in multiple sclerosis. Ann Neurol 10:388–389

Spiro HM (1983) Is the steroid ulcer a myth? (editorial). N Engl J Med 309:45–48

Stefoski D, Davis FA, Schauf CL (1985) Acute improvement in exacerbating multiple sclerosis produced by intravenous administration of mannitol. Ann Neurol 18:443–450

Thompson AJ, Kennard C, Swash M et al. (1989) Relative efficacy of intravenous methylprednisolone and ACTH in the treatment of acute relapses in MS. Neurology 39:969–971

Torbergsen T (1972) The influence of ACTH-treatment on spinal fluid gamma globulins in multiple sclerosis. Acta Neurol Scand Suppl 48:41

Tourtellotte WW, Haerer AF (1965) Use of oral corticosteroids in the treatment of multiple sclerosis. Arch Neurol 12:536–545

Tourtellotte WW, Potvin AR, Mendez M et al. (1980) Failure of intravenous and intrathecal cytarabine to modify central nervous system IgG synthesis in multiple sclerosis. Ann Neurol 8:402–408

Tourtellotte WW, Staugaitis SM, Walsh MJ et al. (1985) The basis of intra-blood-brain-barrier IgG synthesis. Ann Neurol 17:21–27

Troiano R, Hafstein M, Ruderman M, Dowling P, Cook S (1984) Effect of high-dose intravenous steroid administration on contrast-enhancing computed tomographic scan lesions in multiple sclerosis. Ann Neurol 15:257–263

Troiano R, Cook SD, Dowling PC (1987) Steroid therapy in multiple sclerosis: point of view. Arch Neurol 44:803–807

Troiano R, Cook SD, Dowling PC (1990) Corticosteroid therapy in acute multiple sclerosis. In: Cook SD (ed) Handbook of multiple sclerosis. Marcel Dekker Inc, New York, pp 351–369

Trotter JL, Garvey WF (1980) Prolonged effects of large-dose methylprednisolone infusion in multiple sclerosis. Neurology 30:702–708

Van Buskirk C, Poffenbarger AL, Capriles LF, Idea BV (1964) Treatment of multiple sclerosis with intrathecal steroids. Neurology 14:595–597

Warren KG, Catz T, Jeffrey VM, Carroll DJ (1986) Effect of methylprednisolone on CSF IgG parameters, myelin basic protein and anti-myelin basic protein in multiple sclerosis exacerbations. Can J Neurol Sci 13:25–30

Yahr MD, Kabat EA (1957) Cerebrospinal fluid and serum gamma globulin levels in multiple sclerosis: changes induced by large doses of prednisone. Trans Am Neurol Assoc 82:115–119

Zizic TM, Marcoux C (1985) Corticosteroid therapy associated with ischemic necrosis of bone in systemic lupus erythematosus. Am J Med 79:596–604

Chapter 7

Treatment of Multiple Sclerosis with Azathioprine

Richard A.C. Hughes

Introduction

Azathioprine (AZA) has been the immunosuppressant drug most commonly used in multiple sclerosis (MS) and has even been adopted as a standard treatment in some centers, especially in France and Germany (Sabouraud et al. 1984; Lhermitte et al. 1987; Ventre et al. 1985; Kappos et al. 1988). Its use has been based on the hypothesis that MS is an autoimmune disease, a hypothesis which depends on its resemblance to experimental allergic encephalomyelitis (EAE) (see Chap. 8). This hypothesis has been strengthened by the development of chronic relapsing models of EAE in guinea-pigs, rats and mice whose course and clinical features bear a close resemblance to MS (Lassmann 1983). However, although antibodies and T cell responses against myelin antigens that induce EAE in animals have been demonstrated in patients with MS, these responses are also found in normal subjects and in patients with other neurological diseases (Leibowitz and Hughes 1983; Martin et al. 1990; Olsson 1990). Thus the autoimmune hypothesis, although arguably the most likely, has not been established beyond doubt. Consequently trials of immunosuppressive treatment in MS do not have a solid theoretical basis and must be regarded as partly empirical.

Pharmacology of Azathioprine

Azathioprine is a nitroimidazole-substituted form of 6-mercaptopurine. Its chemical formula is 6-(1-methyl-4-nitroimidazol-5-yl-thio)purine. It is readily absorbed orally, reaching its peak plasma level in 2 h and having a plasma half-life of 5 h. It is rapidly converted into 6-mercaptopurine by glutathione in red cells and the liver (de Miranda et al. 1973). The concentration in cerebrospinal fluid is low, only 2% of plasma concentration (Loo et al. 1968). The restricted transport of AZA into the brain is a potential disadvantage in MS, in which there is a marked immune response which is relatively restricted to the intrathecal compartment and which may be the important autoimmune process causing the disease (Warren and Catz 1989; Olsson et al. 1990; Freedman et al.

1990). The actions of AZA are multiple and complex, depending predominantly on its conversion into 6-mercaptopurine which competes with its analogue, hypoxanthine, which occupies a central position in purine and nucleic acid synthesis (Fig. 7.1). Partly as a consequence, AZA has widespread metabolic effects causing partial inhibition of purine, DNA, RNA and membrane glycoprotein synthesis and producing alkylation of sulfhydryl groups (Elion 1967). The action of AZA is prolonged by the xanthine oxidase inhibitor allopurinol: if the two drugs have to be given together the dose of AZA must be reduced by a quarter.

Investigations of the effects of AZA in vitro have shown a wide range of effects, particularly on T-cell function. Thus it inhibits formation of sheep lymphocyte red-cell rosettes, probably by reducing the expression of the CD2 receptor molecule. It also reduces the transformation of lymphocytes in response to phytohemagglutinin or foreign major histocompatability antigens, and the induction of antibody responses (Bach and Bach 1972; Röllinghoff et al. 1973).

Animal experiments have confirmed the wide range of actions of AZA, especially on cell-mediated immunity. Its efficacy is greatest when it is given to prevent the development of immune reactions rather than to suppress established immune responses. Thus it was shown to suppress allograft rejection in dogs when given at the time of the transplant (Calne and Murray 1961). It has also been shown to suppress the development of experimental autoimmune diseases, including EAE, when given at or soon after immunization, but is less effective at treating established autoimmune diseases (Babington and Medeking 1971). Azathioprine suppresses non-specific inflammatory reactions such as that induced by the subcutaneous injection of a non-specific irritant (Perings et al. 1971). Caution must, therefore, be exercised in deducing that a condition which is suppressed by AZA is necessarily autoimmune in origin.

Rationale for Use of Azathioprine

Azathioprine has been widely used in MS beause it is the broad-spectrum immunosuppressant drug most commonly used in autoimmune diseases and prevention of transplant rejection. It can be taken by mouth and is usually well tolerated and relatively safe. Its use is theoretically justified in a condition which is considered to have an autoimmune pathogenesis but in which the detailed mechanisms are unknown. Azathioprine has been reported to be efficacious in organ-specific autoimmune diseases including rheumatoid arthritis (Paulus et al. 1984), myasthenia gravis (Mantegazza et al. 1988), polymyositis (Walton 1991), and chronic idiopathic demyelinating polyradiculoneuropathy (Dyck et al. 1985). The conclusion that it is effective in these conditions has been based on experience with individual patients or in small series and is not based on controlled trials. A small controlled trial of a low dose (2 mg/kg) did not confirm a beneficial effect in chronic idiopathic demyelinating polyradiculoneuropathy but the authors reported anecdotal

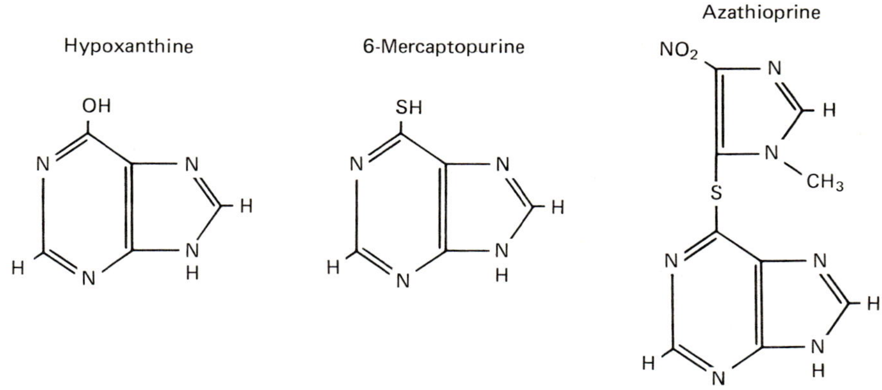

Fig. 7.1. Structures of hypoxanthine, 6-mercaptopurine and azathioprine.

evidence that a dose of 3 mg/kg appeared efficacious in cases not responding to the lower dose. Azathioprine is also considered to be efficacious in non-organ-specific vasculitic disorders including systemic lupus erythematosus (Felson and Anderson 1984), polyarteritis nodosa, Wegener's granulomatosis, and Behçet's syndrome (Yazici et al. 1990). The evidence is based on clinical experience supported in the case of Behçet's syndrome by a controlled trial and in systemic lupus erythematosus by an overview of published trials in lupus nephritis. Patients being treated with AZA show prolonged survival of allografts and suppressed induction of delayed hypersensitivity to DNCB, in keeping with an inhibitory effect on cell-mediated functions. Immunoglobulin concentrations and antibody titres are little changed although systemic IgG and IgM synthesis have been shown to be reduced. Synthesis of IgG in the CSF is also reduced by AZA treatment in MS patients (Caputo et al. 1987). However when AZA was added to prednisone treatment, AZA did not reduce synthesis of IgG in the CSF more than did steroids alone (Staugaitis et al. 1985). The production of IgG by pokeweed mitogen-driven lymphocytes from the blood of MS patients treated with AZA has been shown to be reduced (Oger et al. 1982).

Review of the Use of Azathioprine in Multiple Sclerosis

Uncontrolled Trials

The earlier literature concerning the use of AZA was dominated by uncontrolled trials. In a review of the earliest reports concerning a total of about 200 patients, Ellison and Myers (1978) concluded that the proportion of patients worsening during a year of treatment was 35%, about the same as in the placebo arm of a controlled trial of chronic ACTH treatment (Millar et al. 1967). Authors reporting large series a little later noted apparent reductions in the frequency of relapses or the numbers of patients relapsing, compared with

Table 7.1. Uncontrolled trials of azathioprine in relapsing/remitting multiple sclerosis

Ref.[a]	Daily dose (mg/kg)	Treatment (years)	Observation (years)	No.	Result
Grüninger and Mertens (1973)	2	0.75–4	0.5	101	72% stable or improved
Frick et al. (1977)	2–3	>2	5	66	Relapse rate reduced from 0.65 to 0.12 per year 52% stable or improved
Mertens and Dammasch (1977)	2–3	2.5	>2.5	50	68% no more relapses 75% improved
Aimard et al. (1983)	2–3	4	10	128	46% (vs 13%[b]) no more relapses 36% (vs 35%[b]) relapsed but did not worsen 8% (vs 17%[b]) relapsed and worsened 10% (vs 36%[b]) secondary progression
Lhermitte et al. (1984)	2–5	6.3	10	97	21% no more relapses 42% relapsed but did not worsen 34% relapsed and worsened 14% secondary progression
Fraglioni et al. (1988)	2	>2	3	40	65% stable

Modified from Hughes (1988) with permission.
[a] Six other smaller uncontrolled trials are reviewed by Ellison and Myers (1978).
[b] These percentages refer to 78 patients treated without azathioprine before 1977.

Table 7.2. Uncontrolled trials of azathioprine in progressive multiple sclerosis

Ref.	Daily dose (mg/kg)	Duration (years)		No.	Result
		Treatment	Observation		
Mertens and Dommasch (1977)	2.5	2.5	>2.5	51	30% (P[a]) became stable 36% RP[b] became stable
Rosen (1979)	Variable	10	10	85	<10% of ambulant became non-ambulant
Aimard et al. (1973)	2–3	3	3	31RP 16P	Progression slowed
Lhermitte et al. (1984)	2.5	4.3	8.7	48	35% stable

Reproduced from Hughes (1988) with permission.
[a] P, progressive from onset.
[b] RP, relapsing then progressive.

historical controls or the course of the illness before treatment (Frick et al. 1977; Mertens and Dommasch 1977; Aimard et al. 1983; Lhermitte et al. 1984) (Table 7.1). Similarly the progression of the disease appeared to be somewhat slowed in patients with progressive disease (Table 7.2). The absence of control groups from these reports severely limits their usefulness. The frequency of relapses decreases with the passage of time, even in untreated patients. The frequency of relapses and rate of progression are very variable. Interpretation of symptoms and even signs is subject to placebo effects and observer bias.

Controlled Trials

In the first controlled trial of AZA in MS, 8 of 21 patients worsened over 4 months to 2 years of follow-up and none improved (Cendrowski 1971). However treatment was only given for 1–2 months and such a short treatment period would not now be expected to be effective.

Two trials employing an open study design both showed some evidence of benefit to the AZA-treated group. In the first trial, 22 patients were randomized to receive AZA and only 2 came to require wheelchairs after 6 years compared with 13 of 20 untreated patients (Rosen 1979). This highly significant difference ($p = 0.004$) has to be interpreted cautiously in view of concerns about the potential for observer bias in an unblinded study and possible loss to follow-up of patients who were faring poorly in a single-handed neurological practice. In this trial the dose of AZA was adjusted to produce a slight leukopenia, a regime which may be more efficacious than the fixed-dose regimes more commonly used. In the other (Patzold et al. 1982) 56 patients were randomized to receive a relatively low dose of AZA (2 mg/kg daily) and 51 to receive linoleic acid, a treatment which may itself have a marginal beneficial effect according to an overview analysis (Dworkin et al. 1984). The analysis was complicated because more severely affected patients were randomized to receive AZA than linoleic acid. The main outcome measure was progression on a complex neurological function score, on which the two groups taken as a whole showed no significant difference. Patients were subdivided according to their disease pattern before trial entry. Relapsing/remitting patients with complete remissions between each relapse and patients with chronic/progressive disease deteriorated to the same extent regardless of their treatment group. For patients with an intermittent progressive course, i.e., relapses separated by incomplete remissions, deterioration was significantly slower in the AZA-treated group than in those who received linoleic acid. Even if it were not for the open-trial design and exclusion from analysis of patients who discontinued treatment, little confidence could be placed in this single significant result from analysis of a rather unconventional subgroup when the trial as a whole did not show a significant difference.

In the first single-masked randomized controlled trial of AZA in MS, 25 male patients with relapsing/remitting disease were allocated to receive AZA 2.5 mg/kg daily and 25 to receive ascorbic acid 50 mg as a placebo (Swinburn and Liversedge 1973). The patients were not informed of their treatment group. Four patients withdrew from the AZA group because of gastrointestinal symptoms and one patient from each group moved away from the study area. These patients were not included in the analysis. The overall Kurtzke disability scores were not given but there was no difference between the mean Kurtzke functional scores of the two groups at entry or after 1 or 2 years of treatment. The 24 control patients had an average of 0.52 relapses per year compared with 0.50 in the treated group and the severity of the relapses was also similar between the groups. The authors concluded, reasonably, that this trial showed no evidence of a beneficial effect. However, subsequent estimates of the sample sizes indicate that the trial was too small to detect a moderate effect on reduction of relapse frequency.

In the first double-masked randomized controlled trial 21 patients received AZA 3 mg/kg for 15 months and 22 patients received placebo (Mertin et al. 1982). The AZA treated group were also immunosuppressed with oral prednisolone, starting at 120 mg daily and tapered to zero over 4 weeks, and daily injections of antilymphocyte globulin for 15 days. The randomization process assigned more severely affected patients to AZA, which complicated the analysis. There were slightly fewer relapses and marginally less deterioration in the Kurtzke disability scores in the AZA-treated patients but the differences were nowhere near significant.

In a small Italian trial 40 patients were randomized to receive AZA 2–2.5 mg/kg or placebo and followed for 3 years (Milanese et al. 1988; Milanese 1990 personal communication). There was a high dropout rate, so that only 14 of 19 AZA-allocated patients were still being followed after 3 years and only 7 were still taking AZA. Similarly only 18 of 21 patients allocated to placebo were still being followed and only 12 were still taking their treatment. The mean (SD) change in Kurtzke disability status was 0.25 (0.87) in the AZA-treated group, less but not significantly less than that in the placebo-treated group which was 1.17 (1.47). The proportion of patients avoiding relapse was also greater in the treated group (5 of 14) compared with the control group (2 of 18). These differences may have been biased by the dropouts lost to follow-up and any beneficial effect may have been diluted by the large proportion of patients allocated to AZA who had stopped taking their treatment.

Ellison et al. (1989) compared AZA and placebo, with AZA and steroids, and with double placebo in a meticulous double-masked three-armed study of patients in the progressive phase of MS. The AZA dose was started at 2.2 mg/kg daily and increased to maintain the white blood cell count between 3000 and 4000/μl. The steroid dose was intravenous methylprednisolone 1000 mg daily for 3 days and oral methylprednisolone 96 mg on alternate mornings for the first month, then 72 mg for the second month, 48 mg for the third month, and then a dose reduced by 4 mg every 2 weeks for a total of 36 weeks. After 3 years there was no significant difference between the groups in the rate of progression on Mickey's illness severity score, a weighted score derived from the Kurtzke functional scores, which was used as the major outcome criterion. The outcome may have been affected by the large number of dropouts and by the unexpectedly low rate of progression of the placebo-treated group. Only 81 of 101 patients randomized were followed for 3 years and only 57 completed the trial strictly according to protocol. The mean progression rate of 61 trial patients over the 4 years before trial entry was 1.1 illness severity scale units/year, whereas the progression rate of the placebo group followed for 3 years in the trial was only 0.38 units/year. The authors suggest that the placebo effect of trial participation could have contributed to this difference. Other measures of progression also failed to detect any significant differences between the groups when analyzed on an intention-to-treat basis. These measures included a standardized neurological examination score, Kurtzke disability status scale and a battery of neuropsychological, coordination, and activities of daily living tasks. However there were some measures suggesting a beneficial effect in the AZA-treated patients. Although this was a trial of patients in the progressive phase of MS many experienced relapses during the trial. The relapse rate was half that in the placebo group in each of the groups which received AZA (0.24 relapses per year in each of the AZA groups and 0.48 relapses per year in the placebo group, $p = 0.04$ for the comparison between AZA alone and placebo). Also the subjective impression of the patients and most of their raters was that more of the "strictly evaluable" AZA-treated than of the placebo patients were the same or better at the end of the trial.

During the trial, visual, somatosensory and auditory-evoked potentials were recorded and the results were considered to show treatment-related changes earlier than the standardized neurological examinations scores (Nuwer et al. 1987). The major parameters analyzed were the latency of P100 in the Oz channel for the visual evoked potentials, the main positive peak latency in the cortical channel for the somatosensory-evoked potential, and the I-V interpeak interval for the brainstem-evoked potential. Although these showed significant differences between the 3 treatment groups, the main difference was between the combined AZA-steroid group and the other groups and the changes during the trial were very similar in the AZA alone and placebo groups. The triallists encountered the usual spectrum of side-effects on bone marrow and liver function (see below) and concluded that these outweighed any possible benefits from AZA (Ellison et al. 1989).

Goodkin et al. (1991) conducted a double-masked randomized trial of AZA in patients with relapsing/remitting disease. Fifty-nine patients were randomized to receive AZA 3.0 mg/kg daily with the dose adjusted to maintain the blood white cell count in the range 3500–4000/µl or placebo for 2 years. The authors considered two primary outcome measures – relapse frequency and mean change in Kurtzke expanded disability status scale. There were no significant differences on either of these measures for the trial as a whole. However the frequency of relapses was significantly smaller in the second, but not the first, treatment year in the AZA group (mean rate 0.30/year) compared with the placebo group (0.79/year). There was a non-significant difference in favor of the AZA-treated group in the mean (SD) change in the Kurtzke expanded disability scale which was 0.17 (1.38) in the AZA-treated group compared with 0.42 (1.36) in the placebo group. In addition, there was a trend in favor of the AZA-treated group in each of 9 secondary outcome measures. In particular the time to progression on the Kurtzke expanded disability status scale or on the ambulation index was significantly prolonged in the AZA-treated group compared with the placebo-treated group ($p = 0.04$ and $p = 0.03$ respectively on the log-rank test). This result has to be interpreted in the light of the possibility of bias due to some of the patients being unblinded to the nature of their treatment. Of the 27 AZA patients, 48% did not know their treatment, 44% guessed that they had been taking azathioprine and 7% guessed that they had been taking placebo. The placebo patients were less good at guessing: 64% did not know, 20% guessed placebo and 16% guessed azathioprine. The significance of the difference in these proportions is $p = 0.06$ on a two-tailed chi square test. Breaking of the blind by the patients might have had an effect on their reporting of symptoms. However, in this trial the scoring of relapse required the finding of objective changes in physical signs by the study neurologists.

In the largest trial, a multicenter study in Great Britain and the Netherlands, a trend in favour of the AZA-treated group was observed for all three major outcome criteria – Kurtzke expanded disability status scale, ambulation index and Kurtzke visual functional scale – but this was significant only for the ambulation index (British and Dutch Multiple Sclerosis Azathioprine Trial Group 1988). A fixed dose of 2.5 mg/kg daily was used and 354 patients with relapsing/remitting or progressive disease were randomized. By the end of 3 years 93% of the patients randomized to receive AZA were still being followed and 80% were still taking AZA. This compared with 95% of the placebo patients

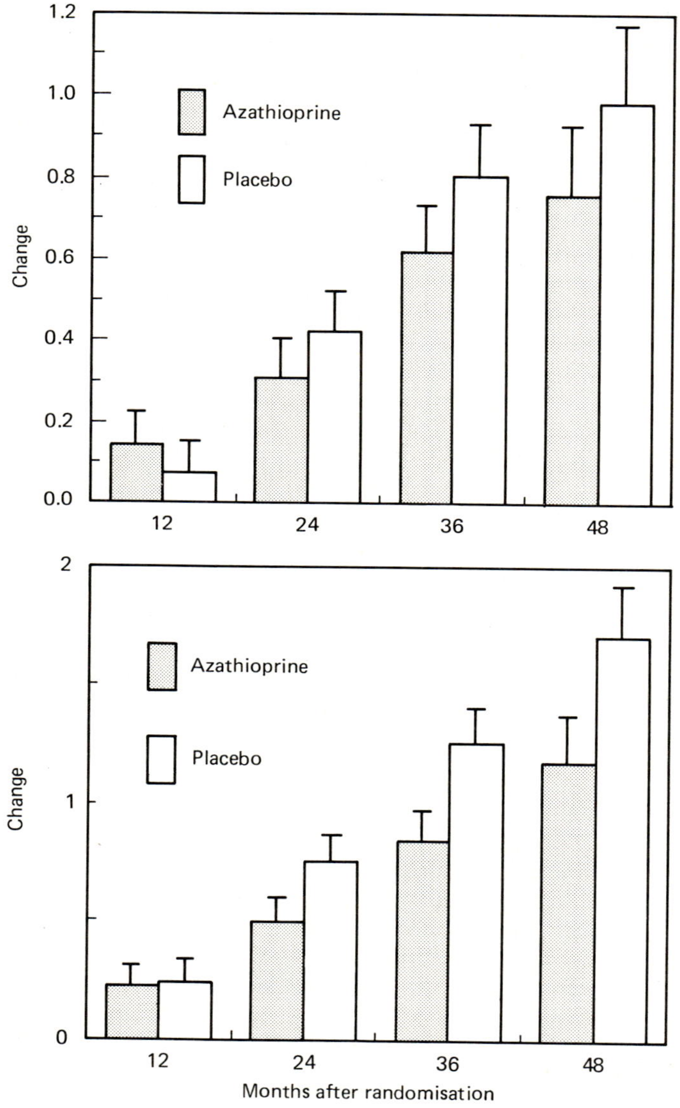

Fig. 7.2. British and Dutch Multiple Sclerosis Azathioprine Trial. Mean (SE) changes in Kurtzke expanded disability status scale (upper) and ambulation index (lower) for patients on azathioprine (solid bars) and placebo (open bars). From British and Dutch Multiple Sclerosis Azathioprine Trial Group (1988), by permission of *The Lancet*.

still being followed and 88% still taking their (placebo) tablets. The randomization process had resulted in balanced groups at entry except that, presumably by chance, there were more females in the AZA group (65%) than in the placebo group (52%). The increase in the Kurtzke disability score after 2, 3 and 4 years was less (in favor of) in the AZA group, but the differences were small and not significant, being only 0.18 (95% confidence intervals −0.15 to +0.52) (Fig. 7.2). There was significantly less deterioration in the ambulation index in the AZA than in the placebo group (0.41 with 95% confidence intervals 0.03 to 0.80) (Fig. 7.2). There was an even smaller difference in the change in the visual function scale scores between the two groups (0.16 with 95% confidence intervals −0.10 to +0.42) which was not significant but did favor the AZA group. In this trial relapse frequency was not planned to be a major outcome criterion but the occurrence of relapses was noted and was less in the AZA-treated patients in each of the 4 years of observation, especially in the fourth. The mean (SE) number of relapses per patient over 4 years was 2.47 (0.26) for the AZA group (n = 98) and 3.38 (0.29) for the placebo group (n = 103) (p = 0.025, two-tailed test). In interpreting these results the possible influence of partial unmasking must be considered: of 279 patients who were asked to guess their treatment allocation after 3 years 117 replied that they did not know, but more (101) guessed correctly than guessed incorrectly (61), a difference in proportions which is slightly greater than chance ($p < 0.05$). However 181 of the assessors replied that they did not know the treatment allocation, 57 guessed correctly and 41 guessed incorrectly (not significant). Of the AZA patients, 11 had to discontinue the trial before 3 years had elapsed because of gastrointestinal intolerance, one because of abnormal liver function, 5 because of leukopenia and 2 because of allergic reactions. No subgroups were identified which showed particular benefit from AZA but subgroups of particular interest were small. For instance there were only about 20 patients in each arm with early disease (within 2 years of onset) and only about 10 with aggressive disease (Kurtzke status 5–6 and within 5 years of onset). The authors considered that the trial demonstrated a small real benefit from AZA but doubted whether this benefit outweighed the undoubted side effects and possible risks of malignancy.

Overview of Controlled Trials

An overview of all the trials of AZA undertaken in MS should be the most powerful method of assessing the efficacy of AZA. Overviews or metaanalyses of treatment effects require that all the trials, published and unpublished, be ascertained and that all patients randomized be followed and included in the analysis. We are preparing such an overview incorporating all the results of the randomized trials mentioned in this chapter (Table 7.3) and retrieving the results for patients who were randomized and followed even if they defaulted from treatment. The only measures which have been common to each trial have been Kurtzke disability score and occurrence of relapse. The overview is nearly complete. The small benefit from AZA in reducing the risk of relapse and in slowing progression as measured by the Kurtzke disability scale is confirmed and shown to be statistically significant, being more easily detected after 2 years of treatment than after 1 year and still being present after 3 years (Yudkin 1990; Yudkin et al. in preparation).

Table 7.3. Controlled trials of azathioprine in multiple sclerosis

Ref.	Daily dose	Sample size[a]	Duration (years)	Kurtzke score mean diff[b]	Relative odds of avoiding relapse in treated vs control group
Swinburn and Liversedge (1973)	2.5	19	2		2.3
Mertin et al. (1982)	3.0[c]	21	1.25	0.09	2.7
British and Dutch Trial (1988)	2.5	160	3	0.18	1.75
Milanese et al. (1988)	2.0–2.5	17	3	0.62	4.0
Ghezzi et al. (1989)	2.5	69	1	0.08	−0.2
Ellison et al. (1989)	2.2[d]	26	3	0.11	2.4
Goodkin et al. (1991)	3.0[d]	27	2	0.25	2.1

[a] Number treated with AZA: the number treated with placebo was always approximately the same.
[b] Difference between the mean changes in Kurtzke disability score of the AZA- treated and placebo-treated groups: a positive difference indicates that the AZA- treated group fared better.
[c] Prednisolone given by mouth for the first 28 days and intravenous anti-lymphocyte globulin for the first 15 days.
[d] Dose adjusted to produce a mild leukopenia.

Table 7.4. Azathioprine: side effects

	Kissel et al. (1986)	Lhermitte et al. (1984)	British and Dutch Trial (1988) first year
Total numbers of patients in trial	64	211	164
Side effects			
Hematological			
macrocytosis	20		
leukopenia	22	6[a]	21
anemia		3[a]	4
thrombocytopenia		1.5[a]	1
Infection (especially viral)		5	
Gastrointestinal			
Nausea, vomiting, abdominal pain	12	8	13
Hepatic dysfunction	9	1	9
Hypersensitivity (erythema nodosum, fever, arthralgia)		2	4
Teratogenicity (theoretical risk)			
Cancer (theoretical risk)	0.7		see text

[a] Another 3% had a combination of hematological abnormalities.

Comparison of Azathioprine and Cyclosporine

Azathioprine has been used as a standard treatment for comparison with cyclosporine in treatment trials without any significant differences emerging between the two treatments in terms of efficacy. One of these trials compared AZA 2 mg/kg daily with cyclosporine 5 mg/kg daily but there were only 17 patients in each group and the trial only lasted a year so that the trial only had a small power to detect a difference (Steck et al. 1990). The other trial undertaken in Germany was more substantial. Ninety-eight patients were randomized to receive cyclosporine 5 mg/kg daily and 96 to AZA 2.5 mg/kg daily (Kappos et al. 1988). After 24 to 32 months there were no differences between the groups in any of the trial measures including the Kurtzke expanded disability status scale and the frequency of relapse. Since cyclosporine has been shown in two randomized controlled trials to confer more benefit than placebo (Rudge et al. 1989; The Multiple Sclerosis Study Group 1990), the failure of the German trial to show any greater benefit than AZA is consistent with a beneficial effect of treatment with AZA. The incidence of side effects from cyclosporine was more than twice those from AZA (Kappos et al. 1988).

Side Effects of Azathioprine

If the benefits of AZA have been difficult to detect, its side effects have been all too obvious (Table 7.4). It characteristically causes a macrocytosis. In myasthenia gravis it has been suggested that the development of macrocytosis might be related to the efficacy of treatment (Witte et al. 1986). This suggestion has not been confirmed and there was no relationship between macrocytosis and treatment effect in the British and Dutch trial of azathioprine in MS (British and Dutch Multiple Sclerosis Azathioprine Trial Group 1988). Dose-related leukopenia is usual during azathioprine treatment and the dose is commonly titrated to produce a leukopenia (Goodkin et al. 1991). While such titration has some theoretical justification there is no hard evidence that such a regime is more efficacious in any condition than fixed dose regimes of 2 to 3 mg/kg. Leukopenia and also anemia and thrombocytopenia may develop unpredictably during continued chronic treatment so that continued vigilance remains necessary. Gastrointestinal intolerance, with nausea, abdominal pain and vomiting, occurs in about 10% of patients and was the commonest medical cause for patients stopping treatment in the British and Dutch trial (British and Dutch Multiple Sclerosis Azathioprine Trial Group 1988). These symptoms can sometimes be avoided by gradually increasing the dose and giving the tablets later in the day. Increased concentrations of liver enzymes in the blood suggesting hepatocellular injury occur in up to 10% of patients and often revert to normal when the dose is reduced. Rare cases of cholestasis have been recorded. Other side effects are rare but include allergic rashes, erythema nodosum, alopecia, pancreatitis, and possibly pneumonitis. Inevitably with an effective immunosuppressant, there will be an increased susceptibility to infections, but in practice this is rarely a problem. In the author's experience there is a possible small increased incidence of warts, herpes simplex and herpes zoster in MS patients taking AZA.

The most worrying potential side effect of AZA is the increased risk of developing malignant disease. This theoretical risk exists in any patient who is immunosuppressed because the immune system normally has a role in detecting and destroying malignant cells which express neoantigens. Renal transplant recipients, most of whom will have received combined prednisolone and AZA, have a markedly increased incidence of skin cancer and non-Hodgkin's lymphoma and a small increase in incidence of other cancers (Kinlen 1985). A retrospective study (Lhermitte et al. 1984) identified 10 cases of cancer among 131 MS patients who had received AZA during a 10-year follow-up period and only 4 cases in 131 patients who had not received AZA. This report is worrying but the difference in proportions is not statistically significant. Furthermore the cancers detected were all solid cancers (5 were carcinoma of the breast) and not the non-Hodgkin's lymphomas which would have been particularly expected. During the follow-up of 161 MS patients treated with AZA in the British and Dutch Trial (of whom 98 were followed for 4 years) there were two fatal cancers (one ovarian carcinoma and one carcinoma of the bronchus) and no non-fatal cancers. In about the same number of patients not treated with AZA there were no cancer deaths and one non-fatal carcinoma of the colon (British and Dutch Multiple Sclerosis Azathioprine Trial Group 1988). The 300 British patients in that trial were flagged with the Office of Population Census and Surveys so that all deaths and cancer notifications are automatically reported to the trial office. As of December 1990 (6–7.5 year follow-up) there had been no cancer deaths but two more cancer notifications in the AZA group and also two more in the placebo group (unpublished information). Thus far this follow-up study has not detected a significant increase in cancer in MS patients treated with AZA nor have any other worrying reports of an increased incidence of cancer emerged from any studies other than the French report just mentioned.

Information from renal transplant recipients and patients with diseases other than MS, especially rheumatoid arthritis, treated with AZA does strongly suggest that azathioprine treatment does cause an increased incidence of non-Hodgkin's lymphoma. For instance 3 cases of non-Hodgkin's lymphoma were encountered in a series of 41 rheumatoid arthritis patients treated with AZA and low-dose steroids for varying lengths of time between 1976 and 1983 (Pitt et al. 1987). In these cases the additional use of steroids may have played a role but the incidence of lymphoma may be increased in rheumatoid arthritis in any case. A prospective study of 1109 patients who had been treated with AZA for medical conditions other than transplants and followed for 1 to 12 years identified 40 cases of cancer compared with 28.6 cases expected in a population of the same age and sex distribution. The only cancer with a strikingly higher incidence than expected was non-Hodgkin's lymphoma, of which there were 5 cases compared with 0.38 expected. This approximately 10-fold increase in risk is consistent with the similar increase in transplant recipients and in patients treated with other immunosuppressants or having immunodeficiency states (Kinlen 1985). Although the increase in risk of non-Hodgkin's lymphoma is large the actual risk to a patient over an approximately 10-year follow-up is only about 0.5%.

There are obvious concerns that the use of cytotoxic drugs such as AZA during pregnancy will cause fetal abnormalities. Teratogenic effects have been reported in rabbits. However many women have had healthy babies following renal transplantation despite continued treatment with steroids and AZA. Rare neonatal leukopenia and thrombocytopenia have occurred. The evidence supporting the use of AZA in MS is not sufficient to warrant its use without practising birth control.

Summary and Conclusions

Each controlled trial has shown a trend suggesting a small benefit from taking AZA compared with placebo. This benefit is statistically significant in an overview analysis but clinically small. The odds of remaining free of relapse appear to be increased about twofold over 3 years and the rate of progression to be reduced by about 0.2 Kurtzke disability units over 2 years. This small benefit can be considered in two ways. On the one hand it is a change smaller than the variation in the performance of some patients on a single day and also within the limits of inter-observer error. On the other hand this change has been detected consistently across all the trials. In the largest trial there was a more significant difference in a more meaningful and reproducible measure, the ambulation index, which appeared to become more marked with longer treatment. If this difference were sustained during treatment for 20 or 30 years benefits might become clinically significant. Trials to test this hypothesis will be problematic since it will now be difficult to randomize patients to receive placebo for such long periods.

Although arguably the safest of the available immunosuppressive drugs, AZA does have significant side effects. About 10% of patients are unable to take the drug because of gastrointestinal intolerance and rare allergic reactions. There is a continued risk of leukopenia and hepatic dysfunction which demands regular blood tests. There is a small risk of malignancy which has been established especially for non-Hodgkin's lymphoma. These risks have to be balanced against the small clinical benefits which may reduce the considerable risk of becoming severely disabled by MS.

There is unfortunately no evidence as to which patients are most likely to benefit from taking AZA. The effects on reducing relapse frequency have been more readily detected than the effect on slowing disease progression, from which it might be argued that AZA is more likely to benefit patients with relapsing/remitting disease. Patients with more aggressive disease, especially those who are having frequent relapses with incomplete recovery from each relapse, are those most likely to consider the risks of side effects and malignancy justified. For these patients, provided they can tolerate the drug, many neurologists, including the author, would consider AZA the best available immunosuppressant. It should only be used after careful discussion of the risks and benefits. The dose is probably best adjusted to maintain a mild leukopenia, and regular blood counts and tests of liver function are mandatory. Although somewhat beneficial, AZA is clearly not the final answer to the treatment of multiple sclerosis. The fact that statistically significant benefits have been detected supports the autoimmune hypothesis of pathogenesis but could also be explained by a non-specific anti-inflammatory effect.

Acknowledgements. The author thanks Prof K. McPherson and Mrs. P. Yudkin for helpful advice and discussion.

References

Aimard G, Confavreux C, Centre JJ et al. (1983) Etude de 213 cas de sclerose en plaques traites par l'azathioprine de 1967 a 1982. Rev Neurol (Paris) 139:509–513

Babington RG, Medeking PW (1971) The influence of cinanserin and selected pharmacologic agents on EAE. J Pharmacol Exp Ther 117:454–460

Bach MA, Back JF (1972) Activities of immunosuppressive agents in vitro. II. Different timing of azathioprine and methotrexate in inhibition and stimulation of mixed lymphocyte reaction. Clin Exp Immunol 11:89–98

British and Dutch Multiple Sclerosis Azathioprine Trial Group (1988) Double-masked trial of azathioprine in multiple sclerosis. Lancet 2:179–183

Calne RY, Murray JE (1961) Inhibition of the rejection of renal homografts in dogs by Burroughs Wellcome 57-322. Surg Forum 12:118–120

Caputo D, Zaffaroni M, Ghezzi A, Cazzullo CL (1987) Azathioprine reduces intrathecal IgG synthesis in multiple sclerosis. Acta Neurol Scand 75:84–86

Cendrowski W (1971) Therapeutic trial of (Imuran) azathioprine in multiple sclerosis. Acta Neurol Scand 47:254–260

de Miranda P, Beacham PL, Creagh TH et al. (1973) The metabolic fate of the methyl nitroimidazole moiety of azathioprine in the rat. J Pharmacol Exp Ther 187:588–601

Dworkin RH, Bates D, Millar JHD, Paty DW (1984) A re-analysis of three double-blind trials. Neurology 34:1441–1445

Dyck PJ, O'Brien P, Swanson C Low P, Daube J (1985) Combined azathioprine and prednisone in chronic inflammatory demyelinating polyneuropathy. Neurology 35:1173–1176

Elion GB (1967) Biochemistry and pharmacology of purine analogues. Fed Proc 26:898–904

Ellison GW, Myers LW (1978) Immunosuppressive drugs in multiple sclerosis: pro and con. Neurology 34:132–139

Ellison GW, Myers LW, Mickey MR et al. (1989) A placebo-controlled, randomized, double-masked, variable dosage, clinical trial of azathioprine with and without methylprednisolone in multiple sclerosis. Neurology 39:1018–1026

Felson DT, Anderson J (1984) Evidence for the superiority of immunosuppressive drugs and prednisone over prednisone alone in lupus nephritis. N Engl J Med 311:1528–1534

Fratiglioni L, Siracusa GF, Amato MP, Sita D, Amaducci L (1988) Effectiveness of azathioprine treatment in multiple sclerosis. Ital J Neurol Sci 9:261–264

Freedman MS, Loertscher R, Cashman NR, Duquette P, Blain M, Antel JP (1990) Immunoregulatory properties of T-cell lines derived from the systemic and intrathecal compartments: A phenotypic and functional study. Ann Neurol 27:258–265

Frick E, Angstwurm H, Blomer R, Strauss G (1977) Immunosuppressive Therapie den Multiplen Sklerose. IV. Behandlungsergebnisse mit azathioprin und antilymphozytenglobulin. Münch Med Wochenschr 119:1111–1114

Ghezzi A, Di Falco M, Locatelli C et al. (1989) Clinical controlled trial of azathioprine in multiple sclerosis. In: Gonsette DR, Delmotte P (eds) Recent advances in multiple sclerosis therapy. Elsevier, Amsterdam

Goodkin DE, Bailly RC, Teetzen ML, Hertsgaard D, Beatty W (1991) The efficacy of azathioprine in relapsing remitting multiple sclerosis. Neurology 41:20–25

Grüninger W, Mertens HG (1973) Uber die immunsuppressive Langzeitbehandlung der Multiplen Sklerose mit Azathioprin. Excerpta Med Int Congr Ser 296:148

Hughes RAC (1988) Use of azathioprine in multiple sclerosis. In: Cazzullo CL, Caputo D, Ghezzi A, Zaffaroni M (eds) Virology and immunology in multiple sclerosis: rationale for therapy. Springer-Verlag, Berlin, pp 153–161

Kappos L, Patzold U, Dommasch D et al. (1988) Cyclosporine versus azathioprine in the long-term treatment of multiple sclerosis – Results of the German multicenter study. Ann Neurol 23:56–63

Kinlen LJ (1985) Incidence of cancer in rheumatoid arthritis and other disorders after immunosuppressive treatment. Am J Med 78 (suppl A):44–49

Kissel JT, Levy RJ, Mendell JR, Griggs RC (1986) Azathioprine toxicity in neuromuscular disease. Neurology 36:35–39

Lassmann H (1983) Comparative neuropathology of chronic experimental allergic encephalomyelitis and multiple sclerosis. Springer-Verlag, Berlin

Leibowitz S, Hughes RAC (1983) Immunology of the nervous system. Edward Arnold, London, pp 1–304

Lhermitte F, Marteau R, de Saxce H (1987) Treatment of progressive and severe forms of multiple sclerosis using a combination of antilymphocyte serum, azathioprine and prednisone. Clinical and biological results. Comparison with a control group treated with azathioprine and prednisone only: 4-year follow-up. Rev Neurol (Paris) 143:98–107

Lhermitte F, Marteau R, Roullet E et al. (1984) Long-term immunosuppression. Rev Neurol (Paris) 140:553–558

Loo TL, Luce JK, Sullivan MP et al. (1968) Clinical pharmacologic observations on 6-mercaptopurine and 6-methylthiopurine ribonucleoside. Clin Pharm Ther 9:180–194

Mantegazza R, Antozzi C, Peluchetti D, Sghirlanzoni A, Cornelio F (1988) Azathioprine as a single drug or in combination with steroids in the treatment of myasthenia gravis. J Neurol 235:449–453

Martin R, Jaraquemada D, Flerlage M et al. (1990) Fine specificity and HLA restriction of myelin basic protein-specific cytotoxic T cell lines from multiple sclerosis patients and healthy individuals. J Immunol 145:540–548

Mertens H-G, Dommasch D (1977) Long term study of immunosuppressive therapy in multiple sclerosis, comparison of periods of the disease before and during treatment. In: Delmotte P, Hommes OR, Gonsette R (eds) Immunosuppressive treatment in multiple sclerosis. Ghent European Press, pp 198–211

Mertin J Rudge P, Kremer M et al. (1982) Double-blind controlled trial of immunosuppression in the treatment of multiple sclerosis. Final report. Lancet 2:351–354

Milanese C, La Mantia L, Salmaggi A et al. (1988) Double blind controlled randomized study on azathioprine efficacy in multiple sclerosis. Preliminary results. Ital J Neurol Sci 9:53–57

Millar JHD, Vas CJ, Noronha MJ, Liversedge LA, Rawson MD (1967) Long-term treatment of multiple sclerosis with corticotrophin. Lancet 2:429–431

Nuwer MR, Packwood JW, Myers LW, Ellison GW (1987) Evoked potentials predict the clinical changes in a multiple sclerosis drug study. Neurology 37:1754–1761

Oger JJ, Antel JP, Kuo HH, Arnason BGW (1982) Influence of azathioprine (Imuran) on in vitro immune function in multiple sclerosis. Ann Neurol 11:177–181

Olsson T, Baig S, Hojeberg B, Link H (1990) Antimyelin basic protein and antimyelin antibody-producing cells in multiple sclerosis. Ann Neurol 27:132–136

Patzold U, Hesker H, Pocklington P (1982) Azathioprine in treatment of multiple sclerosis: Final results of a four and a half year controlled study of its effectiveness covering 115 patients. J Neurol Sci 54:377–394

Paulus HE, Williams HJ, Ward JR et al. (1984) A multicentre study of azathioprine and penicillamine in rheumatoid arthritis. Arthritis Rheum 27:721–731

Perings E, Reisert P-M, Kraft H-G (1971) Untersuchungen über die antiinflammatorische Wirkung von Azathioprin. Int J Clin Pharmacol 5:200–202

Pitt PI, Sultan AH, Malone M, Andrews V, Hamilton EBD (1987) Association between azathioprine therapy and lymphoma in rheumatoid disease. J R Soc Med 80:428–429

Rosen JA (1979) Prolonged azathioprine treatment of non-remitting multiple sclerosis. J Neurol Neurosurg Psychiatry 42:338–344

Röllinghoff M, Schrader J, Wagner H (1973) Effect of azathioprine and cytosine arabinoside on humoral and cellular immunity in vitro. Clin Exp Immunol 15:261–270

Rudge P, Koetsier JC, Mertin J et al. (1989) Randomised double blind controlled trial of cyclosporin in multiple sclerosis. J Neurol Neurosurg Psychiatry 52:559–565

Sabouraud O, Oger J, Darcel F, Madigand M, Merienne M (1984) Immunosuppression au long cours dans la sclerose en plaques: évaluation des traitements commencés avant 1972. Rev Neurol (Paris) 140:125–130

Staugaitis SM, Shapshak P, Myers LW, Ellison GW, Tourtellotte WW, Lee M (1985) Azathioprine and steroids are not more effective in decreasing multiple sclerosis intra-blood-brain-barrier IgG synthesis than steroids alone. Ann Neurol 18:356–357

Steck AJ, Regli F, Ochsner F, Gauthier G (1990) Cyclosporine versus azathioprine in the treatment of multiple sclerosis: 12-month clinical and immunological evaluation. Eur Neurol 30:224–228

Swinburn WR, Liversedge LA (1973) Long-term treatment of multiple sclerosis with azathioprine. J Neurol Neurosurg Psychiatry 36:124–126

The Multiple Sclerosis Study Group (1990) Efficacy and toxicity of cyclosporine in chronic progressive multiple sclerosis: A randomized, double-blinded, placebo-controlled clinical trial. Ann Neurol 27:591–605

Ventre JJ, Guillot M, Confavreux C, Evreux JC, Aimard G (1985) Side effects of azathioprine (Imurel). Apropos of 313 patients treated for multiple sclerosis. Review of the literature. Therapie 40:195–202

Walton JN (1991) Polymyositis. J Neurol Neurosurg Psychiatry 54: in press
Warren KG, Catz I (1989) Cerebrospinal fluid autoantibodies to myelin basic protein in multiple sclerosis patients. Detection during first exacerberations and kinetics of acute relapses and subsequent convalescent phases. J Neurol Sci 91:143–151
Witte AS, Cornblath DR, Schatz NJ, Lisak RP (1986) Monitoring azathioprine therapy in myasthenia gravis. Neurology 36:1533–1534
Yazici H, Pazarli H, Barnes CG et al. (1990) A controlled trial of azathioprine in Behçet's syndrome. N Engl J Med 322:281–285
Yudkin P (1990) An overview of randomised controlled trials of azathioprine in the treatment of multiple sclerosis. In: Cazzullo CL (ed) Immunotherapy of multiple sclerosis. Evaluation of azathioprine treatment. Centro Studi Sclerosi Multipla, Milan, pp 35–41

Chapter 8

Treatment of Multiple Sclerosis with Copolymer I

Murray B. Bornstein and Kenneth P. Johnson

Introduction

The most desirable treatment for multiple sclerosis (MS) would safely arrest the disease process before clinical signs and symptoms had appeared. This has not yet been achieved. Failing this, one would wish safely to arrest or reverse its course as soon as possible after its earliest clinical manifestations. This chapter will present the results of two pilot trials of a synthetic product, Copolymer I (Cop 1), which show promise of attaining the second objective.

Understanding the pathogenetic mechanisms involved in MS and searching for an effective treatment have been intimately associated with the laboratory model, experimental allergic encephalomyelitis (EAE). The validity of EAE as an MS model system has been convincingly presented by Paterson in a series of scholarly publications (Paterson 1977, 1978, 1979, 1980). Our own work in tissue culture (Bornstein and Appel 1961; Appel et al. 1962; Bornstein 1963, 1973) has also served to relate MS, a naturally occurring disorder, to its laboratory counterpart, EAE. Organotypic cultures of mammalian CNS tissue respond with identical patterns of demyelination (Bornstein 1973), swollen myelin sheaths (Bornstein and Raine 1976), and eventual "sclerosis" (Raine and Bornstein 1970) when exposed to serum from EAE (whole white matter)-affected animals or from MS patients. The demyelinating effect is not produced by these EAE sera on cultured peripheral nerve which, nevertheless, are responsive to serum from animals with experimental allergic neuritis (Bornstein and Raine 1977; Raine and Bornstein 1979). The cultures also demonstrate the capacity of mammalian CNS to remyelinate after being demyelinated by antisera (Bornstein 1963; Raine and Bornstein 1970). These laboratory demonstrations provided support for the extension to MS patients of therapeutic possibilities arising from animal studies.

The synthetic polypeptide Copolymer I (Cop 1) is prepared from L-alanine, L-glutamic acid, L-lysine, and L-tyrosine (Table 8.1) and is one of a series of prepared compounds which, alone or in combination with various lipids, might simulate the ability of myelin basic protein (MBP) to induce or suppress EAE (Arnon 1981; Arnon and Teitelbaum 1980; Keith et al. 1979; Lando et al. 1979; Teitelbaum et al. 1971, 1973, 1974; Webb et al. 1973, 1976). None of the series was encephalitogenic, i.e., capable of inducing EAE, but some, particularly Cop 1, did suppress EAE in animals challenged with either whole white

Table 8.1. Composition of copolymer I

Amino acid	*N*-Carboxyanhydride used for reaction	Amount used in the reaction		Molar ratio of amino acid in copolymer
		g	mmol	
Alanine	Alanine	8.6	75	6.0
Glutamic acid	-Benzyl glutamate	6.0	23	1.9
Lysine	*N*-Trifluoroacetyl-lysine	14.0	52	4.7
Tyrosine	Tyrosine	3.0	14	1.0
Molecular weight				23 000

matter or MBP in complete Freund's Adjuvant. The laboratory investigations showing the effectiveness of Cop 1 in preventing or decreasing the severity of EAE involved mice, rats, guinea-pigs, rabbits, monkeys, chimpanzees and baboons and are of particular interest to MS clinical trials (Arnon 1981; Arnon and Teitelbaum 1980; Keith et al. 1979; Teitelbaum et al. 1971, 1973, 1974; Webb et al. 1973, 1976). In addition, extensive laboratory studies failed to demonstrate any toxicological or other undesirable side reactions in experimental animals exposed to Cop 1 under a variety of testing situations (A. Meshorer, personal communication). Finally, Abramsky et al. (1977) first examined Cop 1 for its effect on 3 patients with acute disseminated encephalomyelitis (ADE) and 4 with terminal MS. The 3 ADE patients reportedly recovered rapidly and completely. The MS patients may have demonstrated slight improvements. The absence of any significant undesirable side reactions was important in those first clinical studies.

To date, our clinical trials have included a preliminary trial and two pilot trials, one involving exacerbating/remitting (ER) patients and the second, recently completed, chronic/progressive (CP) patients.

Preliminary Trial

The preliminary trial involved 16 patients (4 ER and 12 CP) and was conducted as an open study (Bornstein et al. 1987) (Table 8.2). The evaluating neurologist was aware that all patients were being treated with Cop 1. The initial dosage schedule was chosen on the basis of previous studies with laboratory animals (Bornstein et al. 1987) at the Weizmann Institute and the brief trial that was conducted by Dr. Oded Abramsky (Abramsky et al. 1977). The Cop 1 was prepared at a concentration of 5 mg/ml in sterile saline solution to be given intramuscularly five times a week for the first 3 weeks, three times a week for the next 3 weeks, twice a week for the next 3 weeks, and, finally, once a week for the balance of a 6-month period, when the trial was to end.

When entered into the study, patients were examined by Dr. A. Miller, the evaluating neurologist, samples of peripheral blood and cerebrospinal fluid were taken, and the Cop 1 injections were started. The first patients were hospitalized at the General Clinical Research Center of the Albert Einstein College of Medicine for the first 3 weeks of treatment to observe for any significant local or systemic effects. No undesirable side reactions of any significance were observed so future participants were hospitalized for only 24–48 h following the lumbar puncture. The patients were followed on an outpatient basis at the Clinical Research Center and their neurological status re-evaluated at various times during the course of the trial.

The specific aims of the preliminary trial were to determine the following: (1) Did Cop 1 produce any apparent significant or undesirable side reactions? (2) Did Cop 1 produce any apparent desirable effects? (3) Could a dosage schedule be established for further (pilot) trials should they appear to be warranted?

During the institution of the treatment with Cop 1, some patients reported and demonstrated improvements in various neurological functions, such as improved bladder control or increased strength. Later, as the dosage of Cop 1 was reduced, as originally planned, these early improvements disappeared and most patients returned to their previous neurological status or continued their chronic/progressive course. To determine whether or not the previously observed effect was dose-related, the dosage was then gradually increased. After the first 18-month period, those patients still in the trial were receiving 20 mg/day in 1 ml saline, 7 days each week. The results of the preliminary trial are presented in Table 8.2.

The patients occasionally reported transient slight pain, discomfort, itching, swelling or redness at the injection sites. No systemic or general reactions of any kind were noted or reported during the preliminary trial. Examinations of urine were unremarkable. Two of the 4 ER patients withdrew from the study

Table 8.2. Results of preliminary trial of copolymer I therapy in 16 patients with multiple sclerosis

Patient	Type	Age	Sex	Date of entry	Date of termin.	Results
I.Y.	CP[a]	46	F	4/25/78	5/27/81	No effect
R.H.	CP	25	M	5/15/78	5/29/79	No effect
G.T.	CP	35	F	5/30/78	9/20/79	No effect
P.P.	ER[b]	30	F	5/30/78	–	No effect
A.T.	CP	23	M	6/27/78	2/08/79	No effect
P.McL.	CP	39	F	7/18/78	–	Arrested – marked improvement
J.P.	ER	39	F	7/18/78	10/27/78	Withdrew at time of exacerbation
J.W.	CP	32	M	6/27/78	6/05/79	No effect
K.J.	CP	33	F	7/31/78	12/30/80	No effect
C.N.	ER	32	M	7/07/78	–	Cessation of characteristic attacks
W.R.	CP	49	M	10/03/78	–	Arrested – slight improvement
S.McC.	CP	42	F	10/16/78	–	No effect
H.W.	CP	36	M	10/24/78	11/13/78	No effect
S.R.	CP	38	F	10/24/78	–	No effect
F.H.	ER	27	F	11/07/78	–	Cessation of characteristic attacks
J.M.	CP	34	F	11/20/78	–	Arrest and improvement

[a] CP = Chronic/progressive.
[b] ER = Exacerbating/remitting.

at the time of an acute attack, one of whom later returned. The other 14 patients remained in the study for at least 6 months as orignially planned. Of the 16 patients, 11 demonstrated no apparent favorable effects in that they either had an exacerbation during the course of the study or continued their chronic/progressive course, and 5 demonstrated a definite improvement such as the cessation of exacerbations or improved balance, strength and gait (see Table 8.2).

Laboratory examinations included a CBC, routine urinalysis and culture, blood chemistry analysis (SMA 6 and 12), VDRL, CSF protein, glucose, and cells. Except for an occasional and transient eosinophilia (reaching 16% in one instance), no significant abnormalities were noted. There was no albuminuria or other evidence of altered kidney function. No pertinent alteration of the patient's serum demyelinating activity on CNS cultured tissues was observed. Several sera have been examined for antibody titers against Cop 1. In general, they have not been elevated. Lymphoblast transformation in response to phytohemagglutinin, myelin basic protein (MBP) and Cop 1 has not occurred.

On the basis of these preliminary results, the evaluation of Cop 1 was extended to rigorous double-blind, randomized, placebo-controlled pilot trials.

It should also be noted that 50 other patients have been treated with Cop 1: 13 for less than 1 year, 25 for 1–3 years, 6 for 3–5 years, 3 for 5–10 years, and 3 for over 11 years. No patient in this group has demonstrated any significant or undesirable local or systemic reactions or late sequelae.

Trial of Patients with Exacerbating/Remitting Multiple Sclerosis

The defined objectives of the pilot trial of the ER patients (Bornstein et al. 1987) were: (1) whether or not the frequency of attacks was different between the Cop 1 and the placebo (bacteriostatic saline)-injected groups; (2) whether there was a difference in the degree of disability developed after two years of participation in the trial; and (3) whether any significant or undesirable side effects occurred.

Methods

The trial was approved by the Committee on Clinical Investigations of the Albert Einstein College of Medicine and by the Federal Food and Drug Administration.

Preparation and Characterization of Cop 1

Cop 1 was first prepared at the Weizmann Institute of Science, Rehovot, Israel, and later by the Bio-Yeda Company in Rehovot (Table 8.1). All batches were analyzed for their amino-acid composition, molecular weight, cross-reactivity with MBP, and suppression of EAE in guinea-pigs. Suppression was expressed as the difference in the percentage of diseased animals treated with Cop 1 and the controls. The 12 batches from the Weizmann Institute had a suppression rate ranging from 10% to 80% (average, 33.5%); the rate for 14 batches produced by Bio-Yeda ranged from 10% to 75% (average 40.6%). In an attempt to reduce inflammatory reactions at injection sites, an in vitro method was used to evaluate cell damage (basophil degranulation) by serotonin release (Barsumian et al. 1981). All the batches in this study produced releases of less than 30%.

Cop 1 was dissolved in bacteriostatic saline at a concentration of 20 mg per ml. Sterile, single-dose vials containing 1 ml of bacteriostatic saline alone or the Cop 1 solution were stored at −20°C. Patients received a monthly supply of 32 vials of the appropriate solution. The preparation and distribution of vials and patient compliance were monitored by a clinical assistant under the direction of the statistician responsible for the randomization of patients (see Study Design below).

Patient Recruitment and Enrollment

Entrance criteria specified that patients have definite multiple sclerosis (Poser et al. 1983), be 20–35 years of age, have at least two well-demarcated and well-documented episodes of exacerbation in the 2 years before entry, have a score no higher than 6 (ambulatory with unilateral assistance) on the Kurtzke Disability Status Scale (DSS) (Kurtzke 1983) and be emotionally stable as determined by psychosocial evaluation.

Questionnaires completed by 932 volunteers were reviewed; 140 of these candidates were evaluated in neurologic and psychosocial examinations, and 90 of these were excluded: 23 because of age, 21 for low frequency of exacerbations, 19 for lack of documentation, 15 for psychosocial inadequacy, 8 for transition to a chronic/progressive course, 3 for distance from the clinic, and 1 for pregnancy. Fifty patients were accepted into the trial (Table 8.3).

Study Design and Data Collection

Study patients were matched according to sex, exacerbation rate per year within one exacerbation, and degree of disability as measured by the DSS in three strata: 0 to 2, 3 to 4, and 5 to 6. The random assignment of the first patient of a pair determined the assignment of both. Treatment assignments were given to the clinical assistant responsible for the production, labeling, and distribution of medication. A second clinic visit was scheduled shortly after acceptance into the study. The patient was formally enrolled after another explanation of the trial, instruction in the method of self-injection, and signing of a consent form.

Eight patients who had an exacerbation after screening were enrolled after their conditions had become stable. One patient was enrolled 1 month after being weaned from corticosteroid therapy.

Data from a personal and disease history, neurologic examination, DSS and FSS were recorded at the time of screening and also at entry. Patients were evaluated 1 month later and then every 3 months for 2 years. At each visit, a blinded neurologist, unaware of the patient's treatment group, completed a neurologic examination and DSS and FSS status evaluation. The patient's self-evaluation of local or generalized side effects and changes in neurologic status were reported to the clinical assistant, who was not blinded to treatment.

Patients were also evaluated when reporting the rapid onset of new symptoms or a worsening of pre-existing symptoms that persisted for 48 h or more. The neurologist verified exacerbations on the basis of study criteria. An event was counted as an exacerbation only when the patient's symptoms were accompanied by observed objective changes on the neurologic examination involving an increase of at least one point in one of the FSS or the DSS. Sensory symptoms unaccompanied by objective findings or transient neurologic worsening were not considered to represent an exacerbation. Patients experiencing an acute exacerbation were evaluated at frequent intervals – usually every 2 weeks – until a new, stable neurologic baseline had been established. Seventy-four percent of 62 exacerbations in the placebo group and 75% of the 16 exacerbations in the Cop 1 group were treated with steroids. Symptomatic medications, such as cholinergic and spasmolytic drugs, were permitted.

Laboratory Tests

Routine urinalyses, blood chemistry (SMA 20) determinations, and complete blood counts were performed at entry and every 3 months thereafter. Aliquots of serum and cells were stored in a deep freezer or in liquid nitrogen (at −90° or −180°C, respectively) for future studies.

HLA typing of HLA-A, B, C, and DR was performed by the tissue typing laboratory of the Department of Surgery, Montefiore Medical Center, Bronx, New York.

Statistical Methods

The baseline characteristics of the two treatment populations were compared by two-tailed *t*-tests for continuous variables and chi-square tests with Yates' correction for discrete variables. Differences in side effects according to treatment arm were evaluated with a chi-square test.

The principal endpoint was the proportion of exacerbation-free patients. The secondary endpoints were frequency of exacerbations, change in Kurtzke DSS from that at baseline and length of time before progression, as defined below.

The study design included planned subgroup analyses according to the disability score of the patients at randomization (DSS 0 to 2, 3 to 4, and 5 to 6). However, only 1 patient entered with a score of 4, and 3 with a score of 5. Therefore, two of the three strata (3 to 4 and 5 to 6), were combined, creating two strata (0 to 2 and 3 to 6) with approximately equal numbers of patients for subgroup analyses.

For the matched-pair analysis, the difference between treatment arms was tested with use of a McNemar's statistic for the 22 matched pairs. A two-tailed Fisher's exact test was used for other two-by-two contingency tables. The chi-square test was used to test two-by-three contingency tables for frequency of exacerbations.

Survival curves were calculated with life-table methods (Anderson et al. 1980) for the length of time before progression, with "progression" defined as an increase of at least one unit in the DSS. Progression was noted at the visit when it was observed; however, it had to be maintained for at least 3 months to be counted. Data on patients lost to follow-up were censored at the time of withdrawal. The log-rank statistic was used to test for comparability of the survival curves for each treatment arm. The curves were also tested for a difference at the discrete point of 24 months (Anderson et al. 1980).

Multiple logistic-regression analyses were undertaken to test the effect of treatment on the outcome, with adjustment for other variables, including sex, the duration of disease, the previous exacerbation rate, disability at the time of entry into the study, and various interactions of these variables. Odds ratios were calculated from the regression coefficients.

Study Population

Fifty patients were enrolled: 48 in 24 matched pairs, and 2 unmatched patients, 1 randomly assigned to each study group. Table 8.3 shows the baseline characteristics of the study population and of the 48 patients included in the analyses. The distributions of these characteristics were similar in the two treatment arms.

To guard against any bias that might be introduced by drop-outs, we tried to include all the randomized patients in the analyses. Seven patients did not complete the 2 years of the trial. Of these, 2 patients in the placebo group were dropped for psychological reasons and were excluded from all the analyses

Table 8.3. Base-line characteristics of the study population

Characteristic	Treatment group		
	Placebo		Cop 1
	Randomized	Included in analysis	
Number entered	25	23	25
Average age (yr)	31.0	31.1	30.0
Average duration of disease (yr)	6.1	6.4	4.9
Sex			
Male	10	10	11
Female	15	13	14
Race/ethnic group			
White	25	23	23
Black or Hispanic	0	0	2
Disability score (Kurtzke scale)			
0–2	11	10	13
3–4	7	7	5
5–6	7	6	7
Average disability score	3.2	3.1	2.9
Prior exacerbation rate (over 2-year period)	3.9	3.9	3.8

because of unusable data. The partial data obtained from the other 5 patients were included in the analyses. One patient taking Cop 1 dropped out during an exacerbation after 2 months of treatment. This patient had a second exacerbation shortly after stopping medication. Both events were counted as study exacerbations in the data analyses.

Results

The study design specified the recruitment of patients in matched pairs, one patient randomly assigned to each treatment arm, with the proportion of exacerbation-free patients as the principal endpoint. The matched analysis of the principal endpoint included 22 pairs. An unmatched analysis permitted the inclusion of an additional 4 patients – 2 who were unmatched and 2 who had been matched to 2 patients who were subsequently excluded (Fig. 8.1). Analyses of exacerbation data are reported both as matched and unmatched. Subsequent analyses were performed on an unmatched basis.

Exacerbations During the 2-Year Study Period

In the 22 matched pairs, there were 12 discordant pairs: 2 patients in the placebo group had no exacerbations, whereas their matches in the Cop 1 group did; 10 patients in the Cop 1 group had no exacerbations, whereas their matches in the placebo group did. The remaining 10 pairs had concordant

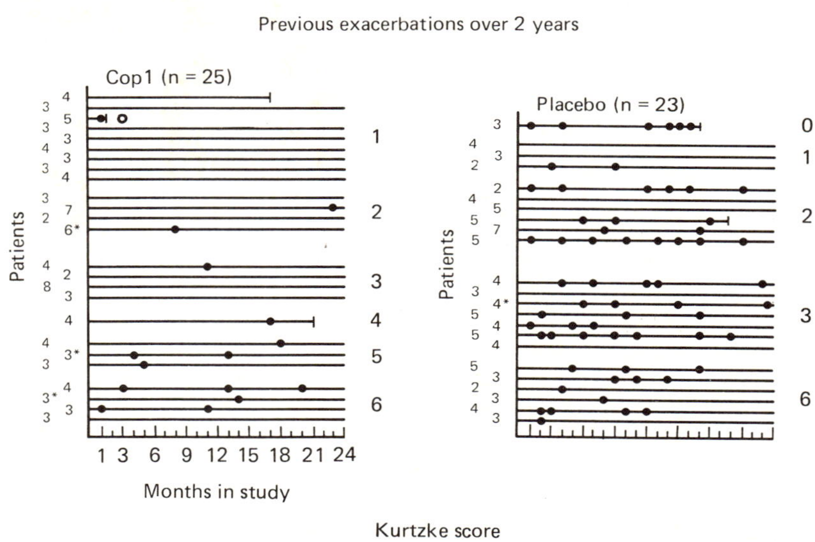

Fig. 8.1. Exacerbations occurring during the 2 years of the ER trial. Each line represents a patient, and each circle an exacerbation. Patients are grouped according to their Kurtzke score on entry. The number of pretrial exacerbations are indicated to the left. Discontinued lines represent patients who withdrew before completion. The open circle indicates an exacerbation occurring after withdrawal that was included as a study event. Patients who were not included in the matched-pair analyses are indicated by an asterisk.

Table 8.4. Exacerbations according to treatment group

Number of exacerbations per patient	Treatment group			
	Placebo		Cop 1	
	Number	%	Number	%
0	6	26.1	14	56.0
1	3	13.1	7	28.0
2	2	8.7	3	12.0
3	5	21.8	1	4.0
4	2	8.7	0	0.0
5	1	4.3	0	0.0
6	2	8.7	0	0.0
7	1	4.3	0	0.0
8	1	4.3	0	0.0
Total	23	100.0	25	100.0

results. The difference in discordant pairs between treatment groups was significant ($p = 0.039$). An unmatched analysis of the presence or absence of exacerbations was also significant ($p = 0.045$).

Fig. 8.1 shows the occurrence and time of exacerbations in each patient during the trial. Over the 2 years, there were 62 exacerbations among 23 patients in the placebo group (average, 2.7) and 16 in the Cop 1 group (average, 0.6). The effect of treatment was also examined according to the entry Kurtzke score. In the 0 to 2 stratum, there were 27 exacerbations over 2 years among 10 placebo-treated patients (average, 2.7) and 4 exacerbations among 13 Cop 1-treated patients (average, 0.3). In the 3 to 6 stratum, there were 35 exacerbations among 13 placebo-treated patients (average, 2.7) and 12 exacerbations among 12 Cop 1-treated patients (average, 1.0).

The distributions of exacerbations for all 48 patients are shown in Table 8.4. Of the 25 patients in the Cop 1 group, 14 (56%) were free of exacerbations, as compared with 6 (26%) of the 23 patients in the placebo group. By contrast, 12 patients in the placebo group (52%) had three or more exacerbations, as compared with 1 in the Cop 1 group (4%). Patients were grouped according to whether they had no exacerbations, one to two, or three or more. The comparison between groups was significant at $p < 0.001$.

Multiple logistic-regression analyses were carried out to evaluate the effect of covariates including treatment, sex, duration of disease, prior exacerbation rate, Kurtzke score at entry, and interactions of these variables. Only the treatment group and Kurtzke score at entry had a significant effect. The multiple logistic-regression analyses showed that treatment with Cop 1 independently increased the likelihood that a patient would be free of exacerbations ($p = 0.036$), as did a lower disability score at entry ($p = 0.003$). An estimate of relative risk with adjustment for sex, disability score at entry, and previous exacerbation rate showed the risk of exacerbations to be 4.6 times greater for a patient taking placebo rather than Cop 1.

There was a decrease in the number of exacerbations among the patients in the placebo group, from 41 in the first year to 21 in the second. The ratio of the number of exacerbations in the placebo group to that in the Cop 1 group was 4.9 for the first year and 3.3 for the second year.

Table 8.5. Changes in disability status over two years according to baseline DSS score strata: ER trial

Change in Kurtzke score	All cases				Baseline DSS stratum 0–2				3–6			
	Placebo		Cop 1		Placebo		Cop 1		Placebo		Cop 1	
	Number	%	Number	%	Number	%	Number	%	Number	%	Number	%
Worse												
4	1	4.4	0	–	1	10.0						
3	3	13.0	1	4.0	1	10.0			2	15.4	1	8.3
2	2	8.7	1	4.0	1	10.0			1	7.7	1	8.3
1	5	21.7	3	12.0	4	40.0	2	15.4	1	7.7	1	8.3
Subtotal	11	47.8	5	20.0	7	70.0	2	15.4	4	30.8	3	24.9
Stable (0)	9	39.1	12	48.0	2	20.0	5	38.4	7	53.8	7	58.4
Improved												
−1	2	8.7	5	20.0	1	10.0	4	30.8	1	7.7	1	8.3
−2	0	0	3	12.0			2	15.4			1	8.3
−3	1	4.4	0						1	7.7		
Subtotal	12	52.2	20	80.0	3	30.0	11	84.6	9	69.2	9	75.0
Total	23	100.0	25	100.0	10	100.0	13	100.0	13	100.0	12	100.0

Fifteen patients were treated throughout the trial with Cop 1 supplied by the Weizmann Institute, and 10 with Cop 1 supplied by Bio-Yeda. Ten of the patients receiving the Weizmann product (67%) were free of exacerbations; there were seven exacerbations among the remaining 5 patients. Of the 10 patients receiving the Bio-Yeda product, 4 (40%) were exacerbation-free; the remaining 6 patients had nine exacerbations. This difference was not statistically significant.

Change in Disability Status

Table 8.5 shows the distribution of the 2-year changes in DSS score according to treatment group. A negative score indicates improvement, a positive score worsening, and zero no change. In the placebo group 11 patients (48%) and in the Cop 1 group 5 patients (20%) had disease progression over the 2-year period. The difference between treatment groups in the proportion who remained stable or improved was of borderline significance ($p = 0.064$). The change in disability status in the patients treated with the Weizmann product was similar to that in the patients treated with the Bio-Yeda product.

Table 8.5 also shows the distribution of the changes in DSS score according to treatment group for each baseline DSS score subgroup. In the 0 to 2 subgroup, Cop 1 had a significant beneficial effect on disability status: 84.6% of patients receiving Cop 1 were stable or improved, as compared with 30% in the placebo group ($p = 0.012$). The average change in DSS score favored Cop 1 by 1.7 units (there was a worsening of 1.2 with placebo and an improvement of 0.5 with Cop 1). In the 3 to 6 subgroup, the proportions of patients whose conditions were stable, improved, and worse were comparable in both treatment groups, as were the average changes in DSS score (there was a worsening of 0.4 with placebo and of 0.3 with Cop 1).

The effect of the previously identified covariates on the comparison of worsening vs. disease stability or improvement was evaluated with the use of multiple logistic-regression analyses and demonstrated a beneficial effect of Cop 1 on disability status ($p = 0.033$). A patient taking placebo was four times more likely to have progression of disease than a patient taking Cop 1, after adjustment for sex, Kurtzke score at entry and previous exacerbation rate.

Fig. 8.2 is a survival curve showing the length of time before progression. Progression was defined as an increase of at least 1 unit in the Kurtzke score maintained for at least 3 months. Over the 2-year period, the curves were significantly different ($p = 0.05$), with the placebo group having progression sooner than the Cop 1 group. Of the patients receiving placebo, 50% had progressed by the end of 18 months, whereas only 20% of those receiving Cop 1 showed progression by the end of 24 months. At 24 months, there was a significant difference ($p < 0.005$) favoring therapy.

Laboratory Studies and Side Effects

The HLA characteristics of the 48 patients were unrelated to the effects of treatment. Patient reactions were monitored during each routine clinic visit by means of urinalysis, blood examination, and the patient's self-evaluation.

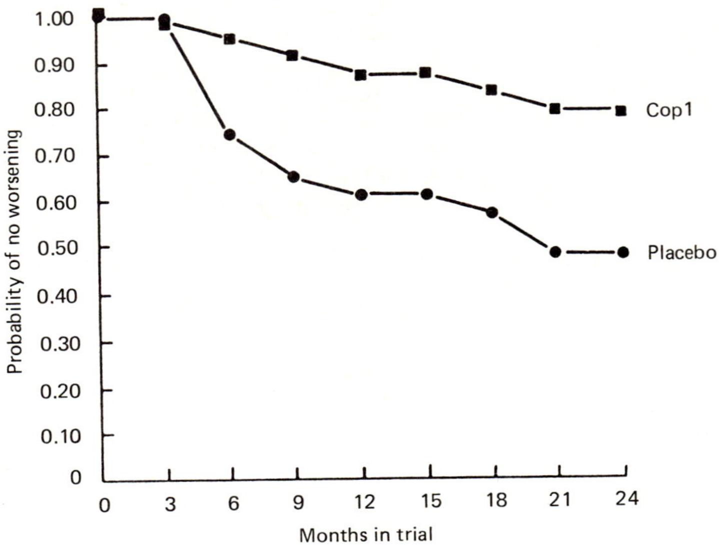

Fig. 8.2. Curves representing the probability of no worsening from the baseline Kurtzke score in ER trial. Worsening was determined when first observed, but was counted only if it continued for 3 months.

Table 8.6. Patients (%) reporting side effects

Symptom	Placebo (n = 23)	Cop 1 (n = 25)
Local		
Soreness[a]	35	92
Itching[b]	22	64
Swelling[a]	17	88
Redness	48	76
Other	35	36
Other		
Headache	39	32
Nausea	17	24
Vomiting	4	4
Dizziness	30	40
Constipation	30	40
Sweating	26	28
Rash	17	24
Palpitations	13	24
Cramps	9	12
Faintness	13	20
Joint pain	39	40
Gastrointestinal discomfort	22	12
Appetite loss	13	20
Drowsiness	26	20
Other	17	28

[a] $p < 0.001$ for the difference between placebo and Cop 1.
[b] $p < 0.01$ for the difference between placebo and Cop 1.

Urinalyses and blood examinations revealed no apparent changes in the functions of the liver, spleen, kidney, bone marrow, gastrointestinal tract, heart or lungs.

Table 8.6 shows the percentage of patients in each group who reported reactions at the injection sites and other reactions. More patients taking Cop 1 reported reactions at the injection site involving soreness ($p < 0.001$), swelling ($p < 0.001$) and itching ($p < 0.01$). In addition, soreness was reported during at least half the visits in 32% of the Cop 1 group as compared with 9% of the placebo group; itching was reported in 40% as compared with 4%; swelling in 56% as compared with none; and redness in 40% as compared with 9%.

Other reactions were reported with comparable frequencies in each group (Table 8.6). No symptom was a persistent problem in more than 12% of either group. Dizziness, constipation, and joint pain were the most common symptoms in the Cop 1 group, whereas headache, dizziness, constipation, and joint pain were the most common in the placebo group.

Two patients had a patterned, transient reaction to Cop 1. It began during or immediately after an injection and consisted of a flush, sweating, palpitations, a feeling of tightness around the chest, difficulty in breathing, and associated anxiety. It lasted from 5 to 15 minutes and passed with no residual difficulties. In 1 patient, the reaction occurred three times in 21 months, and in the other, twice in 17 months. Experimental therapy was discontinued in these 2 patients, who remained under observation for the balance of the trial. The remaining patients were alerted to the possibility of such reactions, informed of precautionary measures, and given a kit containing epinephrine and antihistamine tablets.

After the trial was completed, 1 of the 2 patients who had a reaction volunteered to take Cop 1 in an unblinded manner. This patient reported a hypersensitivity reaction that included urticaria, itching, and marked discomfort. It was controlled with epinephrine and steroids.

Blinding

Considerable efforts were made to maintain blinding. The examining neurologist and the patients did not discuss side effects. Patients reported such effects to the unblinded clinical coordinator.

After the trial, the effectiveness of the blinding was evaluated. The patients and the examining neurologist were asked to guess treatment assignments. Of 18 patients in the placebo group who responded 14 (78%) guessed correctly, as did 15 (68%) of 22 in the Cop 1 group. The blinded neurologist correctly identified 70% of those taking placebo and 78% of those taking Cop 1. He based his evaluation on the clinical status of the patient, as did the majority of the patients (68% of the Cop 1 group and 61% of the placebo group). Approximately 20% of the patients based their guesses on the occurrence or absence of side effects. This suggests that the ability to guess treatment assignment correctly was influenced by the effect of treatment rather than by side effects.

This pilot trial suggests that Cop 1 may be beneficial for patients with the ER form of MS, but the results must be considered preliminary, requiring confirmation by a more extensive clinical trial.

Trial of Patients with Chronic/Progressive Multiple Sclerosis

A second double-blind, randomized, placebo-controlled pilot trial was conducted on the chronic/progressive (CP) MS patients (Bornstein et al. 1991).

Methods

The trial involved a coordinating center, Albert Einstein College of Medicine of Yeshiva University in the Bronx, New York, and Baylor College of Medicine, Texas Medical Center in Houston, Texas. It was approved by the Internal Review Boards at both institutions and by the Federal Food and Drug Administration.

Preparation and Characterization of Cop 1

Cop 1 was prepared and supplied as in the previous ER trial (Bornstein 1987).

Thirty-two shipments of 21 individual batches of Cop 1 were delivered, 13 from Bio-Yeda and 8 from the Weizmann from May 1983 through November 1988. The amounts in each batch varied from 18 to 270 g. Chemical, immunochemical, biological activity and basophil degranulation tests were performed at the Weizmann Institute.

The Cop 1 was packaged and shipped as the sterile, lyophilized product, 300 mg in 50-ml vials. It was stored at −20°C until final preparation when the Cop 1 was dissolved in 15 ml of bacteriostatic saline to yield a concentration of 20 mg per ml. All batches were tested for sterility in thioglycollate medium and tryptic soy broth and observed for 4 weeks. Sterile single-dose vials containing 0.75 ml of bacteriostatic saline alone (placebo) or the Cop 1 solution were prepared and stored at −20°C until use. Random shipments of Cop 1 to the patients were dictated by the patients' date of entry into the trial. Each patient received a month's supply of 64 vials containing 15 mg of Cop 1 in 0.75 ml of bacteriostatic saline or the placebo alone. These were kept frozen until use. The preparation and distribution of vials to both centers and patient compliance at Einstein were monitored by an unblinded clinical assistant. The patients were instructed to self-inject the thawed contents of one vial subcutaneously twice a day. There were no cross-overs during the trial. However, when the supply of Cop 1 was interrupted for 1 month, 16 patients received the placebo rather than the Cop 1. The patients and the evaluating neurologists were unaware of the change. Neither patients nor neurologists reported any significant change in neurological status or side reactions during this period.

Patient Recruitment, Enrollment and Pretrial Observation

Patients were screened at Albert Einstein College of Medicine between December 1981 and October 1985, and at Baylor College of Medicine between March 1983 and July 1985.

The entry criteria for patient selection were: (1) a definite diagnosis of multiple sclerosis (Poser 1983); (2) evidence of a CP course for at least 18 months; (3) no more than 2 exacerbations in the previous 24 months; (4) 20 to 60 years of age; (5) disability between 2.0 and 6.5 inclusive on the Kurtzke Expanded Disability Status Scale (EDSS) (Kurtzke 1983); and (6) emotionally stable and capable of participating in a double-blind clinical trial as determined by psychosocial evaluation.

The EDSS was used to measure degree of neurologic dysfunction at entry and during the study. The overall scale quantifies disability in half units from 0 (no disability) to 10 (death from multiple sclerosis); related scales measure eight functional systems: pyramidal, cerebellar, brainstem, sensory, bowel and bladder, visual, mental, and other.

Interested patients (2270) were screened by phone or questionnaire and 370 were selected for neurological and psychosocial evaluations. From these, 169 eligible patients were selected, gave informed consent, and entered into the pretrial observation period during which the study neurologist examined the patients for evidence of progression every 3 months for a minimum of 6 and a maximum of 15 months. Criteria for entry into the randomized treatment phase of the trial required the demonstration of progression in one of the following ways: (1) a worsening of 2.0 points in one of the functional systems' scores (FSS); or (2) a worsening of 1.0 point in two unrelated functional systems; or (3) a worsening of 2.0 points on the Ambulation Index (Hauser et al. 1983); or (4) a worsening of 1.0 point on the EDSS. Patients who progressed during this 12-month period and maintained the progression for at least 3 months were eligible for entry into the randomized phase of the trial. In addition, patients must not have progressed beyond 6.5 on the EDSS or have experienced more than 1 exacerbation during the pretrial observation period.

Prior to randomization 63 patients were excluded – 2 had a second exacerbation, 8 progressed to an EDSS score of 7 or higher, 10 chose alternate treatments, 31 showed insufficient progression and 12 were otherwise excluded. One hundred and six patients were accepted into the treatment phase of the trial.

Study Design and Data Collection

Patients demonstrating progression in the pretrial observation period entered the treatment phase and were randomized to either the Cop 1 or the placebo treatment arm. Randomization within centers was accomplished by randomized block design with baseline EDSS strata of <5.0 or >5.5. When a patient became eligible, the investigator notified the statistical center which validated the patient's eligibility and assigned a randomization code number. The study was conducted in a double-blind manner. Only the statistician and the clinical assistant at Albert Einstein College of Medicine, who distributed the medication, were aware of patient assignments.

At the time of randomization, patients were again given an explanation of the trial, informed of the side reactions noted by patients in the ER trial, and asked to sign a consent form. They were instructed in the method of self-injection and told to administer study medication on a twice-daily basis.

Statistical Methods

The baseline characteristics of the study population in the two treatment arms were compared with the use of two-tailed *t*-tests for continuous variables, Fisher's Exact Test for dichotomous variables, and chi-square tests with Yates' correction for discrete variables with more than 2 categories. Differences in side effects according to treatment arm were evaluated with a two-tailed Fisher's Exact Test. All tests used an alpha level of 0.05 for significance.

The principal endpoint was the time to reach a confirmed progression. Progression was defined as a worsening of 1 unit over the baseline EDSS for those patients with an entry EDSS of 5.0 or greater, or a worsening of 1.5 units for those with an entry EDSS less than 5.0. To qualify as a confirmed progression, the worsening must have been maintained for at least 3 months. Each patient completed participation in the study when a confirmed progression was reached, or when the patient had been 2 years on study in the absence of a confirmed progression. Other endpoints included: (1) time to unconfirmed progression; (2) time to progression of a half unit in the EDSS score; (3) change in the EDSS score from baseline; and (4) study neurologists' overall evaluation of patients' neurological status.

The study design included planned subgroup analyses by stratum of baseline EDSS score of <5.0 or >5.5, and by center. Contingency tables were tested for statistical significance by Fisher's Exact Test (2 × 2) or for more than 4 cells by a continuity corrected chi-square test.

Survival curves were calculated with life-table methods for the length of time before the endpoint under study, such as confirmed progression, was reached (Anderson et al. 1980). Data on patients lost to follow-up were censored at the time of withdrawal. The log-rank statistic was used to test for comparability of the survival curves for each treatment arm. The curves were also tested for a difference at the discrete points of 12 and 24 months.

Proportional hazards methods and multiple logistic-regression analyses were undertaken to test the effect of treatment on the endpoints. Depending on which endpoint was being evaluated, adjustment was made for other variables, including sex, center, age, baseline Kurtzke score, baseline ambulation score, and various interactions of these variables with treatment.

The blinded neurologist performed a complete neurologic examination, and determined the FSS, EDSS, Ambulation Index (Anderson et al. 1980) and Incapacity Scale Scores at entry and at each subsequent 3-month routine visit. Side effects and problems with injections or compliance were not discussed with the study neurologist but were reported to a clinical assistant. Another blinded neurologist was available to examine patients with severe or unusual side effects. At no time during the trial did it become necessary for this neurologist to request a code break.

Some patients experienced acute worsening of their symptoms or exacerbations. If these persisted for 48 h or more, the patients were seen and evaluated for a possible exacerbation. Steroid treatment was permitted during an exacerbation. The highest daily dosage prescribed was 100 mg of prednisone or 80 units of ACTH for up to 4 weeks. Seven patients (2 placebo and 5 Cop 1) were treated at Einstein and 8 patients were treated (5 placebo and 3 Cop 1) at Baylor. No significant change was reported in the patients' neurologic status at the time of their scheduled evaluations. Symptomatic medications, such as cholinergic and spasmolytic drugs, were permitted.

Patients continued in the study until they had demonstrated either a confirmed progression or had completed 24 months of treatment. An effort was made to examine all patients at 24 months after entry even if they had previously demonstrated a confirmed progression or were no longer participating in the trial.

Laboratory Tests

Blood and urine samples were obtained from each patient upon entry into the trial and at each visit. Routine urinalyses, blood chemistry (SMA 20) determinations, and complete blood counts were performed. Aliquots of serum and cells were stored in a deep freezer or in liquid nitrogen (at −90° or −180°C, respectively) for future studies.

Study Population

One hundred and six patients were randomized into the trial: 55 at Einstein and 51 at Baylor. Table 8.7 shows the baseline characteristics by treatment arm within each center. There were no significant differences between treatment arms for age, sex, race or baseline EDSS score. The mean EDSS at Einstein was 5.7; at Baylor 5.4 ($p = 0.06$).

Of the 106 randomized patients, 86 (81.1%) completed the study requirements. The remaining 20 patients (18.9%, 10 on Cop 1 and 10 on placebo) withdrew: 6 requested removal, 5 for side effects, 3 at the time of demonstrating progression but prior to confirmation, and 6 for various other reasons. An

Table 8.7. Patient baseline characteristics. CP trial. (Percent in each category)

	Einstein		Baylor		Combined	
	Cop 1	Placebo	Cop 1	Placebo	Cop 1	Placebo
Number entered	27	28	24	27	51	55
Age at screening						
20–29	7.4	0	4.2	3.7	5.9	1.8
30–39	37.0	39.3	41.7	51.9	39.2	45.5
40–49	40.7	39.3	20.8	18.5	31.4	29.1
50–60	14.8	21.4	33.3	25.9	23.5	23.6
Average age	40.7	43.4	42.6	41.2	41.6	42.3
Sex						
Male	44.4	50.0	45.8	40.7	45.1	45.5
Female	55.6	50.0	54.2	59.3	54.9	54.5
Race						
White	96.3	100.0	91.7	96.3	94.1	98.2
Black	3.7	0.0	8.3	3.7	5.9	1.8
EDSS at entry						
<5.0	11.1	17.9	33.3	37.0	21.6	27.3
5.0–5.5	14.8	7.9	0.0	11.1	7.8	14.5
6.0–6.5	74.1	64.2	66.7	51.9	70.6	58.2
Mean EDSS	5.8	5.7	5.5	5.3	5.7	5.5

effort was made to obtain a 24-month follow-up on all patients, with success in half of the early withdrawal cases.

Each early withdrawal was reviewed by the principal investigator *prior to the code break*. Based on the data, it was determined that 3 of the withdrawals should be counted as confirmed progressions. One (placebo) stopped taking treatment after progression had been noted, but prior to a 3-month confirmation; one (Cop 1) did not maintain progression at exit from the study, but demonstrated progression 3 months later at a 24-month follow-up visit; and 1 (Cop 1) progressed and was confirmed by the blinded neurologist via telephone information obtained 3 months later. For purposes of statistical analyses, the 20 early withdrawals were counted as follows: 17 patients (8 on Cop 1 and 9 on placebo) who did not meet progression criteria were censored at the time of withdrawal and 3 patients (2 on Cop 1 and 1 on placebo) were counted as confirmed progression at the time of withdrawal.

Results

Time to Confirmed Progression

The major endpoint was time to confirmed progression for all 106 randomized patients. As previously stated, there were 20 early withdrawals from the trial: 3 of these patients were counted as confirmed progressions. There were 23 confirmed progressions, 9 (17.6%) in the Cop 1 treatment arm and 14 (25.5%) in the placebo arm.

Fig. 8.3 shows the probability of progression for each treatment arm. At 9 months, the placebo curve crossed the Cop 1 curve and showed more

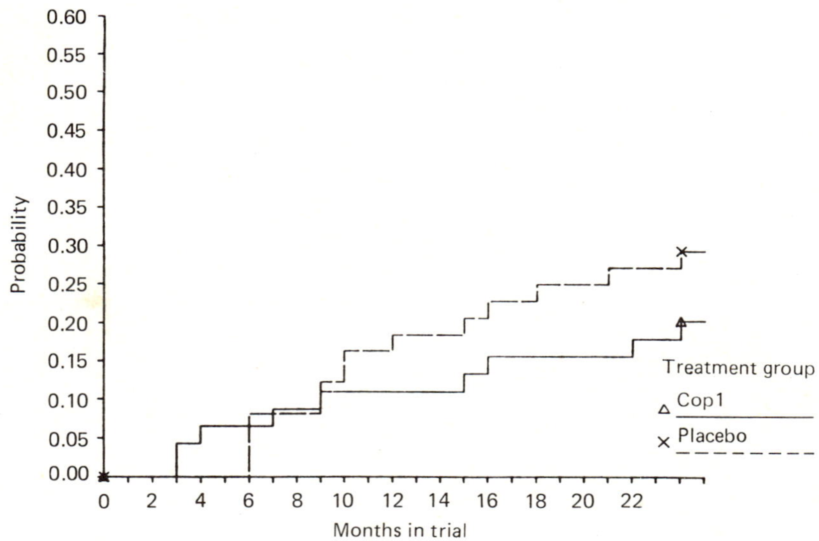

Fig. 8.3. CP trial. Probability of progressing for confirmed progression.

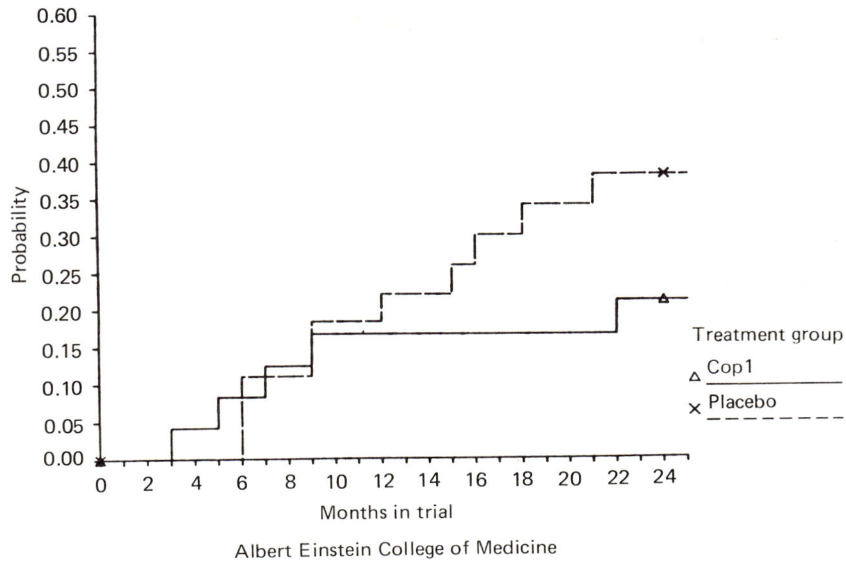

Fig. 8.4. CP trial. Probability of progressing for confirmed progression at Albert Einstein College of Medicine.

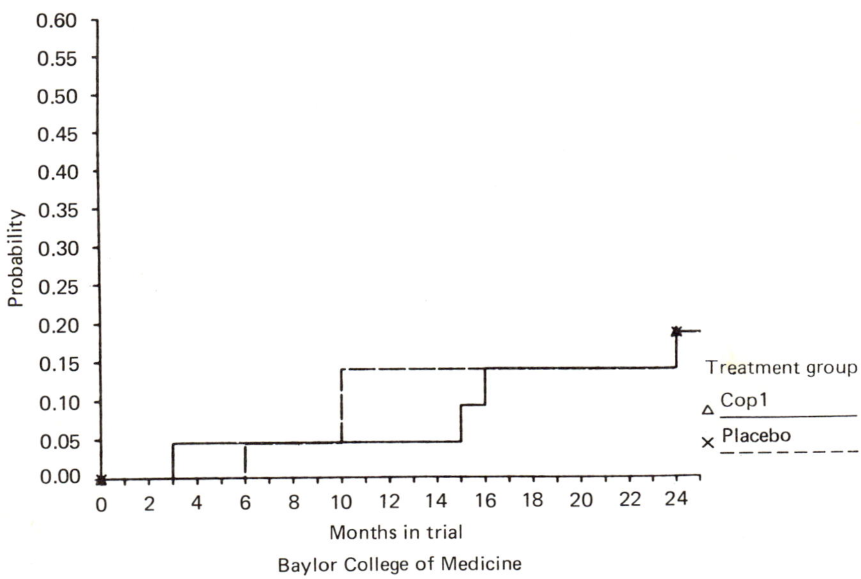

Fig. 8.5. CP trial. Probability of progressing for confirmed progression at Baylor College of Medicine.

progression for the remainder of the trial. The curves were tested in three ways: over the entire 24-month period and specifically at 12 and 24 months. There was no significant difference between the 2 curves over the 24-month study period.

The difference in the survival curves at the time points of 12 and 24 months were evaluated using a one-sided confidence limit. At 12 months, there was an 11.0% probability of progressing for Cop 1 patients as compared to 18.5% for placebo patients ($p = 0.088$). The probability of progressing by 24 months was 20.4% for Cop 1 as compared to 29.5% for placebo ($p = 0.086$).

A proportional hazards model was used to examine the influence of other factors: treatment arm, center, age, baseline EDSS score and their interactions on time to progression. A multiple logistic-regression model was used to examine the influence of these factors on progression. The results were not statistically significant.

Subgroup Analysis by Center

The data were also analyzed by center. Survival curves for the major endpoint, for each center, are shown in Figs. 8.4 and 8.5. For Einstein, the curves are significantly different only at 24 months with a 21.4% chance of progression in the Cop 1-treated arm and a 38.5% chance of progressing in the placebo arm ($p = 0.041$). For Baylor, the curves show no difference in survival. Patients in each treatment arm have a 19% chance of progressing by 24 months in either treatment arm.

For the Cop 1 group, the centers reported similar percentages of patients with confirmed progression, 18.5% (5/27) at Einstein and 16.7% (4/24) at Baylor. For the placebo group, the percentages for patients with confirmed progression at Einstein was 35.7% (10/28) which is more than twice that at Baylor, 14.8% (4/27). Comparing the placebo curves for the 2 centers, the probability of progressing at 24 months for Einstein was significantly higher than Baylor (38.5% vs 19%) ($p = 0.046$, 2-tail).

The interactions between center and treatment effect were not statistically significant.

Time to Unconfirmed Progression

In another analysis, the definition of progression was broadened to include progressions which were not confirmed, providing a total of 30 progressions: 11 in the Cop 1 arm (21.6% progression rate) and 19 in the placebo arm (34.5% progression rate).

Fig. 8.6 shows the probability of progressing for each treatment arm. The curves crossed twice between 2 and 6 months. After 6 months the placebo-treatment arm showed more progression than did the Cop 1. The difference between the two survival curves over 24 months is not statistically significant.

The differences between the survival curves at the specific time points of 12 and 24 months were evaluated. At 12 months, the probability of progression was significantly higher in the placebo group: 27.8%, as compared to 15.4% for Cop 1 ($p = 0.025$). Similarly, at 24 months the probability of progression was

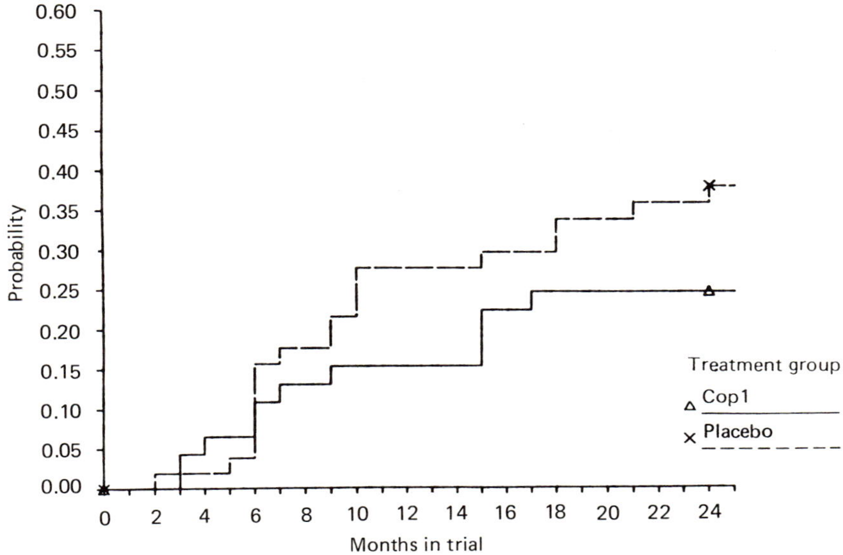

Fig. 8.6. CP trial. Probability of progressing for unconfirmed progression.

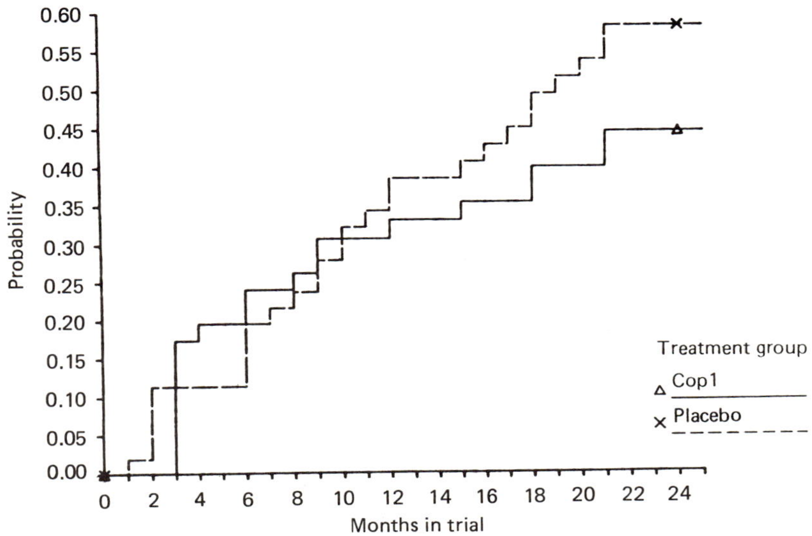

Fig. 8.7. CP trial. Probability of progressing for progression of 0.5 units on EDSS.

significantly higher in the placebo group: 38.1% versus 24.8% for Cop 1 (p = 0.026).

A logistic-regression model and proportional hazards model were used to examine the influence of other factors on progression and time to progression. The results were not statistically significant. The interaction between treatment and centers was not significant.

Time to Confirmed Progression of 0.5 Units on EDSS

Another analysis studied time to confirmed progression of 0.5 units on the EDSS. This endpoint is less demanding for worsening than the major endpoint progression criteria of 1.0–1.5 units. As a result, there were more confirmed progressions for a total of 48 as compared to 23 for the major endpoint. There were 20 confirmed progressions in the Cop 1 treatment arm (39.2% progression rate) and 28 in the placebo arm (50.9% progression rate).

Fig. 8.7 shows the probability of progression for each arm. The placebo curve and the Cop 1 curve were similar for the first 12 months of the trial. Subsequently, the placebo arm showed a higher progression rate. There were no significant differences between the 2 curves over the 24-month study period.

When tested at the specific time points of 12 and 24 months, there was a significant difference at 24 months. The probability of progressing by 24 months was 44.6% for Cop 1 as compared to 58.3% for placebo (p = 0.030).

The treatment center interaction was not significant.

Change in EDSS Score

The change from baseline EDSS score was evaluated for patients who completed 24 months in trial. For those 20 patients who dropped out, the change was calculated for their period on study. For the Cop 1-treatment arm, 19.6% of the patients improved, 37.3% remained stable and 43.1% worsened; on the placebo arm 14.5% improved, 34.6% were stable and 50.9% worsened (Fig. 8.8). Since the patients were expected to continue to worsen over the 24 months in trial, both stabilization and improvement in EDSS scores are considered beneficial effects. Combining these categories, 56.9% of the Cop 1-treatment arm were stable or improved as compared to 49.1% of the placebo. This difference is not statistically significant.

Laboratory Studies and Side Effects

Patients were monitored during each routine clinic visit by urinalysis and blood examination which showed no apparent changes in the functions of the liver, spleen, lymph nodes, kidney, bone marrow, gastrointestinal tract, heart or lungs.

At each routine visit, patients completed a questionnaire on any local or systemic symptoms or side effects that they might have experienced during the previous 3 months.

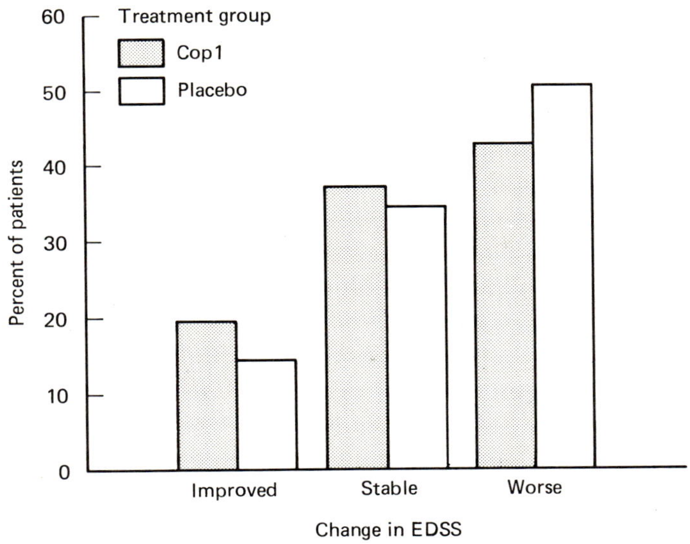

Fig. 8.8. CP trial. Changes in EDSS score from baseline by treatment group.

A much higher percentage of Cop 1 patients ($p = 0.001$) reported soreness (83% versus 47%), itching (61% versus 17%), swelling (80% versus 23%) and redness (85% versus 30%). There were no significant differences in the number of patients reporting various systemic reactions during the trial (Table 8.8).

Twelve Cop 1- and 3 placebo-treated patients reported transient vasomotor responses which included a flush, palpitations, muscle tightness, difficulty breathing, and anxiety. Two Cop 1 and 1 placebo patient reported the full complement of symptoms; the remaining 10 Cop 1 and 2 placebo patients reported only a few of these symptoms. The reactions were transient, lasting from a few seconds to about 1 hour, the median time being 2.5 minutes (mean = 12.4 minutes). One patient reported an allergic (urticarial) response to Cop 1.

Blinding

During the study, precautions were taken to preserve the blinding. The blinded evaluating neurologists and the patients avoided discussing side effects, which were reported to the clinical coordinators. A non-blinded neurologist was available to evaluate and treat any serious side effects or reactions that might be drug-related.

The effectiveness of the blinding was evaluated after the study. The patients were asked to guess treatment assignments and 91 (85.8%) responded. Three said that they believed that they had received both treatments during the study. The rate of correct guesses for the remaining 88 patients was about the same in each treatment arm with about half of the patients (56.2% Cop 1 and 53.6% placebo) making the correct assessment.

Table 8.8. Patient report of side effects. CP trial; collected at each routine visit

Reaction	Percent reporting systemic reactions at any time during the visit		
	Cop 1	Placebo	*p* value[a]
Headache	17.4	24.5	0.464
Nausea	15.2	13.2	0.782
Vomiting	0.0	1.9	1.000
Dizziness	17.4	26.4	0.337
Constipation	28.3	39.6	0.291
Rash	21.7	11.3	0.181
Cramps	19.6	17.0	0.798
Faintness	15.2	11.3	0.767
Joint pain	28.3	24.5	0.819
Abdominal discomfort	15.2	24.5	0.319
Appetite loss	13.0	17.0	0.780
Drowsiness	17.4	24.5	0.464
Sweating[b]	17.4	9.4	0.372
Palpitations[b]	23.9	15.1	0.312
Flush[b]	30.4	17.0	0.153
Difficulty breathing[b]	23.9	11.3	0.115
Tightness in chest[b]	15.2	18.9	0.791
Constriction of throat[b]	21.7	13.2	0.295
Constriction of chest	15.2	11.3	0.767
Anxiety[b]	28.3	20.8	0.482
Other systemic	13.0	18.9	0.586

[a] *p* values obtained with a 2-tailed Fisher's Exact Test.
[b] Symptoms associated with the vaso-motor response.

Discussion

The results of the Cop 1 therapy trial in CP MS fail to reveal a statistically significant difference between the treated and placebo groups for the major endpoint, which is an increase of 1 or 1.5 EDSS units maintained for 3 months. Secondary endpoints, i.e., the time to unconfirmed progression of 1.0 or 1.5 EDSS units or confirmed progression of 0.5 EDSS units, were statistically significant at 12 and 24 months for the former ($p = 0.026$) and at 24 months for the latter ($p = 0.030$), but not significant when the progression curves as a whole are considered. Since all patients were selected for inclusion into the trial on the bais of an observed progressive worsening, there was a remarkable difference in the progression of both the placebo and Cop 1-treated patients when changes observed in the pretrial observation period were compared with those observed in trial. Moreover, the placebo-treated patients at Baylor showed significantly less progression than did those at Einstein. We have no explanation for either the in-trial placebo responses or the differences between the two centers.

The ER pilot trial involved patients whose EDSS scores at entry averaged 3.1 for the placebo and 2.9 for the Cop 1 group. The response to treatment, as shown by the frequency of exacerbations and change in disability status, was greater in the group whose EDSS scores were 2 or less at entry as compared to those of 3 or more. By comparison, the entry EDSS scores in the CP trial averaged 5.5 for the placebo and 5.7 for the Cop 1 group. Thus, the difference in favorable effects between the ER and the CP patients could be interpreted as due to either a difference in the clinical type or a difference in severity of disability at entry, a possibility supported by the greater effect of Cop 1 in the ER patient whose entry DSS was less than 2. In view of the relatively mild side reactions, these pilot studies suggest that treatment with Cop 1 be considered early in the course of the disease.

Acknowledgements. The authors take this opportunity to acknowledge the active participation in the clinical trials of Drs. A. Miller, H. Crystal, A. Merriam, S. Wassertheil-Smoller, Mr. V. Spada, Ms. N.S. Slagle and Mrs. M. Weitzman, at The Albert Einstein College of Medicine, Bronx, New York; Drs. M. Kielson and E. Drexler at Maimonides Medical Center, Brooklyn, New York; Drs. S. Appel, L. Rolak, Y. Harati and Ms. S. Brown at Baylor College of Medicine, Houston, Texas; Drs. R. Arnon, M. Sela, D. Teitelbaum and Mr. I. Jacobsohn at the Weizmann Institutes of Science, Rehovot, Israel and Mr. W. Weiss, Vienna, Virginia.

This work was supported by grants NS-11920 and NS-18879 from the National Institutes of Neurological Communicative Diseases and Stroke and grant GCRC-RR-50 from the National Institutes of Health, Bethesda, Maryland. It is also a pleasure to acknowledge the professional expertise provided by Information Management Services, Inc. and particularly of Drs. Janis Beach and Carol Giffen.

References

Abramsky O, Teitelbaum D, Arnon R (1977) Effect of a synthetic polypeptide (Cop 1) on patients with multiple sclerosis and acute disseminated encephalomyelitis: Preliminary report. J Neurol Sci 31:433–438

Anderson S, Auguier A, Hauck W et al. (1980) Statistical methods for comparative studies. John Wiley and Sons, USA, pp 199–214

Appel SH, Bornstein MB, Seegal BC, Murray MR (1962) The application of tissue culture to the study of experimental "allergic" encephalomyelitis. II. Immunological observations. Proc Int Cong Neuropath 2:283

Arnon R (1981) Experimental allergic encephalomyelitis – susceptibility and suppression. Immunol Rev 55:5–30

Arnon R, Teitelbaum D (1980) Desensitization of experimental allergic encephalomyelitis with synthetic peptide analogues. In: Davison AN, Cuzner ML (eds) The suppression of experimental allergic encepahlomyelitis and multiple sclerosis. Academic Press, New York, pp 105–117

Barsumian EL, Isersky C, Petrino MG et al. (1981) IgE-induced histamine release from rat basophilic leukemia cell lines: Isolation of releasing and nonreleasing clones. Eur J Immunol 11:317–323

Bornstein MB (1963) A tissue culture approach to demyelinative disorders. Nat Cancer Inst Monogr 11:197–214

Bornstein MB (1973) The immunopathology of demyelinating disorders examined in organotypic cultures of mammalian central nerve tissue. In: HM Zimmerman (ed) Progress in neuropathology, vol 2. Grune and Stratton, New York, pp 69–90

Bornstein MB, Appel SH (1961) The application of tissue culture to the study of experimental "allergic" encephalomyelitis. I. Patterns of demyelination. J Neuropath Exp Neurol 20:141–157

Bornstein MB, Raine CS (1976) The initial structural lesion in serum-induced demyelination in vitro. Lab Invest 35:391–401

Bornstein MB, Raine CS (1977) Multiple sclerosis and experimental allergic encephalomyelitis. Specific demyelination of CNS in culture. Neuropathology Applied Neurobiology 3:359–367

Bornstein MB, Miller A, Slagle S et al. (1987) A pilot trial of Cop 1 in exacerbating-remitting multiple sclerosis. N Engl J Med 317:408–414

Bornstein MB, Miller A, Slagle S et al. (1991) A placebo-controlled, double-blind, randomized, two-center, pilot trial of Cop 1 in chronic progressive-multiple sclerosis. Neurology 41:533–539

Hauser L, Dawson DM, Lehrich JR et al. (1983) Intense immunosuppression in progressive multiple sclerosis. N Engl J Med 308:173–180

Keith AB, Arnon R, Teitelbaum D et al. (1979) The effect of Cop 1, a synthetic polypeptide, on chronic relapsing experimental allergic encephalomyelitis in guinea pigs. J Neurol Sci 42:267–274

Kurtzke JF (1983) Rating neurological impairment in multiple sclerosis: An expanded disability status scale (EDSS). Neurology 33:1444–1452

Lando Z, Teitelbaum D, Arnon R (1979) Effect of cyclophosphamide on suppressor cell activity in mice unresponsive to EAE. J Immunol 123:2156–2160

Paterson PY (1977) Autoimmune neurologic disease: Experimental animal systems and implications for multiple sclerosis. In: Talmage N (ed) Autoimmunity: Genetic, immunologic, virologic and clinical aspects. Academic Press, New York, pp 643–692

Paterson PY (1978) The demyelinating diseases: Clinical and experimental studies in animals and man. In: Samter M, Alexander N, Rose B, Sherman WB, Talmage DW, Vaughn JH (eds) Immunologic diseases, 3rd edn. Little, Brown and Company, Boston, pp 1400–1435

Paterson PY (1979) Neurological disorders. In: WJ Irvine (ed) Medical immunology. Teviot Scientific Publications, Edinburgh, pp 361–381

Paterson PY (1980) The immunopathology of experimental allergic encephalomyelitis. In: Davison AN, Cuzner MC (eds) The suppression of experimental allergic encephalomyelitis in multiple sclerosis. Academic Press, New York, pp 11–30

Poser CM, Patty DW, Scheinberg L et al. (1983) New diagnostic criteria for multiple sclerosis: Guidelines for research protocols. Ann Neurol 13:227–231

Raine CS, Bornstein MB (1970) Experimental allergic encephalomyelitis. A light and electron microscope study of remyelination and "sclerosis" in vitro. J Neuropath Exp Neurol 29:552–574

Raine CS, Bornstein MB (1979) Experimental allergic neuritis ultrastructure of serum-induced myelin aberrations in PNS cultures. Lab Invest 40:423–432

Teitelbaum D, Meshorer A, Hirshfeld T et al. (1971) Suppression of experimental allergic encephalomyelitis by a synthetic polypeptide. Eur J Immunol 1:242–248

Teitelbaum D, Webb C, Meshorer A et al. (1973) Suppression by synthetic polypeptides of experimental allergic encephalomyelitis induced in guinea pigs and rabbits with bovine and human basic encephalitogen. Eur J Immunol 3:273–279

Teitelbaum D, Webb C, Bree M et al. (1974) Suppression of experimental allergic encephalomyelitis in rhesus monkeys by a synthetic basic copolymer. Clin Immunol Immunopathol 3:256–262

Webb C, Teitelbaum D, Arnon R et al. (1973) In vivo and in vitro immunological cross-reactions between basic encephalitogen and synthetic basic polypeptides capable of suppressing experimental allergic encephalomyelitis. Eur J Immunol 3:279–286

Webb C, Teitelbaum D, Herz A et al. (1976) Molecular requirements involved in suppression of EAE by synthetic basic copolymers of amino acids. Immunochemistry 13:333–337

Chapter 9

Treatment of Multiple Sclerosis with Cyclophosphamide

Glenn A. Mackin, David M. Dawson, David A. Hafler and Howard L. Weiner

Introduction

Multiple sclerosis (MS) is an inflammatory disease of the central nervous system of presumed autoimmune etiology. A number of immune abnormalities have been described in the disease including loss of suppressor influences and activated T- and B-cells both in the central nervous system and the periphery (Hafler and Weiner 1989). The majority of immunotherapeutic approaches studied over the past 20 years have been designed to suppress the immune system in MS. This has included attempts at both antigen-specific and antigen non-specific suppression (Weiner and Hafler 1988).

Of all the non-specific immunosuppressants studied, cyclophosphamide in combination with some form of corticosteroid has been reported to be one of the more effective drugs in slowing or altering the progression of MS although not all studies have found cyclophosphamide to be effective. Cyclophosphamide has found usefulness for the treatment of other non-malignant inflammatory or autoimmune disease states including minimal change nephrotic syndrome, lupus nephritis, Wegener's granulomatosis, and polyarteritis. The use of periodic intravenous boluses of cyclophosphamide for the treatment of lupus nephritis (Balow et al. 1987) has provided the basis for the periodic intravenous pulse programs that have recently been used in MS. This review will critically assess clinical trials of cyclophosphamide in MS, their implications for the use of immunosuppression to treat the disease, and current status and future directions for the use of cyclophosphamide to treat MS (Table 9.1).

Pharmacology

Cyclophosphamide is a well-known alkylating agent whose principal action is to crosslink DNA. Active metabolites preferentially kill rapidly dividing cells including lymphocytes, certain malignant cells, urothelial, follicular granulosa and scalp hair follicle cells. These actions account for many of the toxicities of cyclophosphamide such as leukopenia, hemorrhagic cystitis, amenorrhea, oligospermia, and transient alopecia. Nausea and vomiting are probably secondary to drug interaction with central nervous system receptors. The primary long-term risks of cyclophosphamide relate to carcinoma of the bladder and

Table 9.1. Studies of cyclophosphamide in multiple sclerosis

Year	Authors	Study size	Follow-up (years)	Comments
1966	Aimard et al.	1	1	First reported use of cyclophosphamide in MS
1967	Girard et al.	30	2	IV cyclophosphamide, 200 mg daily for 4–6 weeks for a total of 4–9 g. Stabilization for 2 years in uncontrolled study
1969	Millac and Miller	16	1	Oral cyclophosphamide, 75–150 mg daily for one year. Unacceptable side effects. No positive effect
1973	Cendrowski	23	1.5	Hydrocortisone plus cyclophosphamide. No positive effects observed
1975	Drachman	6	1 month	IV cyclophosphamide, 4–5 mg/kg (350 mg) daily for 10 days in acute MS, no effects observed
1975–80	Hommes et al.	39	1–5	Oral cyclophosphamide, 400 mg daily plus 100 mg prednisone to induce leukopenia, then retreated for total dose of 8 g. Chronic/progressive MS. Two-thirds of patients stabilized. Unblinded, uncontrolled
1977–80	Gonsette et al.	140	2–10	IV cyclophosphamide to reduce WBC to 1000–2000 for 2 weeks. Relapsing/remitting MS. 75% reduction in relapses. Unblinded, historical controls
1981	Theys et al.	21	2	Regimen of Gonsette and Hommes. Retrospective analysis of 21 patients compared with 21 untreated patients showed no effect
1983	Hauser et al.	58	1	IV cyclophosphamide plus ACTH in progressive MS. 75% stabilization compared to ACTH group in randomized, controlled study
1987	Myers et al.	14	1	Open trial of IV cyclophosphamide pulses designed to affect immune function. 12 of 14 patients stable at 1 year. Adverse side effects reported
1987	Goodkin et al.	51	2	Use of induction plus maintenance boosters. Stabilization in 59% vs. 17% in non-randomized controls. Suggestion that boosters slow progression
1988	Killian et al.	14	1	Double-blind study of monthly IV pulses in relapsing/remitting MS. Decrease in number of attacks
1988	Carter et al.	164	3–5	Unblinded, uncontrolled report of 6 years experience. Reprogression in stabilized patients between 9 and 30 months. No major toxicities with treatment or retreatment

Table 9.1. (Continued)

Year	Authors	Study size	Follow-up (years)	Comments
1988	Likosky	44	1–2	Single-blinded trial in progressive MS. No effect observed. Steroids not used with cyclophosphamide. Placebo group without progression. Final report not yet published
1989	Mauch et al.	21	1	Intravenous low dose cyclophosphamide slows progression. Non-blinded. Non-randomized controls
1990	Noseworthy et al.	168	2	Canadian trial. Single-blind, placebo-controlled study in progressive MS. No boosters given. 75% stabilization in placebo group at 1 year using less sensitive outcome measures than previous trials in progressive MS
1991	Mackin et al.	214	3	Northeast Treatment Group. Single-blind controlled trial in progressive MS. Every 2 month boosters of cyclophosphamide slow progression.

hematologic malignancies. Orally administered cyclophosphamide is relatively well-absorbed with more than 75% bioavailable. The dosage of cyclophosphamide is limited by myelosuppression and excretion is primarily renal. Although cyclophosphamide does not cross the intact blood–brain barrier, unmetabolized drug was found in high concentrations in the cerebrospinal fluid (CSF) (80% of serum levels) in two MS patients treated orally with 400 mg daily for 3 weeks (Bahr et al. 1980). Lamers et al. (1988) showed a significant reduction of elevated CSF levels of myelin basic protein and immunoglobulin G (IgG) in chronic progressive MS patients treated with a similar regimen, indicating an effect on local CNS immunologic processes. These results suggest that in MS active metabolites gain access to the CNS through an abnormally permeable blood–brain barrier.

Early Studies

In 1966, Aimard et al. (1966) described a patient with progressive MS treated with IV cyclophosphamide, who sustained improvement for one year. The following year, Girard et al. (1967) reported their group's experience with 30 patients in an uncontrolled trial. Thirty patients were treated with intravenous (IV) cyclophosphamide (200 mg daily for 4–6 weeks, for a total of 4–9 g). After 2 years, all patients remained stable or improved, and there was an indication that the best responders may have been those who achieved the most profound leukopenia.

The first trial of oral cyclophosphamide in MS was reported by Millac and Miller (1969). Oral cyclophosphamide was administered daily to 16 ambulatory patients with relapsing MS, half of whom completed 1 year. Treated patients were reportedly matched with untreated MS controls by age, sex, and Disability Status Scores (DSS). The only reference to disease activity in the pretreatment year is that relapses had occurred in 5 of the 8 who were subsequently treated, versus only 2 controls. Outcome measures were number of relapses and DSS. The initial plan was to administer enough cyclophosphamide to maintain total white blood cell count (WBC) at about $2000/mm^3$, but the complication rate was deemed unacceptable. Target WBC was raised to $3000/mm^3$, and achieved with doses of 75–150 mg. Seven patients withdrew because of adverse effects including infection, hemorrhagic cystitis, generalized rash and severe nausea. The number of relapses did not differ between the 8 treated for 1 year and their untreated counterparts.

In 1973, Cendrowski treated 23 patients with hydrocortisone plus cyclophosphamide or cytosine arabinoside. Controls consisted of a retrospective group treated only with steroids. No significant benefit was observed. In 1975, Drachman treated 6 patients at the onset of acute attacks with a 10-day course of IV cyclophosphamide. No positive effects were observed at 1 month following therapy.

In one of the most important early studies, Hommes et al. (1975, 1980a) treated 39 consecutive patients with chronic progressive MS, with an induction consisting of high-dose oral cyclophosphamide and prednisone. The study was uncontrolled and results of unblinded evaluations averaging 2.5 years follow-up were reported in 1980. Quantitative CSF and serum immunoglobulins were measured on the final 32 patients entered. Patients received oral high-dose cyclophosphamide to a total of 8 g over 3–4 weeks, with concurrent prednisone 100 mg daily until cyclophosphamide was stopped, tapered by 5 mg daily for 3 weeks.

Cyclophosphamide was administered in two phases, initially 100 mg orally four times daily until the WBC was less than $2000/mm^3$, usually at approximately 2 weeks, held approximately 4–6 days until the WBC recovered to greater than $4000/mm^3$, then given until a total of 8 g were reached in all patients. The entire cyclophosphamide induction required 3–4 weeks, during which lymphopenia was maintained.

Thirteen patients were improved with a DSS decrease of one or more points, 14 were stable, and 12 were worse for an overall response rate of 69%, at a mean follow-up of 2.5 years (range 1–5 years). Three patients were retreated for progression during the course of the study. Patients with improved DSS differed significantly ($p = 0.05$) from those who worsened by being younger at treatment (34.1 vs. 40.9 years), and by having a shorter duration of disease before treatment (5.7 vs. 10.2 years). Patients with a clinical course at pretreatment judged to be malignant were evenly divided between the improved, stable, and worsened groups. Responders showed an abrupt change in clincal course coinciding with treatment.

Hommes concluded that predictors of good response include early onset of disease (mean 28 years) short duration of disease prior to immunosuppression, rapid progression, relatively low initial neurological impairment, improvement during treatment, HLA–DRw2 histocompatability type, and inhibition of CSF IgG synthesis for 3 months or more relative to serum (Hommes et al. 1980b)

The investigators felt they had demonstrated a significant modification of expected progression in terms of published concepts of natural history, which held that improvement is unlikely once the pattern of chronic progressive MS is established.

Gonsette et al. (1977, 1980) reported on a 2–10-year follow-up of 134 patients with frequent relapses, treated as in-patients with high-dose IV cyclophosphamide but no steroids. Primary outcome measures were change in annual relapse rate comparing 2 years after treatment with the 2 preceding years, and length of stabilization compared with pretreatment clinical tempo. The specific dosage regimen was not given, but a quantity was given sufficient to achieve immunosuppression within 1–2 weeks, and to maintain leukopenia $<2000/mm^3$ and lymphopenia $<1000/mm^3$, each for 2–3 weeks. Disability status scores were not assigned. Treated patients were their own controls. The investigators were concerned about the tendency of relapse rates to diminish with time, and referred to a 50% reduction of annual relapse rate in a nonrandomized, untreated comparison group of 91 relapsing patients derived from the outpatient clinic population.

Two years after treatment, there was a 66%–87% decrease in the annual relapse rate, most dramatic in patients with disease durations of 1–5 years, with less of an effect in patients with disease duration of 5–10 years. Mean stabilization interval was 2–3 years. Treatment was ineffective for patients with disease durations more than 10 years, and those already severely handicapped prior to treatment. Approximately 30% did not respond and neurological signs improved in 60%. Side effects were well-controlled, including frequent nausea and vomiting, uniformly reversible hair loss, and infrequent cystitis. No disease exacerbations occurred during treatment. There was no correlation between clinical response and leukopenia or lymphopenia, or on IgG synthesis rates before and after treatment. Predictors of response were not identified, beyond the tendency of patients with shorter durations of relapsing disease to show greater stabilization.

In 1981, Theys et al. reported no significant effect on disability progression, based upon a retrospective analysis of 21 MS patients treated with high-dose cyclophosphamide induction, paired retrospectively with 21 untreated patients. The 42 subjects were selected from among 75 records (of 440 hospital charts reviewed), in which sufficiently regular follow-up disability ratings were recorded for a period of 2 years. Treated patients received a total of 6–8 g of cyclophosphamide over 3–4 weeks, either according to the oral regimen with prednisone of Hommes (Hommes et al. 1975; Hommes et al. 1980a), or the IV regimen without steroids of Gonsette (Gonsette et al. 1977, 1980), and many of the patients in Theys' analysis were reported by Gonsette.

Boston Studies (1983–1991)

In 1983, Hauser et al. reported the first randomized, controlled MS trial designed to confirm the efficacy of short-term intensive immunosuppression with cyclophosphamide plus steroids in severe progressive MS, as suggested primarily by the uncontrolled studies of Hommes et al. (1975) and Gonsette et al. (1977). Three groups were studied. Group 1 (20 patients) received inpatient treatment with synthetic IV ACTH followed by IM ACTH. Group 2 (20 patients) received inpatient treatment with IV cyclophosphamide (400–500 mg daily divided as qid for 10–14 consecutive days, until WBC fell to 4000/mm^3), and ACTH as in Group 1. Group 3 (18 patients) received plasma exchange (4 or 5 exchanges of 1–1.5 plasma volumes, over 2 weeks), oral cyclophosphamide (2 mg/kg daily for 8 weeks, reduced if WBC fell below 4000/mm^3), and ACTH as in Group 1. No group received maintenance booster treatments. The ACTH group served as the control and a new synthetic ACTH was used so patients in this group did not feel they were receiving a treatment that had not helped them in the past.

Evaluations were performed at 6 and 12 months by an unblinded evaluating neurologist for each patient. ACTH was given with cyclophosphamide based on Hommes' use of prednisone. The nature of the treatments, alopecia with cyclophosphamide and the plasma exchange regimen, were too obvious to permit blinding of patient or evaluating neurologists. An ambulation index (AI) was specifically designed for the study to quantitate gait changes and worsening or improvement was defined as a one point change in the DSS or AI.

In group 2, a leukopenia was achieved with a mean WBC nadir of 1800 ± 200/mm^3, and with 55% of these patients below 1600/mm^3, and 15% in the 600–900/mm^3 range. The WBC nadir was reached within 3–5 days of the final cyclophosphamide dose and generally normalized 1 week after nadir. Peripheral blood lymphocyte counts fell a mean of 89% from pretreatment levels to a mean of 213 ± 42/mm^3. There were no infections or febrile episodes during periods of cyclophosphamide-induced leukopenia. IV cyclophophamide induction using this regimen resulted in complete scalp alopecia lasting 4–6 months.

The results showed that in the ACTH group the number of patients stabilized or improved was 8 of 20 at 6 months and 4 of 20 at 1 year; in the IV cyclophosphamide/ACTH group, 18 of 20 at 6 months and 16 of 20 at 1 year; and in the plasma exchange group, 11 of 18 at 6 months and 9 of 18 at 1 year. Physician assessment of stabilization was slightly lower, with 70% of IV cyclophosphamide/ACTH stabilized, versus 10% in the ACTH and 44% of the plasma exchange groups. This discrepancy probably reflects worsening apparent to an evaluating neurologist not reflected in the DSS or AI. Recurrent disease progression in the second year after induction with cyclophosphamide/ACTH occurred in most responders, indicating a short-term benefit without additional treatment. The rate of progression in the ACTH control group is greater than that reported in other trials of progressive MS, probably because a young, very actively progressive subcategory of patients were treated.

Subsequently, Carter et al. (1988) reported on the Boston cumulative 6-year experience in treating 164 patients with high-dose IV cyclophosphamide/ACTH as published in the 1983 study. The report was not a randomized trial and did not involve blinded evaluation but served to provide information on complications of therapy, response to subsequent course of treatment and factors which might predict responders. The major finding was the documentation of reprogression following initial treatment. Virtually all patients began reprogressing by 30 months following treatment. With continued follow-up of those patients who initially responded to treatment with improvement or sta-

Table 9.2. Northeast Cooperative Multiple Sclerosis Treatment Group

	Induction regimen	Maintenance therapy
Group 1	Published[a]	None
Group 2	Published[a]	Yes[c]
Group 3	Modified[b]	None
Group 4	Modified[b]	Yes[c]

[a] 500 mg cyclophosphamide per day in four divided doses for 10 to 14 days; IV ACTH.
[b] 600 mg/m^2 IV cyclophosphamide given in one dose on days 1, 2, 4, 6, and 8; IM ACTH.
[c] 700 mg/m^2 IV cyclophosphamide once every 2 months for 2 years.

bilization, 69% showed evidence of reprogression by 2 years after treatment. The mean time to reprogression was 17.6 months with most patients showing reprogression between 9 and 30 months. In addition, younger patients tended to respond better to treatment. There were no major complications of therapy apart from infections requiring antibiotics in 1%–3% of patients.

Following publication of the 1983 study, the Northeast Cooperative Treatment Group was formed to further investigate use of cyclophosphamide in multiple sclerosis. Two questions were addressed by the group. First, could an alternate induction regimen that was more simple and in which cyclophosphamide was given on a mg/m^2 basis be as effective as the published regimen, and most important, could periodic outpatient booster therapy affect reprogression. For induction, patients were given 600 mg/m^2 intravenously on days 1, 2, 4, 6, and 8 plus IM ACTH which, in pilot studies, had analogous effects on lowering the WBC as the published regimen. This was compared to the published regimen (Hauser et al. 1983) which involved 4 daily infusions of cyclophosphamide and careful monitoring of white blood count to determine when drugs should be discontinued. Outpatient therapy consisted of 700 mg/m^2 intravenously given every 2 months (Table 9.2). The study was single blinded, did not contain a placebo-treated group and involved a total of 256 patients. The results of the study are now available, and although the final results have not yet undergone peer review and publication, the results as presented at the American Academy of Neurology meetings demonstrate that every 2 month booster therapy significantly slows progression as measured at 24 and 30 months (Mackin et al. 1991). No differences were observed between the published and the modified induction regimen. The overall response rate at 1 year of the patients receiving induction only was less than that found in the 1983 study involving 20 cyclophosphamide/ACTH-treated patients and closer to that subsequently reported by Goodkin (Goodkin et al. 1987). Subgroup analysis suggests that patients with relapsing/remitting progressive MS responded better than patients with chronic/progressive MS from the onset. Most dramatic was the finding that older patients did not respond as well as younger patients. For example, in one subgroup-analysis at 30 months 40%–49% of booster-treated patients under 40 were stable whereas only 14%–17% were stable in the over-40 population. Of note is that the average age of patients in the Hauser et al. (1983) study was 30 and in the Northeast Treatment Group was 40. Based on these results, a new treatment program involving more intensive booster therapy is being studied. This program involves induction therapy with cyclophosphamide/ACTH or methylprednisolone followed by a 3-year program of out-patient boosters. Patients receive monthly infusions of cyclophosphamide plus methylprednisolone for 1 year in dosages designed to produce a leukopenia. These treatments are then tapered to every 6 weeks in the second year and every 2 months in the third year. Other patients receive treatment solely with methylprednisolone both as induction and maintenance or cyclophosphamide induction followed by methylprednisolone boosters. The degree to which higher doses will be tolerated by patients and the degree to which high-dose methylprednisolone will be as efficacious as cyclophosphamide remains to be determined. The implications of the over 10 years of work from the Boston group and the Northeast Cooperative Treatment Group is that intermittent outpatient therapy with cyclophosphamide in an analogous fashion to that which has been used with lupus nephritis appears to be the most efficacious way to administer the drug in an attempt to maintain stabilization. Furthermore, younger, actively progressive patients respond better to therapy.

Studies Subsequent to the 1983 Boston Report

In 1987, Myers et al. and Mickey et al. reported results of a preliminary, open, uncontrolled trial of IV cyclophosphamide pulses in chronic progressive MS. Their aims were to use clinical response and immune parameters as guides to monthly dosing of escalating-dose cyclophosphamide treatments. Only 14 patients were treated, as the investigators regarded their method as an efficient way to establish optimum dose and treatment duration without requiring a large number of patients. The investigators felt that low-dose oral cyclophosphamide was too toxic and insufficiently effective in published series. They postulated that changes in peripheral B-cell and helper T-cell populations might be helpful in directing IV therapy, and that changes in helper/suppressor ratios might predict outcome. Patients were begun on 600–800 mg/m^2 doses which were increased by 200 mg/m^2 increments. Although 12 of 14 patients had improved or stabilized by DSS at one year, and correlations existed between rising relative CD8 (suppressor/cytotoxic) and decreasing CD4 (helper) populations and improvements on the standard neurologic examination, these investigators reported what they interpreted as a prohibitively high rate of adverse side effects. In summary, these studies investigate the approach of intermittent IV pulses similar to lupus nephritis studies and that studied by the Northeast Cooperative MS Treatment Group. There is a suggestion of efficacy in this uncontrolled trial.

In 1987, Goodkin et al. reported on the treatment of 27 progressive patients with high-dose IV cyclophosphamide and steroids, and compared them with 24 nonrandomized controls over 2 years, asking three questions. First, does IV cyclophosphamide induction favorably modify disease course as measured by expanded disability status scale (EDSS), functional systems, ambulation index, and an upper extremity index consisting of the 9-Hole Peg Test? Second, is there any difference in efficacy or safety of inpatient versus less-costly outpatient induction? Third, can alternate-month IV cyclophosphamide maintenance treatment extend duration of stabilization or improvement?

All eligible patients were offered treatment, and those that declined became the nonrandomized control group. Those who accepted were randomized between "maintenance" and "non-maintenance" treatment groups. Inpatient induction consisted of IV cyclophosphamide/ACTH using an identical regimen to the 1983 Boston study. Outpatient induction consisted of IV cyclophosphamide (700 mg/m^2 once weekly for 6 weeks) and oral prednisone (daily for 3 weeks, tapering from initial 60 mg). Outpatient maintenance consisted of IV cyclophosphamide at 700 mg/m^2 every other month in a fashion analogous to the Northeast Cooperative Treatment Group.

For treated patients, mean age was 43.8 years, mean duration of disease 5.6 years, mean EDSS 6.33 (vs. 5.71 for controls), and mean AI 5.30 (vs. 5.13 for controls). However, the treated group may have been skewed toward more disabled – and therefore perhaps less likely to progress – patients, since only 1 of 27 treated versus 7 of 24 untreated controls did not require support to ambulate (i.e., EDSS < 6) prior to treatment.

At 12 months, a statistically significant difference in stabilization rates favored cyclophosphamide/ACTH-treated patients over controls (59% vs. 17%), which persisted through 24 months (33% vs. 4%). Treatment outcome was similar for inpatient and outpatient induction. A trend favoring the cyclophosphamide maintenance over non-maintenance was observed between 12 and 24 months, but was not statistically significant. There were no major complications, and no acute exacerbations during or shortly after treatments. Complete scalp alopecia occurred after induction in 100% of inpatients and 71% of outpatients, but not after outpatient maintenance. Nausea and vomiting, at times resistant to varied anti-emetic regimens, occurred in the majority of patients and raised the question of the feasibility of long-term outpatient maintenance therapy. In summary, this study found significant short-term benefits after induction with IV cyclophosphamide/ACTH, the potential for significant cost savings via outpatient treatment, and a trend suggesting but not proving maintenance therapy may extend short-term stabilization.

In 1988, Killian et al. reported on a pilot double-blind trial of monthly intravenous cyclophosphamide pulses in 14 patients with relapsing/remitting MS. Eight patients received placebo and 6 patients received cyclophosphamide. The authors had previously found clinical benefit in an uncontrolled pilot study using monthly IV cyclophosphamide therapy. Cyclophosphamide was given at a dose of 750 mg/m^2. No sustained leukopenia was noted in any of the patients. The cyclophosphamide-treated group showed a definite trend to have less frequent and less pronounced episodes than the placebo group, with a mean number of attacks of 2.3 ± 0.6 vs. 0.5 ± 0.2. Because of the small number of patients, these results were not significant ($p = 0.06$) although a statistically significant result was obtained when all treated patients were compared to pretreatment exacerbation rates and compared to the placebo group. These results suggest that monthly intravenous doses of cyclophosphamide may influence the frequency and duration of episodes of relapsing/remitting MS.

Likosky and a 13-center California Kaiser-Permanente group (Likosky 1988) undertook to confirm the basic premise that high-dose cyclophosphamide could favorably alter the course of chronic progressive MS, as reported by Hauser et al. (1983). Forty-four patients with progressive MS were randomized to receive outpatient IV cyclophosphamide without steroids (400–500 mg 5 times weekly, until WBC was below 4000/mm^3), or IV folic acid (1 mg, 5 times weekly for 2 weeks) in a single-blinded study.

Preliminary data, with results at 12 months, were reported in a 1988 symposium; a final peer-reviewed report has not yet been published. For cyclophosphamide-treated patients, mean age was 43.9, mean years since onset 9.6 years, and mean DSS 5.6. Initial data give the mean total cyclophosphamide dose as 4.8 g, and mean leukocyte nadir as $2045/mm^3$. The study found no difference between treated and control groups at 12 months. A major difference between the Kaiser study and those of investigators who reported a positive effect (Hommes et al. 1975, 1980a; Hauser et al. 1983; Goodkin et al. 1987) was that steroids were not given with the cyclophosphamide, and cyclophosphamide was given in a different dosage schedule. Although ACTH or prednisone alone does not appear to affect the course of progressive MS, steroids are frequently given with cytotoxic agents because of synergistic effects, and in the case of MS may lead to larger doses of cyclophosphamide administered due to elevated white blood counts.

Furthermore, eligibility criteria allowed for inclusion of patients with relapsing/progressive MS, not just chronic progressive, and 70% stabilization at 12 months was observed in folate-treated controls. The Kaiser study reported minimal adverse effects of outpatient IV cyclophosphamide given without steroids for induction of immunosuppression as compared to Goodkin et al. (1987) and Myers et al. (1987), perhaps because lower doses were given.

Mauch et al. in 1989, reported on the treatment of 21 MS patients with chronic progressive MS in which cyclophosphamide (8 mg per kg) was given intravenously at intervals of 4 days until the lymphocyte count was reduced to half the initial value, but not below 1000. The total dose averaged 1.9 g per patient. The control group consisted of 21 patients with progressive MS who received treatment with ACTH or cortisone. The study was not randomized. The authors report 20 out of 21 patients stabilized at 1 year whereas 14 out of 21 were worse in the control group. In reporting on 109 patients treated with cyclophosphamide with relapsing course, the authors find a longer stabilizing effect with cyclophosphamide as opposed to cortisone. The authors propose that since 2 g cyclophosphamide treatment per patient is needed, and that patients begin to deteriorate after 1 year, they advise spacing treatments at intervals of 9 months. The authors also report combining cyclophosphamide treatment with short high-dose methylprednisolone therapy.

Canadian Cooperative Multiple Sclerosis Study

In 1991 the results of the Canadian Cooperative Multiple Sclerosis Study were reported. Because the Canadian study is the only placebo-controlled trial of cyclophosphamide plus corticosteroids in progressive MS, and because of the rigorous manner in which it was performed, it deserves detailed analysis.

In the 9-center single blind trial, 168 patients with progressive MS were randomized into 3 groups to receive either high-dose IV cyclophosphamide and prednisone, oral cyclophosphamide and prednisone with plasma exchange, or two oral placebos with sham plasma exchange. Blinded evaluations were performed every 6 months for 2 years. Eligibility criteria included clinically or laboratory-supported definite MS, pretreatment EDSS 4.0–6.5 and progressive disease defined as a 1.0-point, 2-step increase in the EDSS during the preceding 12 months. Patients were excluded if previously treated with immunosuppressants, or if treated with steroids within 1 month prior to entry. Groups were well matched as to age and pretreatment mean EDSS (approximately 5.7).

Patients in Group 1 received inpatient treatment with IV cyclophosphamide (1 g every other day until WBC fell below 2000/mm^3, an average of 5 g), and oral prednisone (40 mg for 16 days). Group 2 patients received outpatient treatment with oral cyclophosphamide (1.5–2.0 mg/kg daily for 22 weeks, with target WBC 4000–5000/mm^3), oral prednisone (given alternate days for 22 weeks, tapering from 20 mg initially), and plasma exchange (one plasma volume weekly for 20 weeks). Group 3 patients received outpatient treatment, given exactly as in Group 2, consisting of two oral placebo preparations and sham plasma exchanges. After initial treatment, none of the groups received maintenance booster treatments. However, individual patients who worsened could receive methylprednisolone, prednisone or ACTH. Worsening or improvement was defined as an increase in EDSS by at least 1.0 point (2 steps), sustained 6 months or more, and documented by two independent examiners blinded to treatment group and prior EDSS. In a separately published paper, these investigators examined the degree of interrater variability applying both EDSS and Functional Systems (FS) scores to all 168 patients, and recommended that "at least a 2-step change (1.0 point on the EDSS and 2 points on the FS) was needed to be confident of an important change in the degree of disability or response to treatment in this disease." (Noseworthy et al. 1990).

Blinding of the evaluating neurologists was ensured by requiring that all patients wear head coverings at the 6-month point to conceal alopecia, and to wear forearm bandages to conceal plasma exchange venipuncture sites. Double-blinding was feasible only for patients in Groups 2 and 3 because of alopecia noticeable in 75% of patients after treatment with high-dose IV cyclophosphamide. No significant differences were observed between the two active treatment groups and the placebo group as to percent treatment failures, mean time to treatment failure and proportions of patients stabilized or improved at each evaluation point.

Despite the merits of the study, the results of the Canadian study should be viewed with caution, as a number of limitations exist in study design and interpretation that do not allow extension of the Canadian findings to the MS population at large and make direct comparison to other studies difficult. Furthermore, the study did not investigate the effectiveness of periodic retreatment, which has now become a central question in the immunosuppressive treatment of progressive MS. Finally, on careful review of the Canadian study, it appears that an effect was in fact seen at 12 months in the treated groups as compared to the placebo control.

The primary outcome measure employed was insensitive to changes in the disease process. At 1 year following therapy approximately 75% of patients were stabilized or improved in the placebo-treated group and at 2 years 67% were stabilized. Although a component of this stabilization could be related to a placebo effect, a major component may well be due to the outcome measures chosen for the study. The authors required a 2-step change in the Expanded Disability Status Scale (EDSS) to define improvement or worsening. A 2-step change is insensitive for studying progressive MS, especially in the range of

6.0–7.0, an area of the scale that is especially crucial for progressive patients. One-step drops in this range are dramatic: 6.0 (intermittent or constant unilateral assistance required to walk 100 meters); 6.5 (constant bilateral assistance required to walk 20 meters; 7.0 (essentially restricted to wheelchair). The average disability of patients on entry to the Canadian trial was approximately 6 (5.79 ± 0.6) for cyclophosphamide and placebo groups. Thus a patient who entered the Canadian trial using a cane and who then progressed to using a walker, or who progressed from a walker at entry to a wheelchair would be classified as "stable". Of note is that other major trials of immunosuppression in progressive MS defined worsening as one step (0.5 points) on the EDSS or the Ambulation Index. For example, in the placebo group in the double-blind cooperative cyclosporine trial of progressive MS involving 557 patients (274 in the placebo group), 52% had worsened at 1 year and 78% had worsened at 24 months vs. 25% and 33% in the Canadian study (The Multiple Sclerosis Study Group 1990).

The authors argue that 2 steps are required to measure progression on the EDSS because of interrater variability (Noseworthy et al. 1990). While this may be true in the lower EDSS range and is an outcome measure we are utilizing in our double-blind trial of oral tolerization to myelin antigens, it is of limited use for the assessment of progressive MS in the 6.0 to 7.0 range. Furthermore, for reasons that are not clear, there was a marked difference between the evaluating neurologist and monitoring neurologist in assessing patients in this range in the Canadian study. Specifically, of 35 patients found to be wheelchair-bound (EDSS = 7) by the monitoring neurologist, the evaluating neurologist agreed only 14 times, and classified 17 of these 35 patients as requiring only bilateral supports (EDSS = 6.5) (Noseworthy et al. 1990). These results are puzzling since the authors state that in most instances the monitoring and evaluating neurologist observed the patients' gaits simultaneously. One patient was classified by the monitoring neurologist as restricted to a wheelchair and by the evaluating neurologist as able to walk 100 meters with intermittent or constant unilateral support. Such discrepancies should be resolved clinically through more carefully stated criteria if necessary, but not through desensitizing changes in the EDSS scale, especially if the authors wish to compare their results to other trials. It would not seem logical to use different outcome measures when attempting to replicate other trials.

It has become clear that certain categories of patients respond better than others to immunosuppression with cyclophosphamide plus steroids. In the Canadian study, 60% of the cyclophosphamide-treated group, and more than 50% of the study group as a whole, suffered from a purely progressive illness unaccompanied by relapses. Purely progressive MS may represent a distinct subcategory of the disease with different underlying biologic features (Thompson et al. 1990, 1991; Olerup et al. 1989) and be more refractory to immunosuppressive treatment than the relapsing/progressive form. Even more important, it now appears that age is linked to a positive response. The average age of the patients studied in the Canadian trial was 40 whereas that in the 1983 Boston study was 30. Subgroup analysis of the Northeast Cooperative Treatment Group shows a marked difference in response between those who were 40 years old or older as compared to younger patients, a finding consistent with previous work of Hommes (Hommes et al. 1980b) and Gonsette et al. (1980).

The Canadian study employed a different cyclophosphamide-plus-steroids treatment regimen than had been used in earlier studies, making direct comparisons difficult. In addition, the dose of cyclophosphamide might not have been sufficient. The dose of cyclophosphamide chosen was one that the authors state would result in a nadir WBC of $1-2 \times 10^9/l$, yet the authors report that 20% of the cyclophosphamide-treated patients (11/55) did not achieve a target white blood count of less than $2.0 \times 10^9/l$. Also, it is not clear why severe alopecia developed in 16% of placebo patients.

The above limitations notwithstanding, the Canadian study did show a trend in favor of both the cyclophosphamide and plasma exchange study groups at the 6- and 12-month time points. At 6 months, 17% of placebo patients worsened vs. 6% of cyclophosphamide-treated patients, and at 12 months, 25% vs. 15%. No beneficial effect was present at the 18–30 month examination points. Furthermore, at 12 months, if one combines the two immunosuppressive treatment arms (cyclophosphamide/prednisone and plasma exchange/ cyclophosphamide/prednisone) and compares them to the placebo arm, the results show an almost statistically significant effect in favor of immunosuppression ($p = 0.058$; chi square analysis). Thus, our interpretation of the Canadian study is that it actually supports the hypothesis that a short course of intensive non-specific immunosuppression temporarily slows disease progression.

An important caution related to the Canadian study is that it does not address what now appears to be the most crucial issue for the treatment of progressive MS: the need for periodic retreatment or maintenance therapy. In our original description of the effects of short-term cyclophosphamide therapy in progressive MS, we reported that disease stabilization was transient, and that reprogression of disease was present in the majority of patients followed beyond 12 months post-therapy (Hauser et al. 1983). We hypothesized that periodic retreatment or chronic immunosuppression may be required to maintain stabilization, but that the efficacy and toxicity of such regimens were not known. Determination of the efficacy of booster treatment awaits final publication of the results of the Northeast Cooperative Treatment Group and assessment by the neurologic community.

Except for the Canadian trial, all previous studies of cyclophosphamide plus corticosteroids suffer from the lack of a placebo-control group. Given the side effects of the drug and the doses which must be given, it is difficult to design truly blinded placebo-controlled trials. The Canadian study was fortunate in having a true and placebo plasma exchange arm allowing a major intervention to be given as part of the placebo treatment. However, on careful analysis, the placebo group was not "untreated". The placebo group received 22 weekly "sham" exchanges. Repeated stimulation of endogenous corticoid secretion may have occurred due to volume change or stress and some patients were treated with steroids. Because the placebo group was not truly untreated, the results of the placebo regimen raise the question of whether periodic steroid therapy may be of benefit. In this regard, our current studies of cyclophosphamide induction and booster therapy in progressive MS utilize a steroid-only treated control group.

In summary, the Canadian study raises important and appropriate cautions against the unselective use of cyclophosphamide plus steroids in MS. The Canadian results however do not lead to the conclusion that nonspecific immunosuppression is not beneficial in multiple sclerosis. The Canadian study investigated whether 5–9 treatments given every other day for approximately 2 weeks could affect progressive MS over a 30-month period and did, in fact, support a benefit at 12 months as others have reported. (Weiner et al. 1991)

Side Effects and Toxicities

The two major limiting toxicities for the use of cyclophosphamide in patients with multiple sclerosis are those of effects on fertility and increased risk for malignancies. Multiple sclerosis affects young people during their reproductive years and a treatment that affects fertility is unacceptable. Other side effects relate to morbidity and might be acceptable were the treatment to be effective in early stages of the disease. Bladder toxicity is relatively well-controlled with intravenous infusions and hydration, and a modest risk of infection and nausea and vomiting can generally be controlled with anti-emetics and antibiotics. To our knowledge there have been no reports of leukemias in patients treated with pulse cyclophosphamide either in multiple sclerosis or lupus nephritis. Nonetheless even though cyclophosphamide has been cited by Kaldor as substantially less leukemogenic than other alkylating agents (Kaldor et al. 1990), the risk of such leukemogenic effects are real and one would expect late-developing leukemias to be observed if patients are followed long enough and enough patients are treated with cyclophosphamide.

Immunologic Effects of Cyclophosphamide

The immunologic effects of cyclophosphamide are well known and involve decrease of B- and T-cells with more pronounced effect on B-cell function. In animals, low dose cyclophosphamide has been shown to reduce suppressor mechanisms (Fox and McCune 1989). In a study of the clinical and immunologic effects of monthly administration of intravenous cyclophosphamide in severe systemic lupus, a decrease in lymphocytes positive for CD3, CD4, CD8, and B1 occurred during treatment. Thereafter, a return of absolute numbers of B-cells was noted whereas decrease were continually observed in T-lymphocyte subsets. T-cell proliferative responses at follow-up were not significantly different from entry values except that the response to anti-CD2 antibodies was decreased (McCune et al. 1988). In multiple sclerosis, immunologic studies carried out on patients treated as part of the Northeast Cooperative Treatment Group demonstrate a relative decrease of CD4 cells as compared to CD8 cells and linkage of responsive therapy to decrease in spontaneous proliferation and to changes in CD3 and CD4 T cell populations (Hafler et al. 1991). Brinkman et al. (1983) reported decreases of CD4+ but not CD8+ T-cells following daily oral doses of 100–400 mg cyclophosphamide plus prednisone. Moody et al. studied immunologic and clinical effects of increasing monthly pulses of cyclophosphamide in 14 MS patients and found decreases in the percent of CD4+ and increases in CD8+ T cells which were associated with an improved clinical course (Moody et al. 1978; Mickey et al. 1987; Myers et al. 1987). Uitdehaag et al. (1989) showed prolonged depletion of CD4 cells resulting in reduced helper to suppressor ratios in both peripheral blood and CSF.

Summary, Conclusions and Future Directions

1. A clear rationale exists for the use of cyclophosphamide in multiple sclerosis based on its pharmacologic effects, its apparent penetration into the central nervous system and its effectiveness in other non-malignant inflammatory diseases.
2. Cyclophosphamide has major limitations as a therapeutic agent in MS because of its toxicities.
3. The risks from the use of cyclophosphamide are potentially severe and very real. Gastrointestinal upset, amenorrhea, and oligospermia appear to occur in the majority of patients treated. Hemorrhagic cystitis and bladder malignancies are relatively rare. Intercurrent infection occurs in 1%–2% of patients treated. The morbidity of nausea and vomiting makes the treatment unacceptable for many patients. To date, there have been no late-developing malignancies perhaps related to intermittent IV bolus therapy, though until sufficient time has passed the actual rate of cyclophosphamide-induced malignancies cannot be known.
4. The positive effects reported appear to be real and differences between studies are most likely related to patient selection, treatment regimens and outcome measures chosen. Most trials suffer from lack of a placebo-treated group and non-blinded evaluation. However, we feel it is unlikely that the positive clinical effects reported were totally independent of the drug.
5. One treatment with cyclophosphamide over a 2-week period does not induce a permanent remission and some form of repeat treatment or booster therapy is required. Subsequent studies using booster treatments suggest that such therapy may have efficacy in progressive MS. Future trials and use of the drug will require periodic outpatient cyclophosphamide boluses as is given in lupus nephritis. Such outpatient treatment could also be administered at earlier stages of the disease.
6. It appears, though has not been formally proven, that a steroid given concomitantly with the cyclophosphamide may be required and enhances its effect.
7. Further studies by the Boston group and the Northeast Cooperative Treatment Group suggest that the age and characteristics of patients treated may determine which subgroup of progressive patients responds to cyclophosphamide.
8. The Canadian study used different outcome measures and a different treatment regimen than other studies of cyclophosphamide plus steroids in progressive MS. The 75% stabilization rate at 1 year and 67% at 2 years in the placebo group of the Canadian study compared to a stabilization rate of 48% at 1 year and 32% at 2 years in the placebo group of the Cooperative study of cyclosporine in progressive MS made it difficult to demonstrate a positive effect of therapy. Nonetheless, a positive trend was observed in the treated groups at 6 and 12 months.
10. Oral cyclophosphamide over the long term should not be used due to higher incidence of bladder and other malignancies.

11. The total dose of cyclophosphamide that can be given to patients remains unknown though current outpatient booster regimens used by the Boston group approach 50 g total dose over a 3-year period.
12. Short-term intensive immunosuppression appears well-tolerated and could be used as part of a therapeutic armamentarium in which other treatments are then given to maintain remission or for rapidly progressive patients that have not responded to other regimens.
13. An important principle that has been learned from studies of cyclophosphamide in MS is the requirement for some form of periodic treatment if the disease it to remain stable. This principle applies to the use of other immunosuppressant drugs and is clinical verification of what has recently been learned about ongoing disease activity as seen by MRI.
14. Future trials with cyclophosphamide may involve development of outpatient pulse therapy without induction.
15. Because of the side effects associated with the drug, double-blind studies are extremely difficult. The final establishment of regimens using cyclophosphamide plus corticosteroids may await objective MRI monitoring criteria and the acceptance of other treatments for multiple sclerosis against which cyclophosphamide can be tested.
16. In our view, cyclophosphamide plus steroids in combination with a periodic booster program provides an ameliorating effect on the course of a subgroup of multiple sclerosis patients. The toxic side effects preclude its widespread use but it may find use as intermittent therapy in association with other treatments for patients in whom physicians wish to administer immunosuppressive therapy when other regimens have failed.
17. We feel strongly that the major focus of immunotherapy in MS should be the development and use of non-toxic and, to the extent possible, antigen-specific forms of therapy that can be given early in the course of the disease. We and others are involved in testing such approaches including the use of copolymer, beta interferon, T-cell receptor vaccination, and oral tolerization to myelin antigens. Also, potentially less toxic and widely used immunosuppressants such as methotrexate are currently being tested in MS by ourselves and others.

References

Aimard G, Girard PF, Raveau J et al. (1966) Sclerose et plaques et processus d'autoimmunisation. Traitement par les anti-mitotiques. Lyon Med 215:345–352

Bahr U, Schulten HR, Hommes OR, Aerts F (1980) Determination of cyclophosphamide in urine, serum and cerebrospinal fluid of multiple sclerosis patients by field desorption mass spectrometry. Clin Chim Acta 103:183–192

Balow JE, Austin HA, Tsokos GC, Antonovych TT, Steinberg AD, Klipper JH (1987) Lupus nephritis. Ann Int Med 106:79–94

Brinkman CJJ, Nillesen WM, Hommes OR (1983) T-cell subpopulations blood and cerebrospinal fluid of multiple sclerosis patients: effect of cyclophosphamide. Clin Immun Immunopathol 29:341–348

Brinkman CJJ, Nillesen WM, Hommes OR (1984) The effect of cyclophosphamide on T lymphocytes and T lymphocyte subsets in patients with chronic progressive multiple sclerosis. Acta Neurol Scand 69:90–96

Carter JL, Hafler DA, Dawson DM, Orav J, Weiner HL (1988) Immunosuppression with high-dose cyclophosphamide and ACTH in progressive multiple sclerosis: Cumulative 6-year experience in 164 patients. Neurology (Suppl 2) 38:9–14

Cendrowski W (1973) Combined therapeutic trial in multiple sclerosis: hydrocortisone hemisuccinate with cyclophosphamide or cytosine arabinoside. Acta Neurol Belg 73:209–219

Drachman DA (1975) Cyclophosphamide in exacerbations of multiple sclerosis: Therapeutic trial and a strategy for pilot drug studies. Neurol Neurosurg Psychiatry 38:592–597

Fox DA, McCune WJ (1989) Immunologic and clinical effects of cytotoxic drugs used in the treatment of rheumatoid arthritis and systemic lupus erythematosus. Concepts Immunopathol, Basel, Karger 7:20–78

Girard PF, Aimard G, Pellett H (1967) Immunodepressive therapy in neurology. Presse Med 75:967–968

Gonsette RE, Demonty L, Delmotte P (1977) Intensive immunosuppression with cyclophosphamide in multiple sclerosis. Follow up of 100 patients for 2–6 years. J Neurol 214:173–181

Gonsette RE, Demonty L, Delmotte P (1980) Intensive immunosuppression with cyclophosphamide in remittent forms of multiple sclerosis. A follow-up of 134 patients for 2–10 years. In: Bauer HJ, Poser S, Ritter G (eds) Progress in Multiple Sclerosis Research. Springer-Verlag, Berlin, pp 401–406

Goodkin DE, Plencner S, Palmer-Saxerud J, Teetzen M, Hertsgaard D (1987) Cyclophosphamide in chronic progressive multiple sclerosis: Maintenance vs. nonmaintenance therapy. Arch Neurol 44:823–827

Hafler DA, Orav J, Gertz R, Stazzone L, Weiner HL (1991) Immunologic effects of cyclophosphamide/ACTH in patients with chronic progressive multiple sclerosis. J Neuroimmunol 32:149–158

Hafler DA, Weiner HL (1989) MS: a CNS and systemic autoimmune disease. Immunol Today 10:104–107

Hauser SL, Dawson DM, Lehrich JR, Beal MF, Kevy SV, Propper RD, Mills JA, Weiner HL (1983) Intensive immunosuppression in progressive multiple sclerosis: A randomized, three-arm study of high-dose cyclophosphamide, plasma exchange, and ACTH. N Engl J Med 308:173–180

Hommes OR, Prick JJG, Lamers KJB (1975) Treatment of the chronic progressive form of multiple sclerosis with a combination of cyclophosphamide and prednisone. Clin Neurol Neurosurg 78:59–73

Hommes OR, Lamers KJB, Reekers P (1980a) Effect of intensive immunosuppression on the course of chronic progressive multiple sclerosis. J Neurol 223:177–190

Hommes OR, Lamers KJB, Reekers P (1980b) Prognostic factors in intensive immunosuppressive treatment of chronic progressive MS. In: Bauer HJ, Poser S, Ritter G (eds) Progress in Multiple Sclerosis Research. Springer-Verlag, Berlin, pp 396–400

Kaldor JM, Day NE, Pettersson F et al. (1990) Leukemia following chemotherapy for ovarian cancer. N Engl J Med 322:1–6

Killian JM, Bressler RB, Armstrong RM, Huston DP (1988) Controlled pilot trial of monthly intravenous cyclophosphamide in multiple sclerosis. Arch Neurol 45:27–30

Lamers KJB, Uitdehaag BMJ, Hommes OR, Doesburg W, Wevers RA, Geel WJA (1988) The short-term effect of an immunosuppressive treatment on CSF myelin basic protein in chronic progressive multiple sclerosis. J Neurol Neurosurg Psychiatry 51:1334–1337

Likosky WH (1988) Experience with cyclophosphamide in multiple sclerosis: The cons. Neurology 38 (suppl 2): 14–19

Mackin GA, Weiner HL, Orav J et al. (1991) IV cyclophosphamide/ACTH plus maintenance cyclophosphamide boosters in progressive MS: final report of the Northeast Cooperative Treatment Group. Neurology 41 (suppl 1):147

Mauch E, Kornhuber HH, Pfrommer U, Hahnel A, Laufen H, Krapf H (1989) Effective treatment of chronic progressive multiple sclerosis with low-dose cyclophosphamide with minor side-effects. Eur Arch Psychiatr Neurol Sci 238:115–117

McCune WJ, Golbus J, Zeldes W et al. (1988) Clinical and immunologic effects of monthly administration of intravenous cyclophosphamide in severe systemic lupus erythematosus. N Engl J Med 318:1423–1431

Mickey MR, Ellison GW, Fahey JL, Moody DJ, Myers LW (1987) Correlation of clinical and immunological states in multiple sclerosis. Arch Neurol 44:371–375

Millac M, Miller H (1969) Cyclophosphamide in multiple sclerosis. Lancet 1:783

Moody DJ, Fahey JL, Grable E, Ellison GW, Myers LW (1987) Administration of monthly pulses of cyclophosphamide in multiple sclerosis patients: delayed recovery of several immune parameters following discontinuation of long-term cyclophosphamide treatment. J Neuroimmunol 14:175–182

Moody DJ, Kagan J, Liao D, Ellison GW, Myers LW (1978) Administration of monthly-pulse cyclophosphamide in multiple sclerosis patients: effects of long-term treatment on immunologic parameters. J Neuroimmunol 14:161–173

Myers LW, Fahey JL, Moody DJ, Mickey MR, Frane MV, Ellison GW (1987) Cyclophosphamide "pulses" in chronic progressive multiple sclerosis: Arch Neurol 44:828–832

Noseworthy JH, Vandervoort MK, Wong CJ, Ebers GC, and the Canadian Cooperative MS Group (1990) Interrater variability with the Expanded Disability Status Scale (EDSS) and Functional Systems (FS) in a multiple sclerosis clinical trial. Neurology 40:971–975

The Canadian Cooperative Multiple Sclerosis Study Group (1991) The Canadian Cooperative trial of cyclophosphamide and plasma exchange in progressive multiple sclerosis. Lancet 337:442–446

The Multiple Sclerosis Study Group (1990) Efficacy and toxicity of cyclosporine in chronic progressive multiple sclerosis: A randomized, double-blinded, placebo-controlled clinical trial. Ann Neurol 27:591–605

Theys P, Gosseye-Lissoir F, Ketelaer P, Carton H (1981) Short-term intensive cyclophosphamide treatment in multiple sclerosis: A retrospective controlled study. J Neurol 225:119–133

Thompson AJ, Kermode AG, MacManus DG (1990) Patterns of disease activity in multiple sclerosis: clinical and magnetic resonance imaging study. Br Med J 300:631–634

Thompson AJ, Kermode AG, Loicks D (1991) Major differences in the dynamics of primary and secondary progressive multiple sclerosis. Ann Neurol 29:53–62

Uitdehaag BMJ, Nillesen WM, Hommes OR (1989) Long-lasting effects of cyclophosphamide on lymphocytes in peripheral blood and spinal fluid. Acta Neurol Scand 79:12–17

Weiner HL, Hauser SL, Dawson DM, Hafler DA, Mackin GA, Orav EJ (1991) Cyclophosphamide and plasma exchange in multiple sclerosis. Lancet 337:1033–1034

Chapter 10

Treatment of Multiple Sclerosis with Cyclosporine A

Jerry S. Wolinsky

Introduction

Cyclosporine A (cyclosporine) is a cyclic peptide representative of a powerful new class of drugs characterized by semi-selective effects on specific lymphocyte populations. As a prototype agent, cyclosporine has proven effective in preventing host versus graft and graft versus host responses when used as monotherapy or when combined with conventional immunosuppressive agents. As a result, cyclosporine has dramatically altered current approaches to organ transplantation (Kahan 1989). Cyclosporine has increasingly also been reported to be useful in controlling a variety of putative autoimmune diseases of man (reviewed in Bach 1989). Given the proven efficacy of the drug in several model autoimmune diseases of animals, cyclosporine has become an attractive candidate for testing in those human neurological diseases with presumed major immunopathogenic components. This chapter focuses on the pharmacology and immunopharmacology of cyclosporine as applied to man, proposed mechanisms of the immunomodulatory effects of the drug and the known systemic and neural toxicity of the molecule, and reviews the effects of cyclosporines on autoimmune neurological disease models. The results of studies of the use of cyclosporine in multiple sclerosis (MS) are considered in detail.

Mechanisms of Action

Cyclosporine A is a cyclic undecapeptide which was initially recognized as an antifungal metabolite and isolated from *Cylindrocarpon lucidum* Booth and *Tolypocladium inflatum* Gams. The chemical and structural properties of cyclosporine are unusual; several of its amino acids are N-methylated and the amino acid at the C-1 position is unique. The immense interest in cyclosporine and the cyclosporine family of metabolites, derived from these two soil fungi, trace to the efforts of Borel who first described the potent immunosuppressive activity of cyclosporine. Unlike other immunosuppressive agents, cyclosporine was found to be non-toxic to blood-forming elements.

In culture, cyclosporine markedly reduces the proliferative response of human lymphocytes stimulated with the mitogens phytohemagglutin (PHA) and concanavalin A (ConA). Proliferative responses to alloantigens in both primary and secondary mixed lymphocyte reactions (MLR) are also depressed by cyclosporine. The suppressive effects of cyclosporine are not due to lymphocytotoxicity as normal MLR responses obtain when cyclosporine is removed as late as 3 days after initiating the cultures. However, cyclosporine must be present during the early phases of mitogen or alloantigen stimulation. Maximum in vitro suppressive effects appear when cyclosporine is added within the first 2 hours of mitogen stimulation, or within the first 3–4 days of stimulation with alloantigens. While the effects of cyclosporine are most evident on the T-lymphocyte-dependent responses, and particularly those orchestrated by T-helper cells, there is evidence that cyclosporine can inhibit the response of T-independent B-lymphocyte responses to mitogenic antigens (for an extensive review see DiPadova 1989).

The ability of cyclosporine to block the induction of cytotoxic T-cell activity in an allogeneic MLR is dose-dependent. At high concentrations of cyclosporine (>500 ng/ml) no cytotoxic T-cell activity is detected even in the presence of exogenous interleukin 2 (IL-2). In the presence of lower amounts of cyclosporine (100 ng/ml) there is inhibition of cytotoxic T-cell activity, but this activity is reconstituted by the addition of exogenous IL-2. These results suggest that at high doses cyclosporine blocks cytotoxic T-cell IL-2 receptor induction, whereas precursor cytotoxic lymphocytes are activated but are not clonally amplified due to an absence of IL-2 in the low-dose cyclosporine treated cultures (Hess 1985). In contrast to the drug's effects on the T-helper cell, cyclosporine has little effect on the induction of suppressor T-lymphocytes as observed in the allogeneic MLR. Concentrations of cyclosporine up to 1 μg/ml, which totally inhibit cytotoxic T-cell induction, are incapable of affecting cells which suppress in an antigen non-specific manner.

Trough whole blood levels of cyclosporine of 100 to 200 ng/ml are easily obtained in man. Although trough levels of cyclosporine of 400 to 500 ng/ml can be achieved in man, these are often associated with significant toxicity. Thus, with the lower maintenance doses of cyclosporine commonly used in clinical practice, one would expect little blockade of precursor cytotoxic T-lymphocyte activation by cyclosporine and the continued potential for clonal amplification of presensitized cytotoxic T-lymphocytes in the presence of IL-2 production triggered by environmental antigens.

Many of the in vitro effects of cyclosporine can be explained by the lack of production of a number of lymphokines including IL-2, IL-3, migration inhibitory factor (MIF), and gamma interferon, among others. Failure of IL-2 production is probably the result of cyclosporine's inhibition of the induction of IL-2 messenger RNA. The production of other lymphokines appears to be blocked at a similar molecular level (Colombani and Hess 1987). However, cyclosporine appears to spare a T-lymphocyte subpopulation capable of secreting a soluble factor of approximately 21 kilodaltons which is critical for the expansion of non-specific suppressor T-cells (Rich et al. 1984). It is possible that this T-cell subpopulation belongs to a subset of T-cells defined by dual label fluorescence flow cytometry as $CD4^+$, $CD45R^+$.

The effects of cyclosporine on antigen-presenting cell functions are less well understood. However, it is likely that cyclosporine both inhibits IL-1 production and interferes with the expression of receptors for IL-1 to block IL-1 dependent activation of T-cells. It also appears that cyclosporine enhances the synthesis of prostaglandin by monocytes (Whisler et al. 1984). Prostaglandins inhibit IL-2 synthesis, interfere with the expression of Ia antigens on accessory cells, and may selectively activate suppressor T-cells. Such effects would be synergistic to the induction of non-specific and antigen-specific T-cell suppressor mechanisms in the presence of cyclosporine.

At a molecular level, it remains ambiguous as to whether or not there is a specific cell surface receptor for cyclosporine. It is likely that uptake of cyclosporine at the cell membrance and its transport into the cell cytoplasm occurs because of the highly lipophilic nature of cyclosporines. Once having gained access to the cell cytoplasm, cyclosporine appears to associate with at least two protein receptors, calmodulin and cyclophilin (Handschumacher et al. 1984); the latter is now recognized to be peptidyl-prolyl cis-trans isomerase (Fischer et al. 1989).

The association of cyclosporine in an inhibitory manner with calmodulin would prevent a number of calcium-dependent cytoplasmic activation events including the elevation of second messengers such as cyclic GMP. Through this action cyclosporine might also inhibit calmodulin-dependent inducible mRNA transcription. However, the binding of cyclosporine to cyclophilin is much stronger than to calmodulin and only immunologically active metabolites and congeners of cyclosporine bind to cyclophilin; binding of cyclosporine to calmodulin is much more permissive. Thus, a current likely hypothesis is that cyclosporine binding to cyclophilin inhibits the isomerization of molecules involved in the transcriptional activation of specific lymphokine genes (Ryffel 1989). The nuclear factor of activated T-cells (NF-AT) is a candidate target of such an effect (Emmel et al. 1989).

The most dramatic in vivo use of cyclosporine has occurred in certain animal model systems of allogeneic organ transplantation. Under optimal circumstances, pretreatment with cyclosporine or treatment with cyclosporine at the time of engraftment results in long-term graft survival in the absence of continued cyclosporine therapy. Thus, tolerance can be induced in these animal model systems. The results of studies from a number of investigators suggest that tolerance is due to the early induction of a cyclophosphamide-sensitive, nonspecific and eventually antigen-specific suppressor T-cell population. While the use of cyclosporine has effectively revolutionized solid-organ and bone-marrow transplantation programs, actual tolerance induction and prolonged survival of the transplant in the absence of continued cyclosporine therapy is rarely achieved in man.

Immunopharmokinetics

Cyclosporines are highly lipophilic molecules with limited bioavailability. They are insoluble in water, which creates problems in drug administration. Approximately 30% of an oral ingested dose of cyclosporine is absorbed from the small bowel with an absorption half-life of about 1 h. Maximum concentrations in blood occur within 2–6 h of administration with a mean of 4 h. Within the blood compartment, approximately 10% of the drug is bound to white blood cells, 50% is associated with red blood cells and the remainder is free in serum. Elimination is almost entirely by the liver. The beta phase of the biphasic half-life of the drug is between 4 and 10 h. Enterohepatic recycling occurs in about one-quarter of all patients. This contributes to a second peak of cyclosporine in the blood of such individuals nearly 8 h after oral dosing. The drug is well distributed throughout body tissues including brain, but partition into the latter is low.

Because of the high and variable proportion of cyclosporine associated with red blood cells, measurements of plasma cyclosporine levels are prone to error due to problems in the collection and processing of samples. Therefore, whole blood cyclosporine levels have been generally adopted. The most reliable means for monitoring whole blood cyclosporine levels has been by high pressure liquid chromatography (HPLC). However, radioimmunoassays (RIA) which use monoclonal antibodies which are **specific** for cyclosporine or which are **nonspecific** and react with cyclosporine and its metabolites have recently been introduced (reviewed in Quesniaux, 1989). The **specific** monoclonal antibody-based RIA provides reproducibility comparable to HPLC for measurement of parent drug concentrations.

The absorption of cyclosporine is depressed markedly by gastrointestinal disorders, particularly vomiting and diarrhea. Increased gastric emptying time induced by metoclopramide enhances cyclosporine absorption and consequently increases blood levels of the drug. Drug elimination is dramatically influenced by liver disease and biliary tract obstruction. The metabolism of cyclosporine occurs predominantly through mixed function oxidase enzyme systems. Thus, the induction of hepatic cytochrome P450 enzyme systems by drugs such as phenytoin, phenobarbital, carbamazepine, rifampin or isoniazid decreases cyclosporine levels by enhancing drug elimination. An opposite effect related to cytochrome P450 inhibition obtains with erythromycin, ketoconazole and fluconazole and concomitant use of any of these drugs with cyclosporine can induce acute toxicity (Kim and Perfect 1989). Through similar mechanisms, corticosteroids may increase cyclosporine levels and cyclosporine reciprocally decreases the rate of elimination of corticosteroids. Concomitant administration of diltiazem and several other calcium channel blockers may have similar effects. However, there is evidence from animal model studies that verapamil may have synergistic immunosuppressant effects with cyclosporine that are independent of any pharmacological interactions (Scoble et al. 1989). Through independent mechanisms a number of drugs may compound the renal toxicity of cyclosporine due to their own deleterious effects on renal blood flow or direct toxic effects on the proximal renal tubule. Such drugs include the aminoglycosides, amphotericin-B, trimethaprin-sulfamethoxazole, cotrimoxazole and a number of non-steroidal anti-inflammatory agents.

The dose of cyclosporine required in model autoimmune diseases can be reduced greatly when the drug is used concomitantly with bromocriptine (Palestine et al. 1987). Preliminary results suggest that a similar adjunctive effect is also possible following cardiac transplantation (Carrier et al. 1990). The effect of bromocriptine in reducing the required dose of cyclosporine is assumed to be mediated via neural-immune network interactions. Lymphocytes express prolactin receptors on their surface membranes and cyclosporine and prolactin could compete for these surface lymphocyte receptors. However, prolactin may also be a weak modulator of immune activation. Bromocriptine inhibits prolactin release through its action as a dopamine D2 agonist and this is the presumed mechanism for the indirect action of bromocriptine in lowering the effective immunosuppressive dose of cyclosporine.

Data from experimental models also suggest that the formulation of cyclosporine for oral administration in fish oil rich in n-3 polyunsaturated fatty acids may have a synergistic immunosuppressive effect (Kelley et al. 1989). The use of n-3 polyunsaturated fatty acids has been independently shown to produce modest suppression of in vitro measured cellular immune responses in man.

Experimental Allergic Encephalomyelitis (EAE)

Various methods of immunosuppression both prevent induction and modify the course of EAE. Most investigators who have used cyclosporine in EAE report effective prophylaxis and salutary effects in treatment paradigms of both acute and chronic EAE (comprehensively reviewed in Borel, 1989). In addition, $CD4^+$ antigen-specific cells can be recovered by in vitro culture of rat lymph node cells in the presence of cyclosporine and these cells are capable of suppressing the passive transfer of EAE by encephalitogenic T-cell lines (Ellerman et al. 1988). Further, antigen-non-specific macrophages and possibly antigen-specific $CD4^+$ T-cells which facilitate suppression can be induced by in vitro culture of spleen cells from myelin basic protein challenged mice in the presence of cyclosporine (Whitham et al. 1990). Taken together, these findings suggest that cyclosporine is highly effective in modifying EAE, probably by allowing the expansion in vivo of antigen-specific $CD4^+$ T-cells, perhaps of the suppressor-inducer type, and by enhancing non-specific suppressor macrophages.

However, two cautionary notes derive from the animal model studies. First, recent reports suggest that low-dose cyclosporine may actually exacerbate EAE (Pender et al. 1990). Second, tolerance induction seen in organ transplant models is not reproduced in the clinical setting in man and suppression of clinical symptoms of primate EAE requires the continuous use of cyclosporine. These findings suggest caution in considering the use of cyclosporine at doses significantly lower than those evaluated in carefully controlled studies; also, once initiated, cyclosporine therapy may need to be continued indefinitely.

Multiple Sclerosis

Three major clinical trials have assessed the efficacy of cyclosporine in MS. The design of the German study has been well-detailed (Patzold et al. 1985). In brief, patients with clinically defined, definite MS were enrolled from investigative centers in Hanover and Würzburg. Ninety-eight patients were randomized to treatment with cyclosporine (5 mg/kg/day with a mean trough level of 269 ng/ml and levels which ranged from 150 to 750 ng/ml). Another 96 were randomized to treatment with azathioprine (AZA) (2.5 mg/kg/day). Multiple sclerosis patients randomized for treatment included those whose clinical disease ran the spectrum between relapsing/remitting (64% of all cases) to chronic/progressive types. Treatment of exacerbations with an 8-week regime of oral corticosteroids was allowed during this study. About one-third of all patients received one or more courses of such therapy. Eighty-six percent of all patients completed 24 months of continuous drug therapy in accordance with the study protocol.

A variety of clinical endpoints including serial quantified neurological examinations and the expanded disability status scale (EDSS) of Kurtzke were used as outcome measures. Although some trends were recorded which favored cyclosporine-treated patients as showing marginally less progression than their AZA-treated counterparts, no statistically-significant differences between treatment arms could be shown for any of the multiple measures of clinical efficacy (Kappos et al. 1988a). Nor was there a differential effect of either drug on the accumulated cerebral plaque burden as estimated by qualitative or quantitative analysis of magnetic resonance images (MRIs) (Kappos et al. 1988b). Side effects were common in both patient groups and were distinctive for the two drugs. Given the relative toxicities observed, the investigators concluded that cyclosporine used in this manner caused unacceptable toxicity relative to AZA.

The frequency of observed relapses in the German trial proved to be rather low (about 0.3 per patient per year), even though patients were selected in part for relapse rates ≥1 per annum. As might be expected of a primarily relapsing/remitting patient group, progression of at least one point on the EDSS was observed for only 24% of patients who completed the trial. Further, progression of disease as measured by change in EDSS score, ambulation index or other measures was minor in both study arms. Thus, the frequency of measurable events and magnitude of change in disability would make it difficult to detect important differential effects of either drug on the patients' disease course over a study of such relatively short duration. The study design was also unfortunate in that any benefit of either cyclosporine or AZA in altering the natural history of relatively mild and primarily relapsing/remitting MS could not be defined as no placebo-treated control group was included. In this respect it may be pertinent that other recent, well-controlled studies have failed to show any notable benefits of AZA over placebo in a similar MS patient population (Hughes et al. 1988), or one selected for chronic progressive disease (Ellison et al. 1989). For a detailed discussion of the effects of AZA on MS also refer to Chap. 7 by Richard Hughes in this volume.

The second major clinical trial to be completed was a double-blind, placebo-controlled study of patients entered and independently randomized from centers in London (n = 43) and Amsterdam (n = 37) (Rudge 1985). These investigators enrolled MS subjects of both the relapsing/remitting and progressive types with clinically definite and active disease using criteria similar to those used in the German study. Forty patients were actively treated with cyclosporine at an initial dose of 10 mg/kg/day for 2 months. The drug dose was then variably reduced for the final 22 months of observation at the 2 centers. Dosages were adjusted downward to reduce toxicity by an unblinded observer. Blood levels of cyclosporine were measured but the results were not used for dosage control. The mean maintenance doses of cyclosporine were 7.2 mg and

5 mg/kg/day respectively in the London and Amsterdam patients. However, the London patients were maintained at or above a mean dose of 7 mg/kg/day throughout the trial; the Dutch cases were on mean doses below 5 mg/kg/day for most of the second year of the study. Treatment of relapses with short courses of steroids was allowed (Rudge et al. 1989).

A variety of clinical endpoints were used in assessing the outcome. An intention-to-treat analysis was described but 2 patients treated for less than 3 months were arbitrarily withdrawn from the data pool. The Dutch investigators concluded that no beneficial effects referable to cyclosporine occurred at their center and that side effects were a major problem. Early benefit that was statistically significant was, however, seen among cyclosporine-treated patients in London. As a group, the treated patients had fewer relapses and a longer interval to first relapse on treatment over the 2-year study. They also showed significantly better overall functional assessments for the first 6 months of treatment and a trend towards slower progression of disability over the entire trial (Rudge et al. 1989). The combined data showed more stable patients over the first 6 months of treatment and fewer and less severe relapses over the entire study for the cyclosporine-treated subjects. A decrease in total intrathecal IgG and stabilization or decreased light chain synthesis in the cerebrospinal fluid were also observed for treated patients (McLean et al. 1989). However, the major differences in patient disability and drug dosage at entry between the centers rendered results based on the combined data suspect (Rudge 1990).

The final study was an American multi-center cooperative trial (Multiple Sclerosis Study Group 1990). Patients were selected on the basis of having clinically definite, chronic/progressive MS of mild to moderate severity, evidence of progression of at least one point on the EDSS in the year prior to entry and definite progression in the 6 months prior to randomization. Prior treatment with cyclophosphamide was excluded, treatment with other immunosuppressive agents was stopped at least 3 months prior to study entry, and last treatment with corticosteroids was at least 1 month prior to entry. No alteration in symptomatic management or treatment of exacerbations with immunosuppressive drugs including corticosteroids was allowed. In all, 547 patients were randomized to receive either cyclosporine (n = 273) or placebo (n = 274). Treatment groups at entry proved balanced for age, gender, duration of illness and neurological disability. Cyclosporine was started at 6 mg/kg/day and the dose adjusted down or up to avoid toxicity and achieve an adequate trough blood level of the drug. Dose adjustments were made by an unblinded observer who was not involved in rating patient clinical status. A median trough whole blood "**nonspecific**" cyclosporine level of the treated patient group was maintained between 310 and 430 ng/ml. Thus, this study differed from the two European studies by the type of patients selected, a higher targeted dose of cyclosporine, restrictions on other treatments, and a substantially larger cohort of patients randomized.

As in the other trials, multiple measures of neurological status were prospectively obtained on all patients at entry and at 3 month intervals. Prior to initiation of the clinical trial the change in EDSS score was chosen as the primary study end point. However, questions raised during the study on the utility of the EDSS led to adoption of a series of outcome measures before the data were evaluated, which might more reasonably be used for a survival

Table 10.1. Mean changes in EDSS from baseline to exit

Months followed	Cyclosporine			Placebo		
	Total patients	Mean change[a]	% Failed treatment[b]	Total patients	Mean change	% Failed treatment
Withdrawals						
1–6	35	0.14 ± 1.17	29	34	0.78 ± 1.34	79
7–12	29	0.41 ± 1.07	41	26	0.79 ± 0.87	73
13–18	42	0.75 ± 0.85	43	22	1.09 ± 1.37	41
19–23	14	0.54 ± 0.84	50	5	1.30 ± 0.84	80
Completers						
24	153	0.33 ± 1.08		187	0.55 ± 1.01	(p = 0.006)
Total	273	0.39 ± 1.07		274	0.65 ± 1.08	(p = 0.002)

Reproduced with permission from Annals of Neurology (1990) 27:591–605.
[a] Mean increase in EDSS score from entry evaluation ± one standard deviation.
[b] Percentage of those patients who failed to complete the study during a given 6 month interval of the study who were withdrawn as treatment failures.

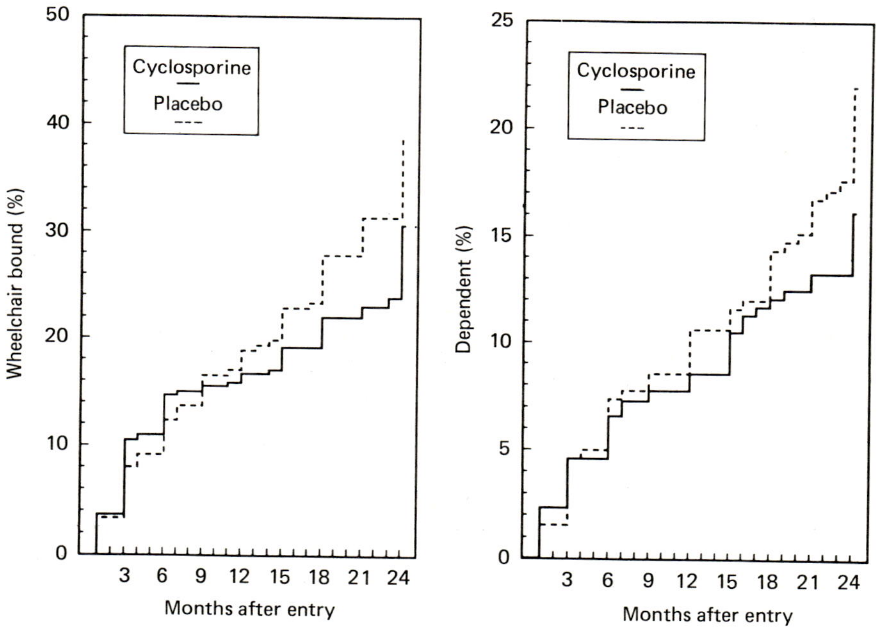

Fig. 10.1. The cumulative probability of becoming wheelchair-bound as defined by an EDSS score of 7.0 or an ambulation index rating of 7 sustained for two visits or at exit from the American cooperative study is shown in the left-hand panel. The survival curves differ at the $p = 0.038$ level. In the right-hand panel is displayed the cumulative probability of becoming dependent on others as defined by an activities of daily living (ADL) score of ≥6. The ADL score was derived from the incapacity status scale items for dressing, grooming and feeding of the Multiple Sclerosis Minimal Record of Disability and is a measure of upper extremity function which is independent of gait assessment. The survival curves failed to reach statistically significant differences ($p = 0.06$). Reproduced with permission from Annals of Neurology (1990) 27:591–605.

analytic statistical approach. The mean increase in EDSS score was 0.39 ± 1.07 units for cyclosporine- and 0.65 ± 1.08 units for placebo-treated patients from entry until the time of early withdrawal or completion of the study (Table 10.1). Of three primary efficacy criteria selected for analysis, cyclosporine delayed the time to becoming wheelchair-bound (Fig. 10.1), was associated with a trend to delayed accumulation of disabling upper extremity deficits which render patients dependent on others as measured by a composite score of "activities of daily living" (Fig. 10.1), but caused no measurable effects for "time to sustained progression" (Multiple Sclerosis Study Group 1990). Active treatment had a favorable effect on several secondary measures of disease outcome, including the change in the "collapsed" EDSS over time. Deterioration also appeared to be slowed as measured by change in ambulation index from baseline with time (Fig. 10.2).

A large and differential withdrawal rate (44% cyclosporine, 32% placebo) complicated the analysis but did not appear to explain the observed effect of cyclosporine in delaying disease progression. Nephrotoxicity and hypertension were common troublesome toxicities that accounted for most of the excess patient loss in the cyclosporine arm of the study. Multivariate analysis did not show any institutional effects but did demonstrate substantial effects of baseline neurological disability on outcome for the primary study outcome measure of time to becoming wheelchair-bound.

Entry and exit head MRI data of adequate quality for quantitative evaluation were available for 162 patients. A weak, but statistically significant, direct correlation was found between the change in EDSS score from study entry and the change in total MRI lesion burden. However, no effect of treatment on

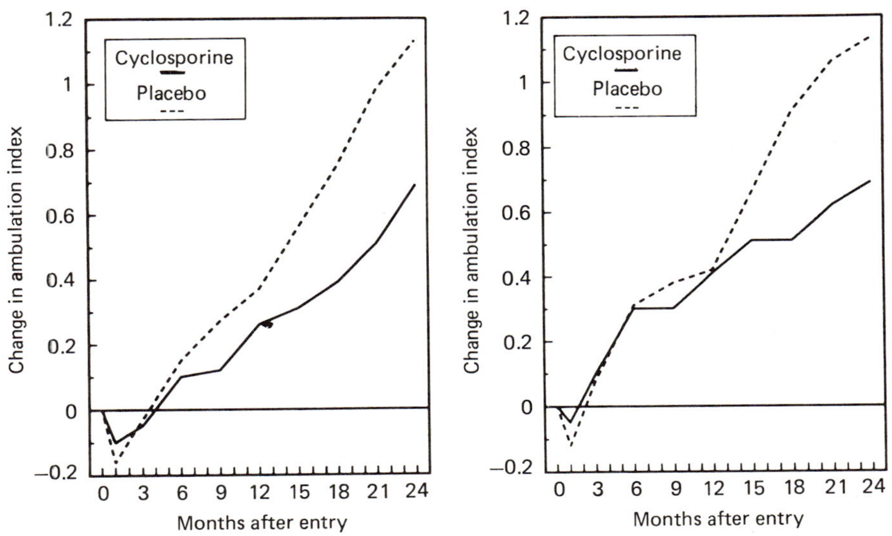

Fig. 10.2. Comparison of the mean change in the ambulation index from entry for those patients who completed the American study (left-hand panel), or for all patients entered into the trial until the time of completion of the 24-month study or their premature exit from the study (right-hand panel). Differences between the groups are significant ($p < 0.01$) for both sets of data at 18, 21 and 24 months.

MRI-defined cerebral lesion burden or the number of MRI-defined lesions was seen (Paty et al., unpublished observations). Paired entry and exit cerebrospinal fluid samples were evaluable from 117 patients. No difference in the intrathecal immunoglobulin (IgG) synthesis rates over time were noted between the study arms (Tourtellotte et al., unpublished observations).

Thus, in the American trial, an apparent effect of cyclosporine in causing modest slowing of progression of clinical disease did not correlate with an effect in a reduced accumulated burden of MRI-defined cerebral disease, or an effect on the intrathecal IgG synthetic rate. Further, the clinical results suggested a possible delay in the appearance of any measurable beneficial effect of cyclosporine on the progression of disability in chronic/progressive MS. Differences between progression rates were only first evident about 15–18 months into therapy. If this observation is valid, it might follow that more striking differences might obtain in a study of longer duration. This conclusion is consistent with theoretical mechanisms of the effect of cyclosporine or other immunomodulators when used relatively late in the course of an established autoimmune disease. As concluded by the American investigators, close supervision by physicians familiar with cyclosporine is clearly mandatory to minimize known adverse effects, particularly nephrotoxicity and hypertension if one is to consider the use of this immunosuppressant in MS or any other putative autoimmune disease.

Immunological Effects of Cyclosporine in MS

During the course of the American trial, a subgroup of patients was serially studied to determine what, if any, effect cyclosporine might have on the phenotypic composition and functional activities of their lymphocytes. Seventy-eight of the chronic/progressive patients randomized at the Health Science Centers of the the University of Texas at Houston and the University of Colorado were serially studied. At entry there were no differences between the placebo and cyclosporine-treated groups. However, the $CD4^+/CD8^+$ ratio, percentages of active T-lymphocytes, and percentages of T-lymphocytes expressing the Ta^{1+} and Ia^+ antigens were all significantly elevated when compared to age-matched controls (Kerman et al. 1988). Over the 24 months of continuous therapy, the chronic/progressive MS patients receiving placebo showed elevations in percentages of helper-T cells ($CD4^+$), active T-cells and T-lymphocytes bearing the Ta^{1+} antigen that were statistically significant, as well as an increased panel allogeneic MLR when compared to the cyclosporine-treated cohort.

Dual label immunofluorescence studies performed approximately 16 months into the trial showed that the placebo-treated MS patients had a reduced percentage of lymphocytes bearing $CD4^+$, $CD45R^+$ antigens. In contrast, the cyclosporine-treated patients had percentages of these dual labeled cells comparable to those seen in an age-matched control group (Table 10.2). These studies suggest the expansion of a helper T-cell subset which appears to contain those lymphocytes that induce suppression. It was also found that patients treated with cyclosporine had a significantly higher frequency of inhibition and

Table 10.2. Cross-sectional immune profiles of chronic/progressive multiple sclerosis patient cohort

	Cyclosporine $n^a = 39/21$	Placebo $n = 39/26$	Control $n = 30$
% $CD4^+$	44 ± 9	58 ± 6^b	40 ± 10
% $CD8^+$	24 ± 9	23 ± 8	24 ± 7
$CD4^+$: $CD8^+$	2.6 ± 1.0	3.4 ± 0.9^b	1.8 ± 0.7
%$CD4^+$, $CD45R^+$	25 ± 7	10 ± 6^b	19 ± 5
% $CD4^+$, $CDw29^+$	16 ± 7	32 ± 9^b	25 ± 5
% $CD8^+$, $CD45R^+$	18 ± 6	6 ± 5^b	14 ± 5
% $CD8^+$, $CDw29^+$	9 ± 9	18 ± 7^b	9 ± 4

[a] n = number of individual subjects tested; several of the MS subjects were tested on more than one visit as reflected by the dual figures for n, the second reflecting the number of distinct subjects tested. All tests were performed at a mean of 16 ± 8 months from entry into the study.
[b] $p < 0.01$ for placebo group versus either the cyclosporine-treated group or the age-matched healthy control group.

mean percentage inhibition in a panel MLR inhibition assay to suggest that the cyclosporine-treated MS patients had expanded their population of nonspecific immunoregulatory cells (Kerman et al. 1987). Thus, cyclosporine appeared to modify the immune system of these MS patients in a theoretically beneficial manner.

In a smaller set of chronic/progressive MS patients evaluated at a single time point early in the course of treatment, Bania and colleagues observed that cyclosporine markedly inhibited $CD8^+$ cell-mediated cytotoxicity to allogeneic targets in vitro. These investigators were unable to find any effect of treatment with the drug on the MS-associated defect in ConA induced suppressor cell activity (Bania et al. 1986). In another subgroup of chronic/progressive MS patients, serum IL-2 levels were found to be elevated when compared with stable or relapsing/remitting MS cases or control individuals, but cyclosporine treatment did not consistently effect the fluctuation of serum IL-2 levels seen over time (Trotter et al. 1990). Finally, the London group has shown that the expression of IL-2 receptors (CD25) on blood but not cerebrospinal fluid obtained lymphocytes is decreased by cyclosporine treatment of a group of mainly relapsing/remitting MS subjects (Calder et al. 1987).

Toxicity

Concern for the use of cyclosporine has centered primarily on nephrotoxicity. Full assessment of the renal toxicity of the drug was initially complicated by the extensive use of cyclosporine in renal transplantation where analyses of drug effects are complicated by rejection phenomena. However, considerable experience outside of renal transplantation and in the absence of pre-existent renal disease has not served to diminish the importance of renal toxicity as a limiting factor for the use of cyclosporine (Palestine et al. 1986; Kappos et al. 1988a; Rudge et al. 1989; Multiple Sclerosis Study Group 1990). Acute renal damage occurs with excessive whole-blood cyclosporine levels. Of greater concern is the nearly universal change encountered with chronic exposure to conventional therapeutic levels of the drug. This consists of irregularly distributed areas of interstitial fibrosis and atrophic tubules in the renal cortex with or without an associated arteriolopathy (Mihatsch et al. 1985). The occurrence of these changes is not strictly dose-related. Serum BUN and creatinine levels are routinely used to monitor for cyclosporine nephrotoxicity but are poor substitutes for the more informative, but more difficult to obtain, measures of glomerular filtration rate. Fortunately, most patients who exhibit deterioration of renal function show return of serum creatinine levels to baseline values within 3 months of discontinuing cyclosporine therapy.

Other non-neurological side effects of cyclosporine recorded in more than 3% of a series of over 3000 treated patients include: hypertension (38.5%), hypertrichosis (32.9%), gingival hyperplasia (14.8%), liver dysfunction (18.4%), gastrointestinal distress (9.4%), hyperuricemia (4%) and increased triglyceride and cholesterol levels (3.6%) (Krupp et al. 1985). Hypertension in MS patients under active treatment with cyclosporine has been associated with the diminished urinary excretion of prostacyclin metabolites (Forstermann et al. 1989). However, increased alpha-adrenergic stimulation via sympathetic nerve fibers may be a more proximal cause of this adverse effect (Scherrer et al. 1990). Coarsening of facial appearance has been seen in both children and adults, which is similar to that seen with chronic phenytoin administration. The incidence of these adverse effects varies considerably from study to study, in part due to the nature of the disease treated and in part due to associated drug usage. For example, in the American study of MS, anemia was common but hepatic dysfunction was rare (Multiple Sclerosis Study Group 1990). Remarkable variation in the perception of side effects has also occurred between the three major trials of cyclosporine in multiple sclerosis patients (Table 10.3). Most side effects of cyclosporine therapy are evident within 3–6 months of initiating treatment and then often remain rather stable in a given patient.

Cancer is also seen with increased frequency with chronic cyclosporine therapy. Non-Hodgkin's lymphoma appears to occur about twice as frequently and more rapidly following organ transplantation with cyclosporine than with conventional immunosuppressive regimes, and the use of cyclosporine in this setting is also associated with about a two-fold higher incidence of renal carcinomas and Kaposi's sarcoma (Cockburn and Krupp 1989). However, it is possible that data from the transplant experience may not be entirely relevant to the use of cyclosporine in neurological disorders of presumed autoimmune etiology.

Neurological complications of cyclosporine therapy have been reported in up to 20% of all patients. An essential-like tremor is predominant. Dysethesias and paresthesias are also frequent but often difficult to ascribe to the drug as opposed to the underlying condition (Rudge et al. 1989). Similarly, seizures, when seen, may be indirectly related to other metabolic derangements which frequent cyclosporine administration, particularly hypomagnesemia (Thompson et al. 1984). However, animal studies suggest that at moderate to high doses cyclosporine may have direct epileptogenic and neurotoxic effects (Famiglio et al. 1989). Of considerable interest is the infrequent occurrence of severe but

Table 10.3. Percentage of patients with adverse effects of cyclosporine as reported in the multiple sclerosis treatment trials. The percentage of affected patients is shown as a range from the lowest to the highest reported for the German, Dutch-English and American studies. The German azathioprine-treated group is excluded from the placebo-treated column

Toxicity	Treated	Placebo
Renal dysfunction	36–"nearly all"	3
Hirsutism	47–94	5–16
Anemia	10–75	–
Paresthesia	11–70	0–10
Gingival hyperplasia	33–64	0–12
Hypertension	35–59	–
Headache	32–52	0–21
Tremor	5–47	0–12
Nausea	16–41	6–15
Arthralgia	6–26	0
Skin changes	0–21	0
Mental disturbance	0–21	5–6
Fatigue	15	13
Seizures	0–10	0

potentially reversible CNS toxicity characterized by confusion, cortical blindness, quadraparesis, seizures and coma attended by low-density white-matter lesions on CT and abnormal signal intensities on MRI (DeGroen et al. 1987; Rubin and Kang 1987).

Prospects

The role for cyclosporine in the neurologist's therapeutic armamentarium for MS remains incompletely defined. However, several tentative conclusions can be offered based on the above studies. First, the results from the American cooperative study and data from patients treated in London suggest that cyclosporine has a beneficial, albeit modest effect in ameliorating clinical disease progression. These two patient populations appear to differ in that the London group was biased towards younger, somewhat less disabled, relapsing/remitting cases and the American subjects were biased to older, more disabled patients with a somewhat longer disease course before treatment and who by definition had chronic/progressive disease. Nonetheless, both patient groups appeared to have been selected for measurably active clinical disease prior to randomization. Thus, it may follow that those patients who are experiencing frequently recurring or significant nearly continuous disease activity are most likely to show measurable slowing of disease progression when treated with cyclosporine. Conversely, the Amsterdam subjects and German patients had less severe disease and showed little progression while under study, suggesting that the narrow benefit–risk ratios for cyclosporine do not favor use of the drug for patients early in their disease course or with relatively benign clinical disease.

Second, multivariate analysis of the American study provided the suggestion that initiation of therapy early into the course of chronic/progressive disease was associated with better outcome. It is quite possible that the effects of cyclosporine on MS are primarily limited to modulation of systemic immune activation; the restricted access of cyclosporine to the central nervous system may markedly impair its influence on preexistent intrathecal immune dysregulation in association with well developed plaques. If so, early treatment of active disease would be more likely to have the greatest impact on disease progression rates.

Third, even if the effect of cyclosporine on disease progression is modest, the observations of the large American study support the currently popular notion that MS is at least in part immune-mediated and that systemic features of immune dysregulation can be partially normalized by this semi-selective immune modulator. This provides the hope that other compounds with mechanisms of action similar to those of cyclosporine but possessing more attractive toxicity profiles might hold promise for this disease. Macrolides such as FK506, rapamycin or rationally designed synthetic molecules based on the immunologically active sites of these compounds (Bierer et al. 1990) are particularly attractive in this regard.

Finally, at present there are few, if any, proven alternatives to cyclosporine for slowing disease progression in MS. Undoubtedly, the relatively narrow profile of MS patients who are likely to benefit from cyclosporine therapy, the high incidence of potentially life-threatening drug-induced toxicities, the need for extremely close monitoring of patients under treatment, and the high cost of the treatment all merge to restrict its use for this disabling neurologic disease. The general use of cyclosporine in MS will undoubtedly be further curtailed by the corporate decision of the drug's manufacturer not to seek a new disease indication for cyclosporine for MS from the United States Food and Drug Administration.

References

Bach, JF (1989) Cyclosporine in autoimmune diseases. Transplant Proc 21:97–113

Bania MB, Antel JP, Reder AT, Nicholas MK, Arnason BG (1986) Suppressor and cytolytic cell function in multiple sclerosis. Effects of cyclosporine A and interleukin 2. J Clin Invest 78:582–586

Bierer BE, Somers PK, Wandless TJ, Burakoff SJ, Schreiber SL (1990) Probing immunosuppressant action with a nonnatural immunophilin ligand. Science 250:556–559

Borel JF (1989) Pharmacology of cyclosporine (Sandimmune). IV. Pharmacological properties in vivo. Pharmacol Rev 41:259–370

Calder VL, Bellamy AS, Owen S et al. (1987) Effects of cyclosporin A on expression of IL-2 and IL-2 receptors in normal and multiple sclerosis patients. Clin Exp Immunol 70:570–577

Carrier M, Wild J, Pelletier LC, Copeland JG (1990) Bromocriptine as an adjuvant to cyclosporine immunosuppression after heart transplantation. Ann Thoracic Surg 49:129–132

Cockburn IT, Krupp P (1989) The risk of neoplasms in patients treated with cyclosporine A. J Autoimmun 2:723–731

Colombani PM, Hess AD (1987) T-lymphocyte inhibition by cyclosporine. Potential mechanisms. Biochem Pharmacol 36:3789–3793

DeGroen PC, Aksamit AJ, Rakela J, Forbes GS, Krom RAF (1987) Central nervous system toxicity after liver transplantation. The role of cyclosporine and cholesterol. N Engl J Med 317:861–866

DiPadova FE (1989) Pharmacology of cyclosporine (Sandimmune). V. Pharmacological effects on immune function – In vitro studies. Pharmacol Rev 41:373–405

Ellerman KE, Powers JM, Brostoff SW (1988) A suppressor T-lymphocyte cell line for autoimmune encephalomyelitis. Nature 331:265–267

Ellison GW, Myers LW, Mickey MR et al. (1989) A placebo-controlled, randomized, double-masked, variable dosage, clinical trial of azathioprine with and without methylprednisolone in multiple sclerosis. Neurology 39:1018–1026

Emmel EA, Verweij CL, Durand DB, Higgins KM, Lacy E, Crabtree GR (1989) Cyclosporin A specifically inhibits function of nuclear proteins involved in T cell activation. Science 246:1617–1620

Famiglio L, Racusen L, Fivush B, Solez K, Fisher R (1989) Central nervous system toxicity of cyclosporine in a rat model. Transplantation 48:316–321

Fischer G, Wittmannliebold B, Lang K, Kiefhaber T, Schmid FX (1989) Cyclophilin and peptidyl-prolyl cis-trans isomerase are probably identical proteins. Nature 337:476–478

Forstermann U, Kuhn K, Vesterqvist O et al. (1989) An increase in the ratio of thromboxane A2 to prostacyclin in association with increased blood pressure in patients on cyclosporine A. Prostaglandins 37:567–575

Handschumacher RE, Harding MW, Rice J, Drugge RJ (1984) Cyclophilin: A specific cytosolic binding protein for cyclosporin A. Science 544–547

Hess AD (1985) Effect of interleukin 2 on the immunosuppressive action of cyclosporine. Transplantation 39:62–68

Hughes RAC, McPherson K, British-Dutch MS Azathioprine Trial Group (1988) Double-masked trial of azathioprine in multiple sclerosis. Lancet 2:170–183

Kahan BD (1989) Cyclosporine. N Engl J Med 321:1725–1739

Kappos L, Patzold U, Dommasch D et al. (1988a) Cyclosporine versus azathioprine in the long-term treatment of multiple sclerosis: Results of the German multicenter study. Ann Neurol 23:56–63

Kappos L, Stadt D, Ratzka M et al. (1988b) Magnetic resonance imaging in the evaluation of treatment in multiple sclerosis. Neuroradiology 30:299–302

Kelley VE, Kirkman RL, Bastos M, Barrett LV, Strom TB (1989) Enhancement of immunosuppression by substitution of fish oil for olive oil as a vehicle for cyclosporine. Transplantation 48:98–102

Kerman RH, Wolinsky JS, Nath A, Sears ES Jr, Franklin GM, Nelson LM (1987) Immune regulation in multiple sclerosis patients treated with cyclosporine. Ann Neurol 22:154

Kerman RH, Wolinsky JS, Nath A, Sears ES Jr (1988) Serial immune evaluation of cyclosporine- and placebo-treated multiple sclerosis patients. J Neuroimmunol 18:325–331

Kim JH, Perfect JR (1989) Infection and cyclosporine. Rev Infect Dis 11:677–690

Krupp P, Timonen P, Gulich A (1985) Side effects and safety of Sandimmune in long-term treatment In: R Schindler (ed) Ciclosporin in Autoimmune Diseases. Springer-Verlag, Berlin, pp 41–49

McLean BN, Rudge P, Thompson EJ (1989) Cyclosporin A curtails the progression of free light chain synthesis in the CSF of patients with multiple sclerosis. J Neurol Neurosurg Psych 52:529–531

Mihatsch MJ, Thiel G, Ryffel B (1985) Ciclosporin-associated nephropathy In: R Schindler (ed) Ciclosporin in Autoimmune Diseases. Springer-Verlag, Berlin, pp 50–58

Multiple Sclerosis Study Group (1990) Efficacy and toxicity of cyclosporine in chronic progressive multiple sclerosis: A randomized, double-blinded, placebo-controlled clinical trial. Ann Neurol 27:591–605

Palestine AG, Austin III HA, Balow JE et al. (1986) Renal histopathologic alterations in patients treated with cyclosporine for uveitis. N Engl J Med 314:1293–1298

Palestine AG, Muellenberg-Coulombre CG, Kim MK, Gelato MC, Nussenblatt RB (1987) Bromocriptine and low dose cyclosporine in the treatment of experimental autoimmune uveitis in the rat. J Clin Invest 79:1078–1081

Patzold U, Dommasch D, Poser S et al. (1985) The effect of ciclosporin versus azathioprine on the course of multiple sclerosis; Design of a long-term follow-up study and side effects In: R Schindler (ed) Ciclosporin in Autoimmune Diseases. Springer-Verlag, Berlin, pp 88–95

Pender MP, Stanley GP, Yoong G, Nguyen KB (1990) The neuropathology of chronic relapsing experimental allergic encephalomyelitis induced in the Lewis rat by inoculation with whole spinal cord and treatment with cyclosporin A. Acta Neuropath 80:172–183

Quesniaux VFJ (1989) Pharmacology of cyclosporine (Sandimmune). III. Immunochemistry and monitoring. Pharm Rev 41:249–258

Rich S, Carpino MR, Arhelger C (1984) Suppressor T cell growth and differentiation: Identification of a cofactor required for suppressor T cell function and distinct from interleukin 2. J Exp Med 1473–1490

Rubin AM, Kang H (1987) Cerebral blindness and encephalopathy with cyclosporin. Neurology 37:1072–1076

Rudge P (1985) The use of ciclosporin (CyA) in multiple sclerosis – Trial design and tolerance. In: R Schindler (ed) Ciclosporin in Autoimmune Diseases. Springer-Verlag, Berlin, pp 83–87

Rudge P (1990) Cyclosporine and multiple sclerosis In: SD Cook (ed) Handbook of Multiple Sclerosis. Marcel Dekker Inc, New York, pp 439–456

Rudge P, Koetsier JC, Mertin J et al. (1989) Randomised double blind controlled trial of cyclosporin in multiple sclerosis. J Neurol Neurosurg Psychiarry 52:559–565

Ryffel B (1989) Pharmacology of cyclosporine. VI. Cellular activation – Regulation of intracellular events by cyclosporine. Pharmacol Rev 41:407–422

Scherrer U, Vissing SF, Morgan BJ et al. (1990) Cyclosporine-induced sympathetic activation and hypertension after heart transplantation. N Engl J Med 323:693–699

Scoble JE, Senior JCM, Chan P, Varghese Z, Sweny P, Moorhead JF (1989) In vitro cyclosporine toxicity the effect of verapamil. Transplantation 47:647–650

Thompson CB, June CH, Sullivan KM, Thomas ED (1984) Association between cyclosporin neurotoxicity and hypomagnesaemia. Lancet 2:116–1120

Trotter JL, van der Veen RC, Clifford DB (1990) Serial studies of serum interleukin-2 in chronic progressive multiple sclerosis patients: Occurrence of 'bursts' and effect of cyclosporine. J Neuroimmunol 28:9–14

Whisler RL, Lindsey JA, Proctor KVW, Morisaki N, Cornwell DG (1984) Characteristics of cyclosporine induction of increased prostaglandin levels from human peripheral blood monocytes. Transplantation 38:377–381

Whitham RH, Vandenbark AA, Bourdette DN, Chou YK, Offner H (1990) Suppressor cell regulation of encephalitogenic T cell lines: Generation of suppressor macrophages with cyclosporin A and myelin basic protein. Cell Immunol 126:290–303

Chapter 11

Treatment of Multiple Sclerosis with Interferons

Lawrence Jacobs and Frederick Munschauer

Introduction and Background

Interferons (IFNs) are a heterogeneous family of naturally occurring glycoproteins first clearly described by Issacs and Lindenmann in 1957 for their capability of blocking or interfering with virus replication and protecting cells against a wide range of viruses (Isaacs and Lindenmann 1957). In addition to their ability to establish an antiviral state in cells, the IFNs activate specific intracellular enzymes, inhibit cell growth, modulate immune responses, activate macrophages, enhance lymphocyte cytotoxicity, and exhibit hormone-like activity (Borden and Ball 1981; Fleischmann et al. 1988; Borden et al. 1982). The mechanisms by which IFNs exert their biological effects are not completely understood. The antiviral, antiproliferative and other biologic effects of IFNs appear to be mediated by de-novo synthesis of a family of proteins.

Three classes of IFN (alpha, beta and gamma) have been distinguished by their antigenic and molecular characteristics. IFN-alpha and IFN-beta (type I IFNs) share considerable nucleotide and amino-acid homology, use a common receptor and share a similar intronless genetic organization. The genes for the family of IFNs-alpha are contained in a multigene cluster on chromosome 9. In close proximity is the single gene including IFN-beta (Borden and Ball 1981; Fleischmann et al. 1988; Borden et al. 1982). Both IFN-alpha and IFN-beta interact with the same cell surface receptors and exert biological effects by nearly identical mechanisms. IFN-gamma (type II IFN) differs from alpha and beta in amino-acid composition and by use of a different cell surface receptor. Moreover, IFN-gamma may exert its antiviral effect by a different mechanism than IFN-alpha and IFN-beta. Although antigenically different from IFN-alpha and beta, IFN-gamma does show some similarity with the other IFNs in its secondary structure (Fleischmann et al. 1988).

During the past 15 years therapeutic trials with IFNs have been conducted mostly in patients with various viral, neoplastic and nervous system disorders. Early clinical trials of IFNs were hampered by the scarcity of natural human IFNs. This problem has been alleviated by IFN production using recombinant techniques. The mixed results of many of the previous studies of different neurologic and non-neurologic disorders have been reviewed elsewhere (Fleischmann et al. 1988; Borden et al. 1982; Smith 1988; Jacobs et al. 1988a).

In this chapter we will limit our review to the experiences and current status of studies on the use of IFNs in multiple sclerosis (MS).

The rationale for testing IFNs in MS derives from the body of evidence for viral and dysimmune pathogenesis of this disease and the known antiviral and immunomodulatory actions of the IFNs (Stewart 1979; Dunnick and Galasso 1979; Cook and Dowling 1980; Leibowitz 1983; Ter Meulen and Stephenson 1983; Salazar et al. 1983). While the earliest testing of IFNs in MS were based on these relatively non-specific premises, a deeper understanding of the immunopathology of MS including putative roles of endogenous IFNs and persisting suspicions of viral infection prompted larger, more carefully designed studies.

Three important recent neuroimmunologic observations substantiate the rational use of IFNs in MS:

1. Barna et al. (1989) demonstrated that human astrocytes obtained from brain biopsy at the time of stereotactic epilepsy surgery do not normally express HLA-DR surface antigen in tissue culture medium. However, when IFN-gamma was added to the medium, the astrocytes responded with a dose-dependent expression of surface HLA-DR. Pre-incubation or co-incubation of the tissue with IFN-beta (natural or recombinant) resulted in a marked inhibition of the IFN-gamma driven HLA-DR expression by these cells. These findings may account, at least partially, for the clinical observations that MS exacerbations are provoked by systemic administration of IFN-gamma, but reduced or prevented by administration of IFN-beta (see Clinical Trials).
2. The studies of Abreu (Abreu 1982; Abreu et al. 1983) and Hertz and Deghenghi (1985) demonstrated that the clinical and pathologic manifestations of experimental allergic encephalomyelitis (EAE), an accepted animal model of MS, could be suppressed or prevented altogether by administration of IFN-beta systemically or intrathecally. IFN-beta was most effective and exerted its beneficial effect at the lowest doses when it was administered directly into the cerebrospinal fluid (CSF). Also, passive transfer of EAE by sensitized lymphocytes could be prevented by treating the lymphocytes with IFN-beta before transfer, an effect which may have been mediated by IFN-beta blocking release of IFN-gamma from T-lymphocytes.
3. Defects in suppressor function have been demonstrated in MS (Antel et al. 1979, 1986; Rose et al. 1985; Morimoto et al. 1988). The non-specific suppressor activity of peripheral blood lymphocytes and the percentage of T-suppressor lymphocytes (CD3+, CD4+, CD45R+) in circulation may be abnormally reduced at the onset of MS exacerbations but normal during remission (Antel et al. 1979; Paty et al. 1983). This abnormal suppression may be linked to the exacerbation-remission cycle seen in MS. In 1983 it was demonstrated that T-suppressor cell function could be increased by exposing mouse cells to IFN-beta in vitro (Schnaper et al. 1983). In a 1990 study by Noronha et al. (1990) these findings were extended to humans in whom the suppressor function defect of MS patients was corrected by administration of IFN-beta.

Some older, but relevant, observations in MS further support IFN trials in MS:

1. In MS the concentration of IgG in the CSF is characteristically increased reflecting elevated immunoglobulin synthesis by abnormally increased numbers

of central nervous system (CNS) plasma cells (Kabat et al. 1942; Tourtellotte et al. 1984). IFN-alpha and IFN-beta influence immunoglobulin synthesis through a direct effect on plasma cells and could influence IgG synthesis in MS patients (Harfast et al. 1981).

2. In approximately 50% of MS patients, peripheral blood lymphocytes produce subnormal amounts of IFN in response to viral and mitogen challenges (Neighbor et al. 1981; Neighbor 1985; Merrill and Targan 1988). In some studies this decreased IFN response was mostly associated with patients expressing the HLA DRW 2 antigen (an HLA type strongly associated with MS) (Merrill and Targan 1988). Exogenously administered IFN might replace the defective endogenous production by lymphocytes or directly stimulate lymphocytes to produce normal amounts of IFN.

3. Natural killer (NK) cell activity is reduced in some MS patients (Neighbor et al. 1981; Neighbor 1985; Vervliet et al. 1983). IFNs can markedly increase NK cell cytotoxicity. Thus, the NK cell activity of MS patients might be stimulated to normal levels by administration of exogenous IFN-beta.

Taken as a whole, the cited neuroimmunologic observations suggest that IFN-beta may exert favorable immunologic effects on MS. In the following sections the results of clinical trials with IFNs in MS are described. The essentials of these trials are also presented in Table 11.1. Much of the data on systemic IFN trials was previously reported by Panitch (1988) and Panitch and Johnson (1988) and that on intrathecal IFN trials by Jacobs et al. (1988b).

Clinical Trials

Systemic Interferon Gamma

Panitch et al. (1987) conducted a pilot study of recombinant IFN-gamma (rIFN-gamma: Immuneron, Biogen) in 18 patients with relapsing disease. The rationale for this treatment was that IFN-gamma had many of the antiviral, antiproliferative, and immunomodulatory activities of the other IFNs and its production appeared to be defective in MS. However, IFN-gamma differs in important ways from IFN-alpha and beta, one of which is in its potency as an immune activator. For example, IFN-gamma activates monocytes and macrophages.

In the Panitch study rIFN-gamma was administered IV at doses of 1, 30, or 1000 μg twice per week for 4 weeks to 3 subgroups of 6 patients each (total 18 patients). During the month of treatment 7 of the 18 patients developed acute exacerbations for an on-study rate of 4.7 exacerbations per year. This was significantly higher ($p < 0.01$) than the pre-study rate (1.4/year). Exacerbation rates returned to pre-study levels during the subsequent 4–12 months (Fig. 11.1). Exacerbations occurred in patients within all three dosage groups.

Side effects, primarily fever, chills, myalgia, headache and fatigue, occurred predominantly in the high-dose group and were not felt to be responsible for the exacerbations; some patients with severe side effects had no exacerbations and others receiving the lowest doses had exacerbations in the absence of clinical side effects.

Table 11.1. Clinical trials of systemic interferon in multiple sclerosis

Investigator	IFN	Dose	Route	Duration of treatment	No. of patients	Clinical type	Design	Results
Ververken et al. (1979)	nB	5×10^4 IU/kg	IM	2 weeks	3	CP	Open	No effect
Fog (1980)	na	$2.5 - 5 \times 10^6$ IU/day	IM	15 months	6	CP	Open	No effect
Montezuma-de-Carallo (1983)	Lymphoblastoid	6×10^4 IU/kg/day then alternate days	IM	3 months	12	CS	Open with ACTH	All patients improved
Knobler et al. (1984)	na	5×10^6 IU/day	SC	6 months	24	15 RR 9RP	DB, PC crossover	Reduced attacks in RR group; no effect on RP
Camenga et al. (1986)	ra_2	2×10^6 IU $3 \times$ week	SC	12 months	98	72 RR 25 RP 1 CP	DB, PC	No difference between IFN and P
Panitch et al. (1987)	r-gamma	1, 30, 1000 μg IU, $2 \times$ week	IV	1 month	18	RR	Single-blind	Attacks in 7 patients during treatment
Austims Research Group (1989)	na	3×10^6 IU $2 \times$ week then $1 \times$ week for 10 months then 1×2 wk	SC	3 years	153	RR, CP	DB, PC	No effect on disability, relapses, VER or CSF
Kastrukoff et al. (1990)	Lymphoblastoid	5×10^6 IU/day	SC	6 months	101	CP	DB, PC	In progress
Johnson et al. (1990)	rB	$4.5 - 90 \times 10^6$ IU, $3 \times$ week	SC	6 months	30	RR	DB, PC	Reduced attacks. Dose-related
Huber et al. (1988)	nB	3×10^6 IU $2 \times$ week, then $2 \times$ month	IV	5 months	9	RR	Open	No effect
Baumhefner et al. (1987)	nB	3×10^6 U $1 \times$ week	IV	3 months	6	CP	Open	Improvement in 4 patients
Johnson et al. (1990)	rB	45×10^6 IU $3 \times$ week 22.5×10^6 IU $3 \times$ week	SC	3 years	330	RR	DB, PC	In progress
Jacobs (1990)	rB	6×10^6 IU $1 \times$ week	IM	2 years	290	RR	DB, PC	In progress
Jacobs et al. (1981, 1982)	nB	1×10^6 IU $2 \times$ week for 1 month then $1 \times$ month	IT	6 months	20	RR, CP	Open	Reduced attacks in RR group
Confavreux et al. (1986)	nB	100×10^3 or 640×10^3 IU $1 \times$ week	IT	2 months	11	CP	Open	No effect
Jacobs et al. (1986, 1987)	nB	1×10^6 IU $1 \times$ week for 1 month, then $1 \times$ month	IT	6 months	69	RR	DB, PC	Reduced attacks

Abbreviations: r, recombinant; IFN, interferon; IU, international units; IM, intramuscular; SC, subcutaneous; RR, relapsing/remitting; RP, relapsing/progressive; CP, chronic/progressive; CS, chronic/stable; DB, double-blind; P, placebo; PC, placebo-controlled; nB, natural IFN-beta; rB, recombinant IFN-beta; na, natural IFN-alpha; ra, recombinant IFN-alpha.

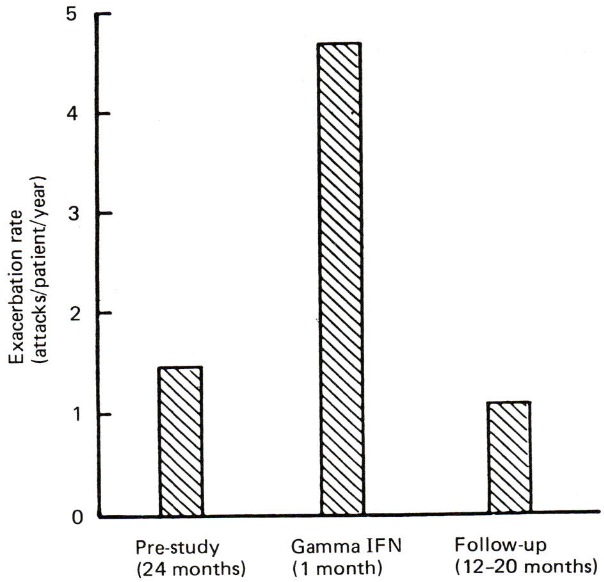

Fig. 11.1. Increase in exacerbation rate during treatment with IFN-gamma compared with pre-treatment and follow-up periods. Data from 18 patients. Prestudy rate increased from 1.42 to 4.7 attacks/patient/year during study ($p < 0.01$); attack rate during follow-up was 1.05 per year. From Panitch et al. (1987), Fig. 1, with permission.

Immunologic studies during treatment showed an increased NK cytotoxicity, no change in cellular responsiveness to IFN-gamma, and normal production of IFN-gamma by patient cells. An important finding which may have contributed to the exacerbations was the induction of HLA-DR2 surface antigen on peripheral blood monocytes indicating activation.

This study clearly demonstrated that systemic IFN-gamma can produce significant deleterious effects on clinical disease activity within the CNS. It also supported the idea that endogenous IFN-gamma plays a role in spontaneous MS exacerbations and that systemically administered IFN-gamma exerts an effect within the CNS. The observed effect of rIFN-gamma in this study was opposite those observed in the IFN-beta studies described below. The fact that IFN-gamma induces MHC Class II (DR) cell surface expression, and IFN-beta inhibits this expression (vida infra) suggests that MS disease activity is influenced by interferon modulation of cell surface MHC markers.

Systemic IFN-alpha

In the earliest study, Fog (1980) administered 2.5 to 5.0 $\times$ 10^6 IU of natural IFN-alpha (nIFN-alpha) intramuscularly (IM) openly to 6 chronic/progressive MS patients for up to 15 months. No benefit was observed.

In 1984, Knobler et al. (1984) reported results of a double-blinded study of nIFN-alpha administered subcutaneously to 24 patients with relapsing disease at a dosage of 5×10^6 IU daily for 6 months. Although subgroup analysis showed a trend toward reduced exacerbations in 15 patients with strictly relapsing disease ($p = 0.08$), no significant improvement could be attributed to nIFN-alpha treatment. Interpretation of this study was complicated by a cross-over design in which patients received 6 months of treatment with either nIFN-alpha or placebo followed by 6 months of washout and then crossed to 6 months of the alternate treatment and another 6 months of washout. There was an increase in serum IgG during treatment and 50% of the treated patients also showed an increase of CSF IgG. Some of the patients in this study also developed a circulating antibody to a contaminant of nIFN-alpha preparation (Sendai derived protein).

Follow-up of 12 patients for 2 years after completion of the trial showed an apparent persisting benefit (without retreatment) in terms of reduction in mean relapse rate (0.92 for 2 years before versus 0.47 for 2 years following the study), although there may have been some variability in how on-study and post-study exacerbations were measured (Panitch 1987).

A much larger multicenter, double-blinded, placebo-controlled study of recombinant IFN-alpha (rIFN-alpha) in MS was reported by Camenga et al. (1986). They treated 98 patients with relapsing disease with 2×10^6 IU administered subcutaneously three times per week for one year followed by a 3-month observation period. In that study a lower dose than previously used by Knobler was administered in order to facilitate double-blinding.

No significant differences in exacerbation rates or clinical profiles were observed between the rIFN-alpha and placebo-treated patients. Thus, this study did not confirm the 1984 observations by Knobler et al. (1984) of reduced exacerbations after nIFN-alpha treatment.

The Camenga et al. (1986) study also showed patterns of NK enhancement and suppression in the placebo group which were basically identical to those in the rIFN-alpha recipient group indicating that placebo administration was accompanied by physiologic effects sufficient to alter immunity. The discrepancy between the results of Camenga et al. (1986) and Knobler et al. (1984) could be that the dose of rIFN-alpha Camenga et al. used was too low, that the preparation was less effective than that used by Knobler et al. or that the original observations were inaccurate.

The Austims Research Group (1989) administered nIFN-alpha to 153 patients with relapsing or chronic/progressive disease in a multicentered, double-blinded, placebo-controlled fashion. In this trial 3×10^6 IU of nIFN-alpha was administered subcutaneously twice per week for 2 months and then once per week for 10 months. The nIFN-alpha treated group was compared with groups of 75 patients each who were treated in an identical fashion with placebo or transfer factor. In this study neither nIFN-alpha nor transfer factor was shown to be of significant benefit to the MS patients (relapsing or chronic/progressive).

Systemic Lymphoblastoid IFN

Montezuma-de-Carallo (1983) reported clinical improvement in 10 chronic/stable patients after 3 months of treatment with lymphoblastoid IFN (a mixture of IFN alpha and beta, mostly alpha) administered IM at a dosage of 6 ×

10^6 IU/kg of body weight daily for 1 month, then every other day for 2 months, but interpretation of results was obscured by multiple methodologic problems.

Kastrukoff et al. (1990) reported the results of a double-blind, placebo-controlled study assessing the efficacy of lymphoblastoid IFN in chronic progressive MS. One hundred patients were included with 50 receiving lymphoblastoid IFN at a dose of 5×10^6 IU and 50 receiving placebo subcutaneously daily for 6 months. After 2 years, there was a trend for the IFN group to be clinically improved at 6 and 18 months, but this did not reach significance. Quantitative MRI analysis of brain plaque burden showed a trend suggesting lower plaque burden in IFN recipients compared to controls at 6 and 18 months. Although the treatments were well tolerated, the authors felt that the results were not compelling enough to recommend lymphoblastoid IFN treatment in chronic progressive MS.

Systemic IFN-beta

In the earliest study Ververken et al. (1979) administered natural IFN-beta (nIFN-beta) intramuscularly openly to 3 patients with chronic/progressive disease at dosages of $2-3 \times 10^6$ IU every other day for 2 weeks. Although no significant toxicity was observed, there was no clinical benefit noted during 9–18 months of follow-up.

Huber et al. (1988) studied the efficacy of nIFN-beta administered intravenously (IV) to 9 patients with chronic/relapsing MS. Patients received 3×10^6 IU of nIFN-beta twice per week for 4 weeks and then twice per month for the next 5 months. These treatments were well-tolerated, but there was no change in exacerbation rates, CSF IgG synthesis or MRI plaque formation during a total follow-up period of 1.2 years.

Baumhefner et al. (1987) reported a beneficial effect of nIFN-beta administered IV in 6 chronic/progressive MS patients. The nIFN-beta dosage was 3×10^6 IU weekly for 12 weeks. Improvement in weekly coded neurological examinations was seen in 4 of the 6 patients. A transient significant reduction of intrathecal IgG synthesis rate was seen in 1 patient. No changes in evoked responses, MRI or other laboratory tests were observed. No significant side effects occurred. It was concluded that IV nIFN-beta even at the low dose tested for a 3-month period could give clinical benefit in some patients with chronic progressive MS. The authors concluded that higher doses by the IV route should be investigated.

Johnson et al. (1990) reported the results of a double-blind, 3-center study of subcutaneously administered rIFN-beta in 30 relapsing MS patients in a dose-escalating, randomized, placebo-controlled, multicenter trial. The interferon used was produced in bacteria by Triton Biosciences, using recombinant DNA technology. This rIFN-beta differs from natural human interferon in certain ways including lack of glycosylation and substitution of a serine residue for cysteine at position 17 (rIFN-beta ser), but Triton rIFN-beta ser has shown antiviral and immunomodulatory effects similar to the natural product. The study was designed to test safety and obtain some information on efficacy and dosing for a full-scale multicenter study of its efficacy in 330 relapsing MS patients. Thirty patients with at least two exacerbations in the 2 years before study entry and Kurtzke EDSS of 0 to 5.5 were randomized into 5 groups.

a

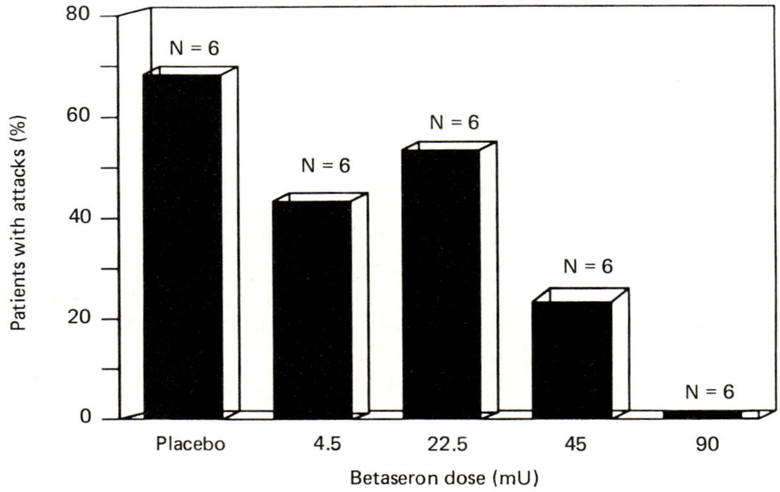

b

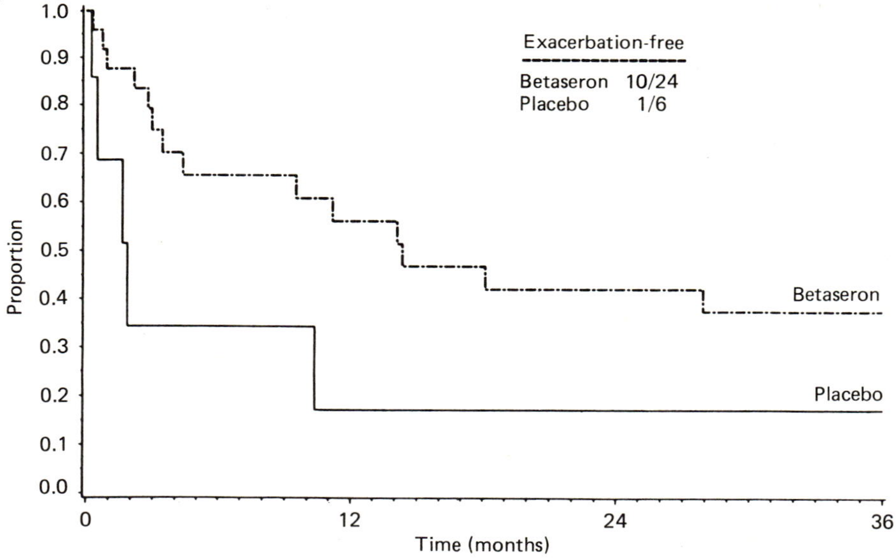

Fig. 11.2. **a** Exacerbations decrease with increasing doses of rIFN-beta ser (Betaseron) until there were no exacerbations at highest dose. There were 6 patients treated in each group for 6 months. Number of patients with exacerbations were: 4 of 6 with placebo, 3 of 7 at 4.5×10^6 IU, 3 of 6 at 22.5×10^6 IU, 2 of 10 at 45×10^6 IU and 0 of 6 at 90×10^6 IU. **b** Proportion of patients who had no exacerbations was greater in the rIFN-beta ser recipients then placebo-treated controls over 6 months. One placebo patient (17%) had no exacerbations, while 10 rIFN-beta ser patients were free of attacks for 3 years. From Johnson et al. (1990) with permission.

Participants self-administered placebo or rIFN-beta ser at doses of 4.5, 22.5, 45 or 90 × 10^6 IU subcutaneously three times weekly. They were evaluated biweekly for 6 weeks, every 6 weeks for the next 18 weeks and then every 3 months for the remainder of the 3-year study period. Analysis of data at 6 months showed a dose-related therapeutic effect on exacerbations, with no relapses in patients receiving the highest dose (Fig. 11.2a). Also, the proportion of patients who were exacerbation-free over time was significantly greater in patients who received rIFN-beta ser than those who received placebo (Fig. 11.2b).

Side effects (injection site erythema, fever, fatigue) were dose-related and profound enough to preclude blinding at 90 × 10^6 IU. Treatments were well-tolerated and blinding was achieved at 45 × 10^6 IU. Therefore, the dose used after 6 months was 45 × 10^6 and this was continued for the remaining 18 months of the study (total 2 years). No exacerbations were precipitated by the rIFN-beta ser. Neutralizing antibodies were identified in approximately 66% of the patients and fluctuated independently of clinical courses. The highest titers appeared in the second year, and tended to fall rapidly in the third year of the study.

This pilot study was too small to determine efficacy but there was a strong trend toward fewer exacerbations in the rIFN-beta ser treated patients. Only 17% of the placebo patients were free of exacerbations, while 42% of the rIFN-beta ser treated patients were exacerbation free over three years.

Intrathecal IFN-beta Administration

The rationale for adminstering IFN intrathecally (IT) rather than systemically was based upon previous research in animals and humans indicating that systemically administered IFN did not effectively cross the blood–brain barrier, but could be safely administered by the IT route (Salazar et al. 1983; Emodi et al. 1975; DeClercq et al. 1975; Habif et al. 1975; Hilfenhaus et al. 1977; Misset et al. 1981; Prange and Wismann 1981; Obbens et al. 1984; Slatkin et al. 1984; Mora et al. 1986). Pharmacokinetic studies in humans indicated that serum to CSF ratio was 30 to 1 after systemic administration (Smith et al. 1985).

That experience included cases of encephalitis, cancer and amyotrophic lateral sclerosis; in several of those studies (Obbens et al. 1984; Slatkin et al. 1984; Mora et al. 1986) the IFN doses administered were substantially greater than in our MS studies. Despite these relatively high doses, the treatments were generally well-tolerated and the side effects similar to those experienced by our patients who received only 1 × 10^6 IU. These experiences provided reassurance as we proceeded with our IT studies.

Jacobs and associates (1981, 1982) reported the results of a trial of IT administration of nIFN-beta in 20 MS patients in an open, unblinded format. Twelve patients had relapsing disease; 8 had stable disease with residua. Patients received approximately 1.0 × 10^6 IU of nIFN-beta by serial LPs semiweekly for the first 4 weeks and then once per month for the next 5 months of the study. There was a significant decrease in the exacerbation rates of the nIFN-beta recipients during the study (mean 0.2/year) compared to prestudy rates (1.8/year) ($p < 0.01$). No change occurred in the exacerbation rates of the untreated controls (prestudy 0.8/year, on-study 0.7/year). Clinically, there was a trend for more recipients than controls to be improved or unchanged but this was not significant. Treatments were generally well-tolerated and side effects (headache, fever, weakness, myalgia) typically cleared within 24 h after treatments. CSF pleocytosis and protein elevations seemed to have no relationship to clinical symptoms and usually cleared within 6–12 months except for slight protein elevations in some patients.

Because of the apparent beneficial response and good tolerance of these treatments, after approximately 2 years of follow-up the initial controls were treated with IT nIFN-beta. They tolerated the treatments as did the original nIFN-beta recipients.

Subsequent follow-up assessments of these patients were conducted after the original recipients had been followed for 4.4 to 5.3 years after nIFN-beta treatment and the controls for a mean of 2.9 years since crossover to rIFN-beta treatment (Jacobs et al. 1985, 1988b). By that time the recipient's prestudy rate of 1.8/year had been further reduced to 0.2/year ($p < 0.001$) and the control mean prestudy rate of 0.68/year, which had been unchanged at the time of crossover, had been reduced to 0.36/year ($p < 0.03$). These observations suggested a persisting, relatively long-term, beneficial effect of IT administered nIFN-beta in the original recipients and a similar pattern of decrease in exacerbation rates in the controls after they were crossed over and began receiving treatment. The treatment phase in these patients only lasted 6 months, after which they were followed without retreatment.

This preliminary study had certain shortcomings including lack of blinding, heterogeneous patient population and different prestudy rates in recipients and controls. Also, the crossover data were analyzed without benefit of concurrent observations on an untreated control group. The decrease in exacerbations in the post-crossover phase of the study could have been due to regression to the mean rather than nIFN-beta treatment. Still, the findings warranted a cautious optimism about the efficacy of IT treatment with nIFN-beta in MS patients and a more definitive study was subsequently undertaken.

In a smaller study Confavreux et al. (1986) assessed the effect of IT-administered nIFN-beta in 11 chronic/progressive patients. The patients received nIFN-beta IT at doses of 100 000 IU (6 patients) or 640 000 IU (5 patients) at weekly intervals for 2 months. The treatments were well-tolerated, but there was no modification in the clinical course of these patients during a 6-month period of observation. The number, motility and intensity of oligoclonal bands in the CSF remained consistent and distinctive for individual patients over serial CSF assessments.

The largest investigation to date of IT IFN in MS was conducted by Jacobs et al. (1986, 1987) in a randomized, double-blinded, placebo-controlled, multicenter study of 69 patients with relapsing disease. All of the patients had an exacerbation rate of at least 0.6/year and there were no differences in age, disease duration, exacerbation rates, and Kurtzke Disability Status Scores between nIFN-beta recipients and controls. The nIFN-beta was administered to 34 recipients by serial lumbar punctures weekly for the first 4 weeks and then once monthly for the next 5 months (i.e., 9 lumbar punctures during first 6 months). The dosage administered at each LP was 1×10^6 IU. The 35 controls underwent placebo treatments according to the same schedule; their treatments consisted of false LPs with needle advanced only into the subcutaneous tissues, where 5 ml of sterile water was injected. Patients received indomethacin (25–50 mg/q 6 hr, for 24 hours) after each treatment to block

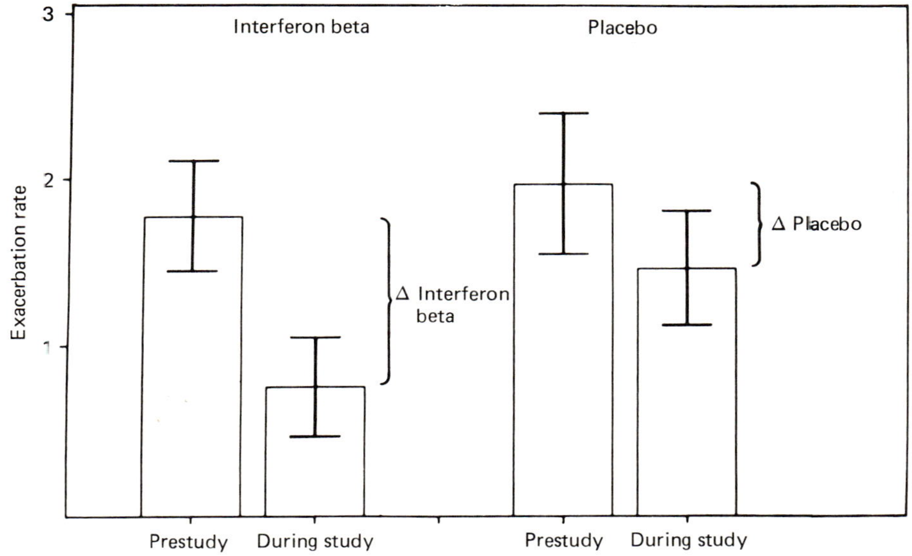

Fig. 11.3. Mean exacerbation rates noted prestudy and during study (exacerbations per year) in patients who received IT IFN-beta and control patients (placebo). Error bars = 2 standard errors of the mean. Changes in rates were expressed by △ IFN-beta and △ placebo. Mean prestudy rates of both groups were nearly identical (patients who received IFN-beta, 1.79; control patients, 1.98). Exacerbation rate during study of patients who received IFN-beta (0.76) was significantly less than that of control patients (1.48) ($p < 0.001$). Change in exacerbation rate of IFN-beta recipients (1.02) was significantly greater than control patients (0.51) ($p < 0.04$). From Jacobs et al. (1987), Fig. 4, with permission.

side effects of IFN-beta to facilitate blinding. The treatment phase of this study lasted only 6 months, but follow-up examinations to assess for exacerbations, Kurtzke scores and overall clinical status continued monthly for the next 18 months.

Fig. 11.3 shows the exacerbation rates on these patients. The prestudy exacerbation rates of the nIFN-beta recipients and controls were nearly identical, but the on-study rate of the nIFN-beta recipients was significantly less than that of control patients ($p < 0.001$). Also, the change in rate of nIFN-beta recipients was significantly greater than that of control patients. Fig. 11.4 shows a correlation analysis of exacerbation rates in these patients. There was a strong direct relationship between prestudy and on-study exacerbation rates in the control patients ($r = 0.51$; $p < 0.001$); control patients with higher prestudy rates tended to have high exacerbation rates during the study while control patients with low prestudy rates had low on-study rates. However, this dependency of on-study rates to prestudy exacerbation rates was not observed in the patients who received nIFN-beta ($r = 0.02$; $p = 0.45$). The nIFn-beta seemed to "uncouple" the relationship of on-study rate to prestudy exacerbation rate in the recipients.

Clinically, the degree of worsening on the Kurtzke scale was greater in the controls (mean 0.80) than in the nIFN-beta recipients (mean 0.32), but this difference was not significant (Table 11.2). Also, more nIFN-beta recipients were clinically improved or unchanged and more controls clinically worse at the end of the study compared with their status at the beginning of the study, but the difference between the groups was not statistically significant.

The clinical side effects of treatments were basically the same in the two groups except for fever which occurred significantly more frequently in nIFN-

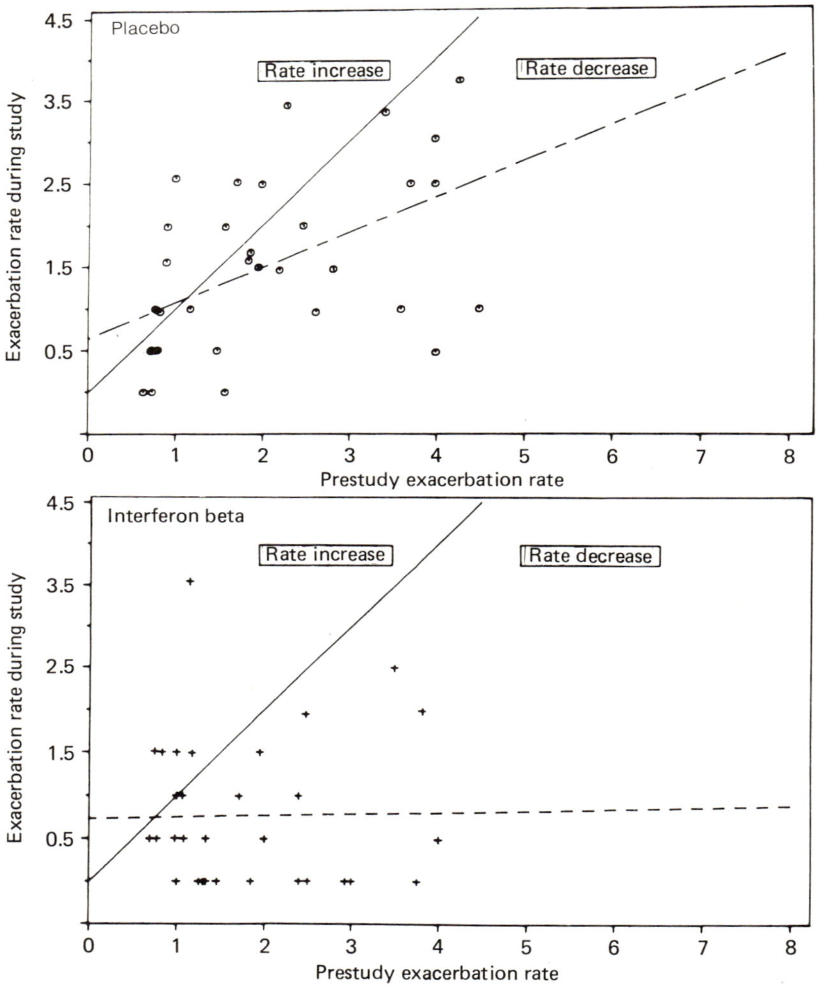

Fig. 11.4. Correlation analyses in control patients (top) and patients who received IFN-beta (bottom). Top panel: hatched line describes strong dependency of exacerbation rate during study on prestudy exacerbation rate ($r = 0.51$; $p < 0.001$). Bottom pannel: hatched line is nearly horizontal, indicating no significant relationship between exacerbation rates during study and prestudy ($r = 0.02$; $p = 0.45$). Solid oblique line in both graphs indicates line of unity (theoretical line produced if each patient's exacerbation rates during study and prestudy were same). Rate increase and rate decrease in both graphs indicate number of patients whose exacerbation rates increased or decreased during study compared with prestudy exacerbation rates. From Jacobs et al. (1987), Fig. 5, with permission.

Table 11.2. Changes in clinical status

Clinical status	Interferon beta (No. (%))	Placebo (No. (%))
Improved/unchanged	26 (76.5)	21 (60)
Worsened	8 (23.5)	14 (40)
Degree of worsening	0.32	0.80

From Jacobs (1987), Table 2, with permission.
More patients who received IFN-beta were improved or unchanged and more control patients worse at the end of the study compared with their status at the beginning of the study; difference between the two groups was not significant ($p = 0.23$). Mean degree of worsening in the control patients (0.80) was greater than that of those who received IFN-beta (0.32) on modified Kurtzke scale; difference was not significant ($p = 0.32$).

beta recipients than in controls. The CSF changes observed were less severe than in the predecessor study and the abnormalities improved during the study. By the end of the study there was no difference in the CSF protein levels or cell counts in the nIFN-beta recipients and controls. We also observed an increase in IgG index and synthesis rate and a decrease in CSF kappa light chains in the nIFN-beta recipients compared to the controls (Rudick et al. 1987), documenting an intrathecal immunologic response accompanying IT administration of nIFN-beta.

This study demonstrated that nIFN-beta, adminstered IT, significantly reduces exacerbation rates in patients with relapsing MS and thus confirmed the findings of the predecessor preliminary study. While changes in exacerbation rate were significant, there was only a trend toward concomitant improvement in clinical status. The overall impact of reducing or eliminating exacerbations in such patients can only be determined by continued follow-up clinical assessments over more protracted periods of time.

Ongoing Clinical Trials

The clinical trials outlined above suggest that IFN-beta is the most promising IFN for use in future clinical trials in MS. Recent research indicates that systemically administered IFN does cross the blood–brain barrier to produce direct effects within the CNS. The interferon specific C-56 inducible protein was detected in the brains of healthy monkeys following systemic as well as IT administration of nIFN-alpha (Smith et al. 1987). Also, the interferon-induced enzyme 2′,5′-oligoadenylate synthetase (2′,5′-AS) was induced in rat brain following systemic administration of IFN-beta (Hovanessian et al. 1988). Furthermore symptoms of EAE were prevented or reduced by systemic administration of IFN-beta (Abreu 1982; Abreu et al. 1983; Hertz and Deghenghi 1985) in rats. Others found that systemically administered IFNs (alpha, beta) were effective in certain CNS disease in humans such as encephalitis (Panitch 1988). These results, coupled with the inherent difficulties and potential morbidity of repeated IT administration, compel further assessment of the efficacy of systemically-administered IFN-beta in MS. Currently two independent prospective, double-blinded, clinical studies are under way to test the efficacy of rIFN-beta adminstered systemically in MS.

In the first, Johnson et al. (1990) are studying relatively high-dose frequent subcutaneous injections of rIFN-beta ser in 330 relapsing MS patients at several centers in the United States and Canada. Three treatment groups have been included: (1) rIFN-beta ser at 45 × 10^6 IU, (2) rIFN-beta ser at 22.5 × 10^6 IU and, (3) placebo. Treatment doses are administered three times per week and the primary outcome measure of the study is change in exacerbation rate during the study. Clinical disability and immunologic parameters will also be assessed as secondary outcome measures. Results of the pilot study segment of this trial were described above; those of the full trial will probably be known in late 1991.

In the second study, Jacobs et al. are conducting a randomized, double-blinded, placebo-controlled, multicenter study assessing the efficacy of IM administration of low dose rIFn-beta in 290 patients with relapsing MS. The rIFN-beta used in this study is produced by recombinant technology using Chinese Hamster Ovary (CHO) cells (Bioferon Inc., Laupheim, Germany; Biogen, USA). This mammalian cell line generates a glycosylated human rIFN-beta which is identical in amino-acid content and sequence to naturally occurring human IFN-beta. There is evidence that glycosylation may be important in influencing the extent and duration of IFN-beta biologic activity. The rIFN-beta will be administered IM at a dose of 6 × 10^6 IU once per week for 2 years.

This treatment regimen was determined in a pilot study demonstrating that 6 × 10^6 IU was the highest dosage that could be administered under double-blinded conditions when acetaminophen was administered to facilitate blinding. Higher doses of 9.5 and 18.0 × 10^6 IU caused side effects that were not adequately suppressed by acetaminophen and were sufficiently severe to break double-blinding. The dosage interval of one week was determined from the

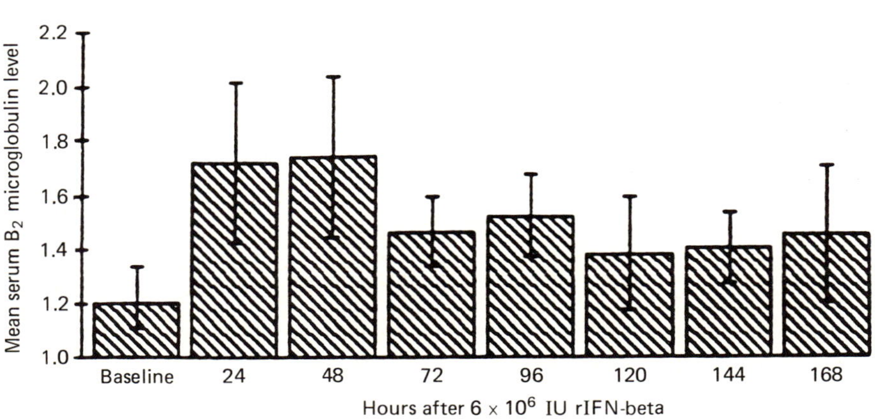

Fig. 11.5. Mean serum B2 microglobulin levels following single IM injections of 6 × 10^6 IU rIFN-beta. There is significant elevation of levels above baseline from 24 to 96 h (4 days) (p = 0.007); elevation of lesser degree (p = 0.09) persists for 168 h (7 days). Data is from 5 patients; error bars = ±1 SD.

observation that a single IM dose of 6×10^6 IU resulted in a significant increase from baseline serum B2 microglobulin (an indirect market of IFN-beta activity) that persisted for 6 days (Fig. 11.5). The change from baseline for B2 microglobulin was of approximately the same magnitude as seen with the next higher dose (9.5×10^6 IU). The next lower dose tested (3×10^6 IU) resulted in significant elevation of B2 microglobulins for only 48 h after injection. It was, therefore, determined that the optimum dosage for the study was 6×10^6 IU administered IM once per week.

The primary aim of the Jacobs study is to test the hypothesis that rIFN-beta treated patients will show a significantly longer time to progression in disability defined as a deterioration of at least 1.0 EDSS unit that persists for at least 6 months. Only patients with active relapsing disease and minimal disability (EDSS <3.5) will be accessed to the study. Patients will be treated weekly for 2 years and followed for 1–2 years following therapy. The studies of Bornstein et al. (1987) and Goodkin et al. (1988) indicate that 67% to 88% of untreated relapsing patients will have entry EDSS scroes of 1.0 to 3.5 , so the present study should capture the majority of relapsing patients for inclusion. Statistical analysis of the primary end point will be carried out using a stratified log-rank test with the Type I error rate set to 0.05. The only stratification will be by the four clinical institutions and the sample size of 290 will provide a power of 80% to detect a difference between rIFN-beta recipients and placebo controls. The Kurtzke EDSS was used as the primary outcome measure because it has been well-validated as a measure of neurologic impairment in MS. It has been shown that approximately 50% of placebo-treated control patients with DSS of 1–4 inclusive progressed at least 1.0 DSS unit over a 2-year period (Bornstein et al. 1987). Based upon these data, the study was designed to detect an increase in median time to progression from 2 years to 3 years and this is the difference expected to be observed if rIFN-beta slows the on-study progression of EDSS.

Subsidiary aims of the study are to determine whether rIFN-beta treated patients differ from controls in several parameters of exacerbation, functional status (physical, cognitive, social), upper and lower extremity disability, global assessment of worsening, and amount of brain-plaque load determined by MRI. Certain potentially important viral and immunologic markers in the serum and CSF will also be analyzed. This study, supported and monitored by the NIH, began in June 1990. The final analysis for efficacy is planned for June 1994.

Conclusion

Certain conclusions can be drawn from the experience with IFNs in MS to date. Interferon gamma provokes exacerbations and IFN-beta reduces them. The pathophysiologic basis of these opposing phenomena is unknown, but may relate to the expression of MHC Class II molecules by human astrocytes, which is up-regulated by IFN-gamma and down-regulated by IFN-beta. The previous belief that IFNs administered systemically do not cross the blood–brain barrier has been contradicted by studies showing IFN bioactivity in monkey brain after systemic administration. This, and certain less direct observations have prompted two new studies of systemically administered rIFN-beta in MS. The results of these studies are not yet known, but preliminary pilot results suggest a beneficial effect on exacerbations, quite similar to those observed after intrathecal administration of IFN-beta. What is not known is whether IFN-beta can effectively reduce clinical disability in MS patients. It is possible that IFN-beta reduces exacerbations without modifying the progression of disability in MS. Future research on the efficacy of IFNs in MS must consider disability in a broad sense and requires stringent double-blinded, placebo-controlled prospective designs.

References

Abreu SL (1982) Suppression of experimental allergic encephalomyelitis by interferon. Immunol Invest 11:1–7

Abreu SL, Tondreau J, Levine S et al. (1983) Inhibition of passive localized allergic encephalomyelitis by interferon. Int Arch Allergy Appl Immunol 72:30–33

Antel JP, Arnason BGW, Medof ME (1979) Suppressor cell function in multiple sclerosis: correlation with clinical disease activity. Ann Neurol 5:476–482

Antel JP, Bania M, Noronha A et al. (1986) Defective suppressor cell function mediated by T8+ cell lines from patients with progressive multiple sclerosis. J Immunol 137:3436–3439

Austims Research Group (1989) Interferon and transfer factor in the treatment of multiple sclerosis: a double-blind, placebo controlled trial. J Neurol Neurosurg Psychiat 52:566–574

Barna BP, Chou SM, Jacobs B et al. (1989) Interferon-B impairs induction of HLA-DR antigen expression in cultured human astrocytes. J Neuroimmunol 23:45–53

Baumhefner RW, Tourtellotte WW, Syndulkok et al. (1987) Effect of intravenous natural beta-interferon on clinical neurofunction, magnetic resonance imaging plaque burden, intrablood-brain barrier IgG synthesis, blood and cerebrospinal fluid cellular immunology and visual evoked responses. Ann Neurol 22:171

Borden EC, Ball LA (1981) Interferons: Biochemical, cell growth inhibitory and immunological effects. In: EB Brown (ed), Progress in hematology, vol III. Grune & Stratton Inc, New York, pp 299–339

Borden EC, Edwards BS, Hawkins MJ, Merritt JA (1982) Interferons: Biological response modification and pharmacology. In: Mihich E (ed), Biological responses in cancer: progress toward potential applications, vol 1. Plenum Publishing, New York, pp 169–218

Bornstein MB, Miller A, Slagle S et al. (1987) A pilot trial of COP 1 in exacerbating-remitting multiple sclerosis. N Engl J Med 317:408–414

Camenga DL, Johnson KP, Alter M et al. (1986) Systemic recombinant alpha-2 interferon therapy in relapsing multiple sclerosis. Arch Neurol 43:1239–1246

Confavreux C, Chapuis-Cellier C, Arnaud P et al. (1986) Oligoclonal "fingerprint" of CSF IgG in multiple sclerosis patients is not modified following intrathecal administration of natural beta-interferon. J Neurol Neurosurg Psychiatry 49:1308–1312

Cook D, Dowling PC (1980) Multiple sclerosis and viruses: An overview. Neurology 20:80–91

DeClercq E, Edy VG, de Vlieger H et al. (1975) Intrathecal adminstration of interferon in neonatal herpes. J Pediatr 86:736–739

Dunnick JK, Galasso GJ (1979) Clinical trials with exogenous interferon: Summary of a meeting. J Infect Dis 139:109–123

Emodi G, Just M, Hernandez R et al. (1975) Circulating interferon in man after administration of exogenous human leukocyte interferon. J Natl Cancer Inst 54:1045–1049

Fleischmann WR, Ramamurthy V, Stanton JG, Baron S (1988) Interferon: mode of action and clinical applications. In: RA Smith (ed), Interferon treatment of neurologic disorders. Marcel Dekker, New York, pp 1–42

Fog T (1980) Interferon treatment of multiple sclerosis patients: A pilot study. In: Boese A (ed). Search for the cause of multiple sclerosis and other chronic diseases of the nervous system. Verlag Chemie, Weinheim, pp 491–493

Goodkin DE, Rudick RA, Hertsgarrd D (1988) Exacerbation rate and adherence to disease type in a prospectively followed MS population: Implications for clinical trials. Arch Neurol 46: 1107–1112

Habif DV, Liptin R, Cantell K (1975) Interferon crosses the blood-cerebrospinal fluid barrier in monkeys. Proc Soc Exp Biol Med 149:287–298

Harfast B, Huddlestone JR, Casali P et al. (1991) Interferon acts directly on human B-lymphocytes to modulate immunoglobulin synthesis. J Immunol 127:2146–2150

Hertz F, Deghenghi R (1985) Effect of rat and beta human interferon on hyperactute experimental allergic encephalomyelitis in rats. Agents Actions 16:397–403

Hilfenhaus J, Weinman E, Major M et al. (1977) Administration of human interferon to rabies virus-infected monkeys affer exposure. J Infect Dis 135:846–849

Hovanessian AG, Marcovistz R, Rivere Y et al. (1988) Production and action of interferon in rabies virus infection. In: Smith RA (ed), Interferon treatment of neurologic disorders. Marcel Dekker, New York, pp 157–186

Huber M, Bamborschke S, Assheuer J, Heib WD (1988) Intravenous natural beta interferon treatment of chronic exacerbating-remitting multiple sclerosis: clinical response and MRI/CSF findings. J Neurol 235:171–173

Isaacs A, Lindenmann J (1957) Virus interference. I. The Interferon. Proc R Soc Lond (Biol) 147:258–267

Jacobs L, O'Malley J, Freeman A et al. (1981) Intrathecal interferon reduces exacerbations of multiple sclerosis. Science 214:1026–1028

Jacobs L, O'Malley J, Freeman A et al. (1982) Intrathecal interferon in multiple sclerosis. Arch Neurol 39:609–615

Jacobs L, O'Malley JA, Freeman A et al. (1985) Intrathecal interferon in the treatment of multiple sclerosis: Patient follow-up. Arch Neurol 42:841–847

Jacobs L, Salazar AM, Herndon R et al. (1986) Multicenter double-blind study of effect of intrathecally administered natural human fibroblast interferon on exacerbations of multiple sclerosis. Lancet 2:1411–1413

Jacobs L, Salazar AM, Herndon R et al. (1987) Intrathecally administered natural human fibroblast interferon reduces exacerbations of multiple sclerosis: results of a multicenter double-blind study. Arch Neurol 44:589–595

Jacobs L, Salazar AM, O'Malley JA (1988a) The use of interferons in the treatment of certain diseases of the central nervous system. In: S Baron (ed), The interferon system, a current review to 1987. Marcel Dekker Inc., New York, pp 241–264

Jacobs L, Salazar A, Herndon RM et al. (1988b) Intrathecal interferon in the treatment of multiple sclerosis. In: Smith RA (ed), Interferon treatment of neurologic disorders. Marcel Dekker, New York, pp 241–262

Johnson KP, Knobler RL, Greenstein JI et al. (1990) Recombinant human beta interferon treatment of relapsing-remitting multiple sclerosis. Neurology 40 (Suppl 1):261

Kabat EA, Moore OH, Landow H (1942) An electrophoretic study of the protein components in the cerebrospinal fluid and their relationship to the serum proteins. J Clin Invest 21:571–577

Kaskrukoff LF, Oger JJ, Hashimoto SA et al. (1990) Systemic lymphoblastoid interferon therapy in chronic progressive multiple sclerosis. I. Clinical and MRI evaluation. Neurology 40:479–486

Knobler RL, Panitch HS, Braheny SL et al. (1984) Systemic alpha interferon therapy in multiple sclerosis. Neurology 34:1273–1279

Leibowitz S (1983) The immunology of multiple sclerosis. In: Hallpike JF, Adams CWM, Tourtellotte WW (eds), Multiple sclerosis. Williams and Wilkins, Baltimore, pp 379–412

Merrill JE, Targan SR (1988) The immunologic basis for the use of interferons. In: Smith RA (ed), Interferon treatment of neurologic disorders. Marcel Dekker, New York, pp 65–101

Misset JL, Mathe G, Horoszewica JS (1981) Intrathecal interferon in meningeal leukemia. N Eng J Med 304:1544

Montezuma-de-Carallo MJ (1983) A treatment for the chronic disabilities of stable multiple sclerosis. Acta Medicotechnica 31:155–160

Mora JS, Munsat TL, Kao KP et al. (1986) Intrathecal administration of natural human interferon alpha in amyotrophic lateral sclerosis. Neurology 36:1137–1140

Morimoto C, Hafler DA, Weiner HL (1988) Selective loss of suppressor inducer T cell subset in progressive multiple sclerosis: analysis with anti-2H4 monoclonal antibody. N Engl J Med 316:67–72

Neighbor PA (1984) Studies of interferon production and natural killing by lymphocytes from multiple sclerosis patients. Ann NY Acad Sci 436:181–191

Neighbor PA, Miller AE, Bloom BR (1981) Interferon responses of leukocytes in multiple sclerosis. Neurology 31:561–566

Noronha A, Toscas A, Jensen MA (1990) Interferon beta augments suppressor cell function in multiple scelerosis. Ann Neurol 27:207–210

Obbens EAMT, Feum LG, Leavens ME et al. (1984) Interferon in the treatment of intracranial malignancies: A pilot study. Neurology 34 (Suppl 1):232

Panitch HS (1987) Systemic alpha-interferon in multiple sclerosis: long-term patient follow-up. Arch Neurol 44:61–63

Panitch HS (1988) Treatment of subacute sclerosing panencephalitis with interferon. In: Smith RA (ed), Interferons in the treatment of neurologic disorders. Marcel Dekker, New York, pp 187–208

Panitch HS, Johnson KP (1988) Treatment of multiple sclerosis by systemic administration of interferon, In Smith RA (ed), Interferon treatment of neurologic disorders. Marcel Dekker, New York, pp 209–232

Panitch HS, Heracl RL, Schindler J, Johnson KP (1987) Treatment of multiple sclerosis with gamma interferon: exacerbations associated with activation of the immune system. Neurology 37:1097–1120

Paty DW, Kastrukoff L, Morgan N et al. (1983) Suppressor T-lymphocytes in multiple sclerosis: Analysis of patients with acute relapsing and chronic progressive disease. Ann Neurol 14: 445–449

Prange H, Wismann H (1981) Intrathecal use of interferon in encephalitis. N Engl J Med 305: 1283–1284

Rose LM, Ginsberg AH, Rothstein TI et al. (1985) Selective loss of a subset of T helper cells in active multiple sclerosis. Proc Natl Acad Sci USA 82:7389–7393

Rudick RA, Jacobs L, Reese PA et al. (1987) Changes in the humoral immune response accompanying intrathecal natural human fibroblast interferon in patients with multiple sclerosis. Neurology 37 (Suppl 1):305

Salazar AM, Gibbs CJ, Gajudsek DC et al. (1983) Clinical use of interferons: Central nervous system disorders. In: Came P, Carter WA (eds), Handbook of Experimental Pharmacology: vol 71. Springer-Verlag, New York, pp 472–497

Schnaper HW, Aune TM, Pierce CW (1983) Suppressor T cell activation by human leukocyte interferon. J Immunol 131:2301–2306

Slatkin NE, Jaeckle KA, Lukes SA et al. (1984) Treatment of leptomeningeal gliomatosis with human leukocyte interferon: Results in two patients. Neurology 34 (Suppl 1):151

Smith RA, Norris F, Palmer D et al. (1985) Distribution of alpha interferon in serum and cerebrospinal fluid after systemic administration. Clin Pharmacol Ther 1:85–88

Smith RA, Landel CP, Cornelius CE, Revel M (1987) Mapping the action of interferon on primate brain. In: Cantell K, Schellekens H (eds), The biology of the interferon system. Martinus Nijhoff, Boston, pp 563–566

Stewart WE II (1979) The interferon system. Springer-Verlag, New York

Ter Meulen V, Stephenson JR (1983) The possible role of viral infections in multiple sclerosis and other related demyelinating diseases. In: Hallpike JF, Adams CWM, Tourtellotte WW (eds), Multiple sclerosis. Williams and Wilkins, Baltimore, pp 241–274

Tourtellotte WW, Walsh MJ, Baumhefner RW et al. (1984) The current status of multiple sclerosis intra-blood-brain barrier IgG synthesis. Ann NY Acad Sci 436:52–67

Ververken D, Carton H, Billiau A et al. (1979) Intrathecal administration of interferon in MS patients. In: Karcher D, Lowenthal A, Strosberg AD (eds), Humoral immunity in neurological disease. Plenum, New York, pp 625–627

Vervliet G, Claeys H, Van Haver H et al. (1983) Interferon production and natural killer cell (NK) activity in leukocyte cultures from multiple sclerosis patients. J Neurol Sci 60:137–150

Wills R, Smith RA (1988) Pharmacokinetics of interferons, In: Smith RA (ed) Interferon treatment of neurologic disorders. Marcel Dekker, New York, pp 103–134

Chapter 12

Treatment of Multiple Sclerosis with Plasma Exchange

John H. Noseworthy

Introduction

The initial studies of plasma exchange (formerly plasmapheresis) as a possible therapy for multiple sclerosis (MS) were published 10 years ago (Dau et al. 1980; Weiner and Dawson 1980). This technique had been shown to be a life-saving procedure in patients with Goodpasture's syndrome (Lockwood et al. 1975; Rossen et al. 1976; Walker et al. 1977; Kincaid-Smith and d'Apice 1978; Rosenblatt et al. 1979). Plasma exchange was technically feasible and generally well-tolerated. Although cumbersome and expensive, it could be administered over several weeks, generally in combination with a low dose of an immunosuppressive drug, and was being considered a candidate therapy for a large number of putative autoimmune diseases. As MS was felt to be immunologically mediated, it seemed highly reasonable to commit the resources needed to determine if this treatment approach could be tailored to benefit patients with MS (van den Noort and Waksman 1980). In this chapter I will review the reasons for this early enthusiasm as well as the results of this decade of study.

Pharmacology

Plasmapheresis was initially developed as a technique to collect anti-tetanus antiserum from horses and subsequently from human plasma to treat soldiers wounded in World War II. The term plasma exchange is preferred for the therapeutic removal of plasma and replacement with a suitable colloid solution. Lymphocytapheresis, the therapeutic removal of circulating blood lymphocytes, is an experimental treatment which was tested briefly and discarded when the preliminary experience suggested little benefit in patients with progressive MS (Giordano 1981; Hauser et al. 1984; Rose et al. 1983; Hocker et al. 1984; Medaer et al. 1984).

Indications and Mechanisms of Action

The Clinical Applications Committee of the American Society of Apheresis divided the medical disorders in which plasma exchange has been attempted into four broad categories: (1) acceptable therapy under appropriate circumstances, (2) sufficient data to warrant a preliminary position, (3) requires further investigation, and (4) adequately tested and found to be of no benefit (Klein et al. 1986). Chronic inflammatory demyelinating polyneuropathy, Guillain–Barré syndrome, and myasthenia gravis were assigned to Category 1 in 1986 and paraproteinemic peripheral neuropathy and MS were grouped with other indications in Category 2.

As discussed below, there are a number of possible ways in which therapeutic plasma exchange might influence the course of MS. In a number of other neurological and systemic diseases, plasma exchange is presumed to assert its therapeutic effect through the removal of soluble substances. In both fulminating myasthenia gravis (reviewed by Klein et al. 1986) and anti-glomerular basement membrane disease (Goodpasture's syndrome: Lockwood et al. 1975; Rossen et al. 1976; Walker et al. 1977; Kincaid-Smith and d'Apice 1978; Rosenblatt et al. 1979; reviewed in Klein et al. 1986), it is possible to achieve prompt clinical stabilization after one or several plasma exchange treatments. The presumed mechanism of action in myasthenia gravis and Goodpasture's syndrome is removal of circulating IgG directed against the acetylcholine receptor and lung and glomerular basement membrane antigens, respectively. Similarly, alloantibodies against coagulation Factors VIII and IX and ABO antigens can be removed successfully in patients with Factor VIII and Factor IX unresponsiveness (Slocombe et al. 1981; Cobcroft 1977) and in patients with ABO incompatibility prior to bone marrow transplantation (Berkman et al. 1978). Patients with both acute and chronic hyperviscosity syndrome due to Waldenström's macroglobulinemia, light-chain disease, multiple myeloma, cryoglobulinemia, and cold agglutinin disease can be treated with repeated plasma exchange (Schwab and Fahey 1960; Russell et al. 1977). In disease states associated with an abnormal level of circulating IgM (e.g., hyperviscosity syndrome), the plasma exchange-derived lowering of the circulating concentrations of immunoglobulin is more prolonged than in conditions where IgG is present in excess. This is because IgM is restricted to the intravascular compartment and, as such, there is no rapid return to pre-exchange levels from equilibration between intra- and extra-vascular compartments as is seen with IgG. It is assumed that the mechanism of action of plasma exchange in Guillain–Barré syndrome (The Guillian-Barré Syndrome Study Group, 1985) and chronic inflammatory demyelinating polyneuropathy (Dyck et al. 1986) may be through the removal of antibodies or other soluble substances (e.g., complement) that are damaging to peripheral nerve myelin. There is some evidence to suggest that patients with a paraprotein associated neuropathy may benefit from therapeutic plasma exchange (reviewed in Klein et al. 1986; Dyck et al. 1990). Repeated plasma exchanges could reduce levels of circulating immune complexes both directly and indirectly by plasma exchange-derived removal of reticuloendothelial blockade. Circulating immune complexes may be responsible for such complications as cerebritis, nephritis, vasculitis, cryoglobulinemia, and the pulmonary hypersensitivity syndrome seen in rheumatoid arthritis and systemic lupus erythematosus (Wallace et al. 1979; Rothwell et al. 1980; Brubaker and Winkelstein 1981; Jones et al. 1979; Schildermans et al. 1979; Schlansky et al. 1981). Plasma exchange in conjunction with immunosuppressive drug therapy may be followed by clinical improvement in these patients but the mechanism of this improvement is not clear. It is also possible to remove toxins (Paraquat, methyl parathion; Dearnaley and Martin 1978; Luzhnikov et al. 1977), metabolic products (e.g., phytanic acid in Refsum's disease; Gibberg et al. 1979), delta amino levulinic acid in acute intermittent porphyria (Spiva et al. 1981), and low-density lipoprotein in patients with homozygous familial cholesterolemia (Thompson 1981). Patients with thrombotic thrombocytopenic purpura can be treated effectively with therapeutic plasma exchange using fresh-frozen plasma as the replacement fluid (Lian et al. 1979; Rock et al. 1991), although the specific plasma factor responsible for the response has not been definitively identified.

Techniques

A detailed review of the different techniques used in therapeutic plasma exchange is beyond the mandate of this review (see Silvergleid 1983; Klein et al. 1986; Kennedy and Domen 1983; Shumak and Rock 1984; Patten 1986; Reimann and Mason 1990). Discontinuous or continuous flow centrifugation systems are used in most centers where neurological patients are treated. Although a single vascular access site can be used for a discontinuous flow system, plasma exchange takes less time and hemodynamic control is better when two sites are used (simultaneous blood removal and infusion). There is almost certainly a lower risk of complications from unwanted thrombosis and infection when access is achieved by using superficial arm veins rather than double-lumen dialysis catheters inserted into either the femoral or large central veins (internal jugular and subclavian veins). In neurologic patients, it is rare to have to resort to an arteriovenous fistula, shunt, venous cutdown, or arterial catheter. Decisions about the volume of plasma to be exchanged (usually 1 plasma volume (40 ml/kg) per exchange) and the frequency and total number of plasma exchanges per patient are more often dictated by individual experience or prior protocols than by clear scientific rationale. In Goodpasture's syndrome and myasthenia gravis, for example, where evidence strongly suggests a pathogenic role for circulating antibodies, an initially intensive (daily or alternate day) regimen seems appropriate whereas less frequent exchanges are usually recommended for more slowly progressive, chronic conditions (e.g., chronic inflammatory demyelinating polyneuropathy, chronic cutaneous vasculitis). Similary, the type of anticoagulation used (acid citrate dextrose infusion versus systemic or local heparinization) differs from center to center. Five percent albumin is currently regarded as the replacement fluid of choice because of the low risk of an allergic response or transmission of infection (viral hepatitis, HIV infection). Fresh-frozen plasma is now perhaps only indicated when deficient proteins must be replaced (e.g., clotting factors, thrombotic thrombocytopenic purpura).

Complications

MS patients who are free of serious concomitant medical illnesses (e.g., cardiac or renal disease) generally tolerate therapeutic plasma exchange quite well (Valbonesi et al. 1981; Tindall et al. 1982; Hauser et al. 1983; Guarnieri et al. 1985; Gordon et al. 1985; Khatri et al. 1985a; Weiner et al. 1989; Noseworthy et al. 1989b). The most common side effect with repeated plasma exchange is difficulty achieving venous access. Patients who are judged by experienced plasma exchange personnel to have adequate antecubital veins are generally able to have at least weekly plasma exchange using the superficial arm veins (Noseworthy et al. 1989b), although approximately 20% of treatments will be complicated by problems in obtaining access (e.g., more than one venipuncture, low flow rates, clotting of intravenous tubing, incomplete exchange, etc.). In our experience (Noseworthy et al. 1989b), fewer than 5% of plasma-exchange treatments were complicated by problems with clotting, hypotension, circumoral paresthesia (citrate toxicity), light-headedness, or nausea. Fewer than 1% of exchanges were associated with muscle cramping, bradycardia, vomiting, and bleeding. Care must be taken to avoid hypovolemia and fluid overload, particularly in elderly patients and in those with a history of hypotension, renal or cardiac disease. In most of the protocols described below, plasma exchange is not repeated sufficiently often (e.g., more than 3 times per week) to be complicated by a depletion in platelets, clotting factors, complement, immunoglobulins, cholinesterase, other enzymes (transaminases, lactate dehydrogenase, amylase, etc.) or blood levels of medications. Smith and colleagues (1986) attributed thrombosis of an axillary and subclavian vein to plasma exchange-induced plasminogen deficiency in an MS patient who had received 8 exchanges in a period of only 16 days. Allergic reactions are most frequently observed when fresh-frozen plasma is used as the replacement fluid. These patients may develop urticaria, bronchospasm, pulmonary edema, and hypotension. Recently, two examples of possible plasma exchange-related MS exacerbations have been reported (Wirguin et al. 1989). Death related to plasma exchange is uncommon (Huestis 1986), and, to my knowledge, has not been reported in MS.

Rationale

The etiology and pathogenesis of MS remain unknown. A large amount of information (reviewed in Chap. 5) suggests that a disturbance in the immune response either causes the disease or contributes to the central nervous system injury (Rationale for immunomodulating therapies of multiple sclerosis 1988). Plasma exchange could theoretically favorably influence the course of active MS by a number of mechanisms.

The most appealing rationale for the use of plasma exchange in MS is that this treatment approach is beneficial in other putative autoimmune diseases (see above). Although the mechanism of action is not entirely clear, plasma exchange is thought to act in several of these settings by rapidly lowering the level of circulating immunoglobulins. Although MS patients have elevated levels of IgG in brain and cerebrospinal fluid (CSF), there is no convincing evidence for a pathogenically important circulating immunoglobulin in this disease. It remains possible, however, that unidentified immunoglobulins or immune complexes contribute either to the injury to myelin or somehow regulate an immune-mediated change in the immune response. Although circulating immune complexes may be detected in up to 30% of MS patients (reviewed in Salmi et al. 1982), there is little evidence implicating either immune complex formation or reduced reticuloendothelial function in the pathogenesis of the MS lesion. Alternatively, soluble mediators or products of the immune response (e.g., interferon-gamma, tumor necrosis factor, IL-4) may be removed by repeated plasma exchange resulting in down-regulation of the inflammatory response. Repeated plasma exchange could similarly reduce the level of an unidentified circulating antigen. Triggering peptides or other poorly catalyzable molecules which bind to MHC and T-cell receptors resulting in T-cell activation could theoretically be reduced or eliminated by plasma exchange.

There is an extensive body of evidence suggesting that MS is a T-cell mediated autoimmune disease. Kiprov (1983) has reported that repeated plasma-exchange treatments result in normalization of previously increased OKT4/OKT8 ratios in patients with MS, myasthenia gravis, scleroderma, and SLE. Another isolated observation in a single SLE patient suggested improvement of suppressor cell function following plasma exchange (Abdou et al. 1981). The significance of observations such as these awaits clarification of the degree of functional suppression of the immune response in MS. It seems unlikely that MS patients are deficient in some factor which could be replenished by the use of either fresh-frozen plasma or albumin as the replacement fluid. Theoretically, plasma exchange could lead to enhanced conduction by somehow altering the microenvironment of the demyelinated axon particularly at sites of recent blood–brain barrier disruption.

Clinical Trial Experience

In reviewing the published literature on the use of plasma exchange in MS, one is reminded of the many challenges faced by those attempting to design clinical trials of experimental therapy in this disease (Brown et al. 1979; Herndon and Murray 1983; Kurtzke 1986; Noseworthy 1988; Noseworthy et al. 1984, 1989a). None of the trials completed to date are above criticism although the designs of the more recently completed studies reflect the advances which have occurred in clinical trial methodology in the last decade. For the purposes of this review, it should be emphasized that no published trial has adequately addressed whether plasma exchange alone is worthwhile. This presumably stems from anecdotal experience and preliminary evidence in MS and other presumed autoimmune diseases that corticosteroids and/or immunosuppressive drugs must be used concomitantly with plasma exchange to prevent a "rebound" in immunoglobulin production and T-cell activation. Many of the early trials were uncontrolled, nonrandomized, and unblinded. Protocols differed between investigators and sometimes within these same series. Many of the early studies included severely disabled patients in whom the potential for meaningful improvement was presumably minimal.

The early reports suggested that plasma exchange might have a role in the management of patients with progressive MS (Table 12.1). The modest results of these nonrandomized, unblinded, and largely uncontrolled pilot studies can be compared with the four randomized studies which have now been completed (Table 12.2). Hauser and colleagues (1983) reported a significantly

Table 12.1. Nonrandomized clinical experience with plasma exchange in progressive multiple sclerosis

Investigator	Treatment[a]	Patients[b]	Trial design[c]	Follow-up	Results[d]
Dau et al. (1980)	Aza, P, PE	8 CP	–	2–15 months	Modest improvement[e] 7/8; 5/8 stable at 2–15 months
Weiner et al. (1980)	Aza, P, PE	8 CP	–	≤6 months	6 mild initial improvement. 2/6 responders still stable at 6 months
Tindall et al. (1982)	Aza, PE vs. Aza	10 CP, 10 CP	C	12 months	No difference. Continued progression in 5/7 Aza & PE at 1 year. Continued progression in 4/7 Aza treated at 1 year
Guarnieri et al. (1985)	Aza & PE	20 CP, 1R, 12 inactive	–	Unstated	Initial improvement in 14/21 CP (5 objective (3 DSS improved), 9 subjective)
Trouillas et al. (1986)	PE	12 CP	–	Weeks	Brief (≤8 weeks) improvement of DSS in 4/12 CP
Miller et al. (1985)	CY, P, PE	33 CP	–	Unstated	None worse, mean EDSS improved from 6.53 to 6.0. 10/33 stable. 23/33 better: 17/23 EDSS improved by 0.5, 3/23 EDSS improved by 1.0, 2/23 EDSS improved by 1.5, 1/23 EDSS improved by 2.5
Khatri et al. (1991)	CY, P, PE	200 CP	–	Up to 6 years	Unblinded observations of percent stable (improved ≥1.0 DSS): 1 year 59% stable (39% improved), 2 year 52% (36%), 3 year 48% (35%). 43 patients retreated.

[a] Aza = azathioprine; P = prednisone; PE = plasma exchange; CY = oral cyclophosphamide.
[b] CP = chronic/progressive MS; R = relapsing MS.
[c] Trial design: R = randomized, C = controlled, SB = single blinded, DB = double blinded, – = neither randomized, controlled, or blinded.
[d] DSS = Disability Status Scale: EDSS = Expanded DSS.
[e] Unable to determine if clinical change would have altered the DSS or EDSS score.

Table 12.2. Randomized clinical trials assessing plasma exchange in progressive multiple sclerosis

Investigator	Treatment[a]	Patients[b]	Trial design[c]	Follow-up	Results
Hauser et al. (1983)	CY & ACTH vs. CY*, ACTH, PE vs. ACTH	20 Prog, 18 Prog, 20 Prog	R, C	12 months	1 year stable or improved: 16/20 (CY), 9/18 (PE), and 4/20 (ACTH)
Gordon et al. (1985)	Aza, P, PE vs. Aza, P, Sham-PE	10 CP, 10 CP	R, C, DB	3–6 months	Modest, transient initial improvement 7/10 PE (no change DSS). 3/10 Sham-PE; no change DSS
Khatri et al. (1985a)	CY*, P, PE vs. CY*, P, Sham-PE	26 Prog, 29 Prog	R, C, DB	11 months	23/26 stabilized (12) or improved (11) in PE group vs. 23/29 stabilized (18) or improved (5) in Sham-PE group
Canadian Cooperative Study (1991)	CY*, P vs. CY*, P, PE vs. CY*-Placebo, P-Placebo, Sham-PE	55 Prog, 57 Prog, 56 Prog,	R, C, SB^+	30.4 months	Nonsignificant differences in stabilized/improved, "treatment failures," or degree of worsening

[a] Aza = azathioprine; P = prednisone; PE = plasma exchange; CY = IV cyclophosphamide; CY* = PO cyclophosphamide.
[b] CP = chronic/progressive MS; Prog = progressive MS.
[c] Trial design: R = randomized, C = controlled, DB = double blinded, SB^+ = partially double blinded (see text).

different rate of stabilization or improvement in patients treated with an intensive course of intravenous cyclophosphamide and ACTH compared with either oral cyclophosphamide (8 weeks), intravenous ACTH, and repeated plasma exchange (4–5 exchanges over 14 days) or ACTH treatment alone. The authors deemed a patient "improved" if either the Ambulation Index or the Disability Status Scale (DSS; Kurtzke 1955) decreased by one or more points compared with the entry value. If one recalculates their data using only the DSS, their results are even more favorable with stabilization or improvement seen in 18 of 20 intravenous cyclophosphamide ($p < 0.001$ compared with ACTH; Fisher's exact), 11 of 18 plasma exchange ($p = 0.047$) and 5 of 20 ACTH-treated patients. This report stimulated the development of additional protocols to confirm and extend these observations that cyclophosphamide (Carter et al. 1988; Mackin et al. 1990) and plasma exchange (The Canadian Cooperative Multiple Sclerosis Study Group 1991) may have a role in the treatment of progressive MS. Gordon and colleagues (1985) terminated their double-blinded trial at the 6-month follow-up when they could not detect that plasma exchange added significantly to the outcome obtained with the combination of azathioprine and prednisone. Khatri and colleagues (1985) performed a controlled and double-blinded study in which 55 progressive patients were randomized to receive daily oral cyclophosphamide (6 months), alternate day oral prednisone, and either 20 weekly plasma-exchange or sham plasma exchange treatments. At the 11-month follow-up, 23 of 26 plasma exchange treated patients were rated as either stabilized (12) or improved (11) compared with 23 of 29 stabilized (18) or improved (5) sham treated patients. This group continues to recommend a combination of immunosuppressive drug treatment and plasma exchange to progressive MS patients (Khatri 1988). This enthusiasm for plasma exchange is not universally shared by other clinical investigators (Weiner 1985; Noseworthy et al. 1989a) despite a recent report of the nonblinded observed clinical behavior of patients treated with this protocol in an open-label study (Khatri et al. 1991, Table 12.1) and this treatment approach has not received wide acceptance in North America.

Following the preliminary presentation of the Hauser and Khatri data, members of the Canadian multiple sclerosis research community joined with the Canadian Apheresis Study Group to perform the Canadian Cooperative trial of cyclophosphamide and plasma exchange in progressive MS (Noseworthy et al. 1990a; The Canadian Cooperative Multiple Sclerosis Study Group 1991). These investigators felt that the promising reports by Hauser and Khatri needed to be confirmed in a placebo-controlled study. One hundred and sixty-eight patients whose illness had progressed by at least 1.0 on the EDSS in the preceding year were randomized into one of three treatment limbs: (1) intravenous cyclophosphamide and prednisone (hospital setting), (2) oral cyclophosphamide (22 weeks), alternate day prednisone (22 weeks), and 20 weekly plasma exchanges, or (3) placebo cyclophosphamide, placebo prednisone, and sham plasma exchange. The trial was single-blinded for all patients and double-blinded for patients in groups 2 and 3. The clinical characteristics were well matched between groups at entry (sex, age, disease duration, mean EDSS). The primary analysis compared the cumulative treatment failure rates in each of the three treatment groups using survival analysis (treatment failure definition: worsening of the blinded evaluating neurologist's score of ≥ 1.0 points [two-step change] on the EDSS on two consecutive examinations separated by at least 6 months). There was no difference in the number of treatment failures between groups (intravenous cyclophosphamide 19/55 (34.6%), plasma exchange 18/57 (31.6%), and placebo 16/56 (28.6%). Only very minor differences were seen in the time to treatment failure (cyclophosphamide 24.8 months, plasma exchange 29.3 months, and placebo 20.6 months). At the 12-, 18-, and 24-month assessments, the proportion of patients stabilized or improved was greatest in the patients randomized to the plasma exchange group. Similarly, minor differences (less than 0.5 EDSS points) in the EDSS scores in the first 2 years after randomization suggested a small treatment advantage to the plasma exchange limb over the placebo group. Each of these secondary analyses of efficacy failed to reach statistical significance using a two-tailed analysis of the data, however. These minor trends were no longer apparent at the final follow-up (30.4 months following randomization). The degree of apparent clinical improvement seen at 1 year (11 months in the study by Khatri et al.) in the active treatment groups from these trials is compared in Table 12.3. As illustrated, both the proportion of patients showing improvement and the degree of improvement seen in the Canadian study were far less than that which had been reported previously. Following completion of this study, the Canadian investigators have abandoned these treatments.

How can one explain these conflicting results? There were some differences in the treatment protocols and measurements of disability (DSS versus EDSS). In the Hauser study, intravenous cyclophosphamide was given on a daily basis (400–500 mg/d for 10–14 days) and ACTH was used, whereas in the Canadian trial a higher dose of intravenous cyclophosphamide was given on alternate days (1 g) and prednisone was administered. It is probably unlikely that either of these protocol differences explains the discrepancy in the results in that the total amount of cyclophosphamide administered was similar (80–100 mg/kg in the Hauser study versus 5.0 ± 1.2 g in the Canadian trial). It is also doubtful that this marked difference in the proportion of patients improved at 1 year can be attributed to the use of ACTH (versus prednisone). Khatri's plasma exchange treated patients received both a higher dose of prednisone (1 mg/kg alternate days versus 20 mg on alternate days in the Canadian study) and

Table 12.3. Degree of clinical improvement at one-year[a]. Active treatment groups

Investigator	Protocol[b] (n)	DSS[c] improvement			
		1.0	2.0	3.0	4.0
Hauser et al. (1983)	CY, ACTH (20)	3	2	1	–
	CY*, ACTH, PE (18)	1	2	–	–
Khatri et al. (1985a)	CY*, P, PE (26)	4	4	2	1
Canadian Cooperative Study (1991)	CY, P (48)	3	–	–	–
	CY*, P, PE (48)	4	–	–	–

[a] One year = 11 months in study by Khatri et al.
[b] CY = IV cyclophosphamide; CY* = po cyclophosphamide; P = prednisone; PE = plasma exchange; n = number of patients.
[c] DSS = EDSS in the Canadian Cooperative Study.

Table 12.4. Progressive multiple sclerosis clinical trials. Clinical behavior of the control group

Trial (Year published)	Control group	1 Year		3 Year	
		↑ ≥ 1.0 DSS[a]	Δ $\overline{\text{DSS}}$[b]	↑ ≥ 1.0 DSS	Δ $\overline{\text{DSS}}$
Hauser et al. (1983)	ACTH group	75%	0.7 ± 0.3	–[c]	–
Rudge et al. (1989)	Placebo	42.5%	–	–	–
Ellison et al. (1988)	Placebo	12%	–	46%	0.46 ± 0.2
Miller et al. (1988)	Placebo	29.5%	–	–	–
Canadian (1991)	Placebo	25%	0.39 ± 0.09	39.2%	0.50 ± 0.014

[a] DSS = disability Status Score (EDSS for the Canadian Study).
[b] Δ $\overline{\text{DSS}}$ = mean change in DSS.
[c] – = information unavailable from the published reports.

pooled human immune serum globulin (40 ml in four divided IM injections over 48 h after each plasma exchange procedure). When one considers that in the Canadian experience there was no significant treatment advantage to the combination of oral cyclophosphamide, alternate-day prednisone (in a relatively low dose) and weekly plasma exchange in comparison with a double-placebo, sham-plasma exchange protocol, it is tempting to speculate that the apparent beneficial response seen in both limbs of the trial by Khatri and colleagues might be largely attributable to the prolonged administration of high-dose prednisone. The importance of observer blinding in MS clinical trials is illustrated by the observation that the unblinded examiners in the Canadian trial (and Khatri et al. in their 1991 report) recorded a treatment advantage to the plasma exchange protocols, but this was not the case for the blinded examiners who evaluated the patients simultaneously (Noseworthy et al. 1991).

The most striking difference between the Hauser report and the Canadian study is found in the behavior of the control group (Table 12.4). As illustrated, the ACTH-treated "controls" in the Hauser study did very poorly with 75% experiencing worsening of at least 1 full point on the DSS 1 year after randomization. In contrast, only 25% of the placebo-treated patients in the Canadian study progressed by a comparable degree on the EDSS (1.0 point) at 1 year, and at 3 years progression of at least a full point was seen in only 39.2%. As we have discussed (The Canadian Multiple Sclerosis Study Group 1991), if the "control group"(ACTH) in the Hauser study had progressed at a rate similar to that experienced in the placebo-controlled trials summarized in Table 12.4, the authors would not have been able to detect a treatment advantage from either of their two active protocols. The placebo-treated Canadian patients had a "stabilization rate" (as determined by the EDSS) similar to the intravenous cyclophosphamide stabilization rate in the Hauser and Canadian trials and similar to the clinical behavior of other placebo-treated progressive patients in recently reported treatment trials (Table 12.4 (Rudge et al. 1989; Ellison et al. 1988; Miller et al. 1988)) and natural history studies (Weinshenker et al. 1989, 1991). Although the DSS and EDSS scales are not perfectly comparable (the EDSS scale defines one-half step changes between each point in the scale), the degree of change required to define worsening is the same in this comparison of control groups (Table 12.4: one full point, e.g., a two-step change on the EDSS). Recent evidence suggests that the EDSS (DSS) is not a uniform scale and that changes of a similar degree (e.g., 1.0 point) are not comparable across the range of the scale (Weinshenker et al. 1991). Given the relatively small numbers of patients at each DSS (EDSS) level in each of the studies summarized in Table 12.4, it is not possible to make a definitive statement about the risk of progression at 1 year for each step of the DSS (EDSS). This analysis, however, shows clearly that progressive MS patients who have worsened significantly in the year prior to randomization into a controlled clinical trial do not invariably continue to progress in the subsequent year. Although all of the patients in the Canadian trial had worsened by at least a full 1.0 EDSS point in the year prior to randomization, in the next year patients progressed by only 0.14 ± 0.1 (plasma exchange group), 0.18 ± 0.09 (intravenous cyclophosphamide), and 0.39 ± 0.09 (placebo group) EDSS points, respectively.

There is very little published information on the use of plasma exchange in the setting of acute exacerbations of MS (Table 12.5). Dau and colleagues (1980) administered prednisone and plasma exchange to 3 patients in the midst of an MS attack. A beneficial clinical response was seen in all 3 in the weeks following this treatment. In a small, uncontrolled and unblinded study, Valbonesi and colleagues (1981) reported moderate to marked improvement in 4 of 6 relapsing patients treated with plasma exchange either alone or in combination with cyclophosphamide and corticosteroids. In the largest study of plasma exchange in the setting of an acute MS exacerbation, Weiner and colleagues (1989) randomized 116 relapsing and progressing patients to receive oral cyclophosphamide, ACTH, and either 11 plasma exchange or sham plasma exchange treatments over a period of 8 weeks. They reported that the plasma exchange treated relapsing/remitting patients had "accelerated improvement and recovery" when compared with the control group. Unfortunately, however, there was no clear long-term benefit from this intervention. The authors recommended "that plasma exchange in conjunction with ACTH plus cyclophosphamide, may be indicated when the physician judges an attack in a relapsing-remitting patient to be so severe that the lessened morbidity associated with a more rapid recovery over the ensuing 1 to 12 months warrants it". Others have disagreed with these conclusions (Goodin 1990; Noseworthy et al. 1990b,c; Weiner et al. 1990). The actual role, if any, for plasma exchange in the management of acute attacks of MS will require further clarification. A study comparing plasma exchange, cyclophosphamide, and ACTH (or prednisone or methylprednisolone) against ACTH (or prednisone or methylprednisolone), placebo cyclophosphamide and sham plasma exchange would make it possible to determine if the combination of measures proposed by Weiner and colleagues are superior to the "standard treatment for acute attacks" (e.g., ACTH or corticosteroids).

Summary, Conclusions and Future Directions

Published evidence suggests that, with rare exceptions, patients with MS tolerate repeated plasma exchange treatments essentially as well as other patients who do not have serious systemic disease. The clinical trials completed to

Table 12.5. Clinical trial experience with plasma exchange in relapsing multiple sclerosis

Investigator	Treatment[a]	Patients[b]	Trial Design[c]	Followup	Results
Dau et al. (1980)	PE, P	3	–	Weeks	All responded
Valbonesi et al. (1981)	PE ± CY ± corticosteroids	6	–	Unstated	4/6 moderate to marked improvement
Weiner et al. (1989)	CY, ACTH, PE vs. CY, ACTH, Sham-PE	59 (39 RR, 20 CP), 57 (37 RR, 20 CP)	R, C, DB	2 years	PE treated RR patients "increased improvement at one month" only. No long term benefit

[a] PE = plasma exchange; CY = oral cyclophosphamide; P = prednisone; RR = relapsing-remitting MS.
[b] CP = chronic progressive MS.
[c] R = randomized; C = controlled; DB = doule blinded; – = neither randomized, controlled, or blinded.

this point have not demonstrated definitively that plasma exchange has an important place in the treatment of either acute exacerbations or progressive MS. The remarkable findings from Khatri's group were unfortunately not confirmed by the only randomized, placebo-controlled, and blinded study performed to this point using a comparable plasma exchange protocol. The plasma exchange group in the Canadian Cooperative Trial consistently fared marginally better than either the cyclophosphamide or the placebo group, but none of these secondary assessments of efficacy achieved statistical significance. Dr. Weiner and colleagues have reported a treatment advantage with their combination of oral cyclophosphamide, ACTH, and repeated plasma exchange in the setting of acute MS attacks in their subgroup of relapsing MS patients (again, a secondary analysis). Interesting trends such as these which emerge from secondary and subset analyses traditionally generate new hypotheses and enthusiasm for further rigorous clinical studies.

It seems unlikely that plasma exchange alone will significantly change the natural history of active MS. Perhaps there is enough evidence from published studies to suggest that an alternative approach would be worthwhile, however. It is conceivable that repeated plasma exchange could be effectively combined with an agent which is less toxic than either azathioprine or cyclophosphamide and yet which has been shown to modify either the inflammatory response, a secondary immune reaction, or the integrity of the blood–brain barrier. Published experience suggests that it is possible to blind patients and examining physicians effectively using sham plasma exchange in the context of a controlled clinical trial. If there are to be future trials of plasma exchange, they should be randomized, blinded, placebo-controlled (sham plasma exchange), and of sufficient duration to be definitive.

References

Abdou NI, Lindsley HB, Pollack A et al. (1981) Plasmapheresis in active systemic lupus erythematosus. Effects on clinical serum and cellular abnormalities. Case Report. Clin Immunol Immunopathol 19:44–54

Berkman EM, Caplan S, Kim GS (1978) ABO-incompatible bone marrow transplantation: preparation by plasma exchange and in vivo antibody absorption. Transfusion 18:504–508

Brown JR, Beebe GW, Kurtzke JF et al. (1979) The design of clinical studies to assess therapeutic efficacy in multiple sclerosis. Neurology 29:3–23

Brubaker DB, Winkelstein A (1981) Plasma exchange in rheumatoid vasculitis. Vox Sang 41: 295–301

Carter JL, Hafler DA, Dawson DM, Orav J, Weiner HL (1988) Immunosuppression with high-dose IV cyclophosphamide and ACTH in progressive multiple sclerosis: cumulative 6-year experience with 164 patients. Neurology 38 (Suppl 2):9–14

Cobcroft R (1977) Serial plasmapheresis in a hemophiliac with antibodies to factor VIII. Proc HRI Adv Comp Semin, London, England

Dau PC, Petajan JH, Johnson KP, Panitch HS, Bornstein MB (1980) Plasmapheresis in multiple sclerosis: preliminary findings. Neurology 30:1023–1028

Dearnaley DR, Martin MFR (1978) Plasmapheresis for paraquat poisoning. Lancet 1:162

Dyck PJ, Daube J, O'Brien P et al. (1986) Plasma exchange in chronic inflammatory demyelinating polyneuropathy. N Engl J Med 314:461–465

Dyck PJ, Pineda A, Low PA et al. (1990) Sham controlled trial of plasma exchange in monoclonal protein associated neuropathy. Peripheral Neuropathy Association Meeting, Oxford, England, pp 17

Ellison GW, Myers LW, Mickey MR et al. (1988) Clinical experience with azathioprine: The pros. Neurology 38 (Suppl 2):20–23

Gibberg FB, Billimoria JD, Page NGR (1979) Heredopathia atactica polyneuritiformis (Refsum's disease) treated by diet and plasma exchange. Lancet 1:575–578

Giordano GF (1984) Lymphocytapheresis results of treatment in 50 patients with multiple sclerosis. Plasmatherapy 2:654–658

Goodin DS (1990) Letter to the Editor. Neurology 40:864–865

Gordon PA, Carroll DJ, Etches WS et al. (1985) A double-blind controlled pilot study of plasma exchange versus sham apheresis in chronic progressive multiple sclerosis. Can J Neurol Sci 12:39–44

Guarnieri BM, Capparelli R, Fratiglioni L et al. (1985) Plasma exchange in multiple sclerosis. Int J Artif Organs 8:215–220

Hauser SL, Dawson DM, Lehrich JR et al. (1983) Intensive immunosuppression in progressive multiple sclerosis. N Engl J Med 308:173–180

Hauser SL, Fosburg M, Kevy SV, Weiner HL (1984) Lymphocytapheresis in chronic progressive multiple sclerosis: immunologic and clinical effects. Neurology 34:922–926

Herndon RM, Murray TJ (1983) Proceedings of the International Conference on therapeutic trials in multiple sclerosis. Arch Neurol 40:663–710

Höcker P, Stellamor V, Summer K, Mann M (1984) Plasma exchange (PE) and lymphocytapheresis (LCA) in multiple sclerosis (MS). Int J Artif Organs 7:39–42

Huestis DW (1986) Complications of therapeutic apheresis. In: Valbones M, Pineda A, Briggs JC (eds) Therapeutic hemapheresis. Wichting Editore, Milan, pp 179–186

Jones JV, Cummings CH, Pacon PA (1979) Evidence for a therapeutic effect of plasmapheresis in patients with systemic lupus erythematosus. Q J Med 48:555–576

Kennedy MS, Domen RE (1983) Therapeutic apheresis applications and future directions. Vox Sang 45:261–277

Khatri BO, McQuillen MP, Harrington GL et al. (1985a) Chronic progressive multiple sclerosis: double-blind controlled study of plasmapheresis in patients taking immunosuppressive drugs. Neurology 35:312–319

Khatri BO, McQuillen MP, Harrington GJ et al. (1985b) Plasmapheresis in progressive MS. Neurology 35:614

Khatri BO (1988) Experience with use of plasmapheresis in chronic progressive multiple sclerosis. Neurology 38 (Suppl 2):50–52

Khatri BO, McQuillen MP, Hoffman RG, Harrington GJ, Schmoll D (1991) Plasma exchange in chronic progressive multiple sclerosis: A long-term study. Neurology 41:409–414

Kincaid-Smith P, d'Apice AJF (1978) Plasmapheresis in rapidly progressive glomerulonephritis. Am J Med 65:564–566

Kiprov DD (1983) Influence of plasmapheresis on cellular immunity. In: Lysaght MJ, Gurland HJ (eds) Plasma separation and plasma fractionation: current status and future directions. Karger, Basel, pp 48–63

Klein HG, Balow JE, Dau PC et al. (1986) Clinical applications of therapeutic apheresis. Report of the Clinical Applications Committee, American Society for Apheresis. J Clin Apheresis 3:1–92

Kurtzke JF (1955) A new scale for evaluating disability in multiple sclerosis. Neurology 5:580–583

Kurtzke JF (1986) Neuroepidemiology. Part II: Assessment of therapeutic trials. Ann Neurol 19:311–319

Lian ECY, Harkness DR, Byrnes JJ et al. (1979) Presence of a platelet aggregating factor in the plasma of patients with thrombotic thrombocytopenic purpura (TTP) and its inhibition by normal plasma. Blood 53:333–340

Lockwood CM, Boulton-Jones, JM, Lowenthal RM (1975) Recovery from Goodpasture's syndrome after immunosuppressive treatment and plasmapheresis. Br Med J 2:252–254

Luzhnikov EA, Yaraslavsky AA, Molodenov MN (1977) Plasma perfusion through charcoal in methylparathion poisoning. Lancet 1:38–39

Mackin GA, Weiner HL, Orav JA et al. (1990) IV cyclophosphamide/ACTH plus maintenance cyclophosphamide boosters in progressive MS: Interim report of the Northeast Cooperative MS Treatment Group. Neurology 40 (Suppl 1):260

Medaer R, Eeckhout C, Gautama K, Vermijlen C (1984) Lymphocytapheresis therapy in multiple sclerosis, a preliminary study. Acta Neurol Scand 70:111–115

Miller A, Drexler E, Keilson M et al. (1988) Spontaneous stabilization in patients with progressive MS. Neurology 38 (Suppl 1):194

Miller RG, Filler-Katz A, Kiprov DD (1985) More on plasmapheresis in chronic progressive MS. Neurology 35:1261

Noseworthy JH, Seland TP, Ebers GC (1984) Therapeutic trials in multiple sclerosis. Can J Neurol Sci 11:355–362

Noseworthy JH (1988) There are no alternatives to double-blind, controlled trials. Neurology 38 (Suppl 2):76–79

Noseworthy JH, Vandervoort MK, Hopkins M, Ebers GC (1989a) A referendum on clinical trial research in multiple sclerosis: the opinion of the participants at the Jekyll Island workshop. Neurology 39:977–981

Noseworthy JH, Shumak KH, Vandervoort MK, The Canadian Cooperative Multiple Sclerosis Study Group (1989b) Long-term use of antecubital veins for plasma exchange. Transfusion 29:610–613

Noseworthy JH, The Canadian Cooperative Multiple Sclerosis Study Group (1990a) The Canadian Cooperative Study of cyclophosphamide and plasma exchange in progressive multiple sclerosis. Neurology 40 (Suppl 1):284

Noseworthy JH, Vandervoort MK, Ebers GC (1990b) Plasma exchange in MS. Neurology 40:864

Noseworthy JH, Vandervoort MK, Ebers GC (1990c) Plasma exchange in MS. Neurology 40:1153

Noseworthy JH, Vandervoort MK, Penman M et al. (1991) The Lancet 337:1540–1541

Patten E (1986) Therapeutic plasmapheresis and plasma exchange. CRC Crit Rev Clin Lab Sci 23:147–175

Rationale for immunomodulating therapies of multiple sclerosis (1988) Neurology 38 (Suppl 2):1–89

Reimann PM, Mason PD (1990) Plasmapheresis: technique and complications. Intensive Care Med 16:3–10

Rock GA, Shumak KH, Buskard NA et al. (1991) Comparison of plasma exchange with plasma infusion in the treatment of thrombotic thrombocytopenic purpura. N Engl J Med 325:393–397

Rose J, Klein H, Greenstein et al. (1983) Lymphocytapheresis in chronic progressive multiple sclerosis: results of a preliminary trial. Ann Neurol 14:593–594

Rosenblatt SG, Knight W, Bannayan GA, Wilson CB, Stein J (1979) Treatment of Goodpasture's syndrome with plasmapheresis. Am J Med 66:689–696

Rossen RD, Duffy J, McCredie KB et al. (1976) Treatment of Goodpasture's syndrome with cyclophosphamide, prednisone and plasma exchange transfusions. Clin Exp Immunol 24: 218–222

Rothwell RS, Davis P, Gordon P et al. (1980) A controlled study of plasma exchange in the treatment of severe rheumatoid arthritis. Arth Rheum 23:785–789

Rudge P, Koetsier JC, Mertin J et al. (1989) Randomised double blind controlled trial of cyclosporin in multiple sclerosis. J Neurol Neurosurg 52:559–565

Russell JA, Toy JL, Powles RL (1977) Plasma exchange in malignant paraproteinemias. Exp Hematol 5:105–116

Salmi A, Ziola B, Reunanen M, Julkunen I, Wager O (1982) Immune complexes in serum and cerebrospinal fluid of multiple sclerosis patients and patients with other neurological diseases. Acta Neurol Scand 66:1–15

Schildermans F, Dequeker J, Van de Puthe I (1979) Plasmapheresis combined with corticosteroids and cyclophosphamide in uncontrolled active SLE. J Rheum 6:687

Schlansky R, DeHoratius RJ, Pincus T, Tung KSK (1981) Plasmapheresis in systemic lupus erythematosus: a cautionary note. Arthritis Rheum 24:49–53

Schwab PJ, Fahey JF (1960) Treatment of Waldenstrom's macroglobulinemia by plasmapheresis. N Engl J Med 263:574–579

Shumak KH, Rock GA (1984) Therapeutic plasma exchange. N Engl J Med 310:762–771

Silvergleid AJ (1983) Applications and limitations of hemapheresis. Annu Rev Med 34:69–89

Slocombe GW, Newland AC, Colvin MP, Colvin BT (1981) The role of intensive plasma exchange in the prevention and management of haemorrhage in patients with inhibitors to Factor VIII. Br J Haematol 47:577–585

Smith CD, Latortue R, McFarland JG, Menitove JE (1986) Plasminogen deficiency and thrombosis after plasmapheresis therapy for multiple sclerosis. Neurology 36:1410–1411

Spiva DA, Lewis C, Langley JW (1981) New treatment for the porphyrias: porphyria (AIP) and variegate porphyria (VP). Blood 58:186a

The Canadian Cooperative Multiple Sclerosis Study Group (1991) The Canadian Cooperative trial of cyclophosphamide and plasma exchange in progressive multiple sclerosis. Lancet 337: 441–446

The Guillain-Barré Syndrome Study Group (1985) Plasmapheresis and acute Guillain-Barré syndrome. Neurology 35:1095–1104

Thompson GR (1981) Plasma exchange for hypercholesterolaemia. Lancet 1:1246–1248

Tindall RSA, Walker JE, Ehle AL et al. (1982) Plasmapheresis in multiple sclerosis. Prospective trial of pheresis and immunosuppression versus immunosuppression alone. Neurology 32: 739–743

Trouillas P, Neuschwander Ph, Tremisi JP (1986) Modification rapide par les échanges plasmatiques de la sémiologie de formes progressives de la sclérose en plaques. Rev Neurol (Paris) 142: 689–695

Valbonesi M, Garelli S, Mosconi L, Zerbi D, Forlani G (1981) Plasma exchange in the management of patients with multiple sclerosis: preliminary observations. Vox Sang 41:68–73

van den Noort S, Waksman BH (1980) Plasma exchange: aid to therapy of multiple sclerosis? Neurology 30:1111–1112

Walker RG, d'Apice AJ, Becker GJ et al. (1977) Plasmapheresis in Goodpasture's syndrome with renal failure. Med J Aust 875–879

Wallace DJ, Goldfinger D, Gatti, et al. (1979) Plasmapheresis and lymphoplasmapheresis in the management of rheumatoid arthritis. Arthritis Rheum 22:703–710

Weiner HL, Dawson DM (1980) Plasmapheresis in multiple sclerosis: Preliminary study. Neurology 30:1029–1033

Weiner HL (1985) An assessment of plasma exchange in progressive multiple sclerosis. Neurology 35:320–322

Weiner HL, Dau PC, Khatri BO et al. (1989) Double-blind study of true vs. sham plasma exchange in patients treated with immunosuppression for acute attacks of multiple sclerosis. Neurology 39:1143–1149

Weiner HL, Khatri BO, Dau PC, (1990) Reply from the authors. Neurology 40:865

Weinshenker BG, Bass B, Rice GPA et al. (1989) The natural history of multiple sclerosis: A geographically based study. I. Clinical course and disability. Brain 112:133–146

Weinshenker BG, Rice GPA, Noseworthy JH et al. (1991) The natural history of multiple sclerosis. A geographically based study. IV. Applications to planning and interpretation of clinical therapeutic trials. Brain 114:1057–1067

Wirguin I, Shinar E, Abramsky O (1989) Relapse of multiple sclerosis following acute allergic reactions to plasma during plasmapheresis. J Neurol 236:62–63

Chapter 13

Total Lymphoid Irradiation in Multiple Sclerosis

Stuart D. Cook, Corinne Devereux, Raymond Troiano, Christine Rohowsky-Kochan, Amiram Sheffet, Annette Jotkowitz, George Zito and Peter C. Dowling

Introduction

Immunosuppressive drugs have been increasingly used in both uncontrolled and controlled studies in an attempt to modify the relentless deterioration in neurologic function which commonly occurs in patients with chronic/progressive multiple sclerosis (CPMS) (The Multiple Sclerosis Study Group 1990; Rudge et al. 1989; Hauser et al. 1983; British and Dutch Multiple Sclerosis Azathioprine Trial Group 1988; Ellison et al. 1988). Unfortunately, no unequivocal long-term clinical benefits have been documented with immunosuppressive drugs in carefully controlled trials of CPMS. Further, many immunosuppressive drugs must be given at frequent intervals or even daily to sustain remissions in autoimmune disorders, which obviously increases their potential for toxic side effects including infection and neoplasia.

An alternative method for effective immunosuppression is total lymphoid irradiation (TLI). TLI produces sustained suppression of the immune response, prolongs organ transplant survival, and can induce long-term remissions in both natural and experimental autoimmune disorders (Slavin et al. 1977; Kotzin and Strober 1979; Kotzin et al. 1981; Tanay et al. 1987; Trentham et al. 1981; Strober et al. 1987). TLI has been extensively utilized as a primary therapeutic modality in Hodgkin's disease (Kaplan 1980), in which it was associated with a relatively low risk of severe bacterial infections. Unlike some cytotoxic drugs, TLI has not been associated with a high risk of hematologic neoplasias in long-term follow-up of patients with Hodgkin's disease. For example, in 3000 patients with Hodgkin's disease, second tumors were no more common than expected by chance alone during a 10-year follow-up period (Calin 1985; Bookman et al. 1988). Because of the safety of TLI in Hodgkin's disease and the effective as well as protracted immunosuppressive effects of treatment, we have used TLI as a therapeutic modality in patients with CPMS. In this chapter, we will review the mechanisms of immunosuppression with TLI, the effect of TLI in other human autoimmune diseases, and our experience with TLI in CPMS.

Immunosuppressive Effects of Total Lymphoid Irradiation

TLI has profound immunosuppressive effects on humoral and cell-mediated immune responses in man and laboratory animals. In Hodgkin's-disease patients treated with TLI, there was relative T-cell lymphocytopenia and B- and null-cell lymphocytosis (Fuks et al. 1976). There were also dramatic decreases in the number of total $CD3^+$, helper/inducer $CD4^+$ and suppressor/cytotoxic $CD8^+$ T-cells (Lauria et al. 1983). Approximately 6–8 months post-TLI, CD8-reactive T-cells returned to pretreatment levels whereas $CD4^+$ T-lymphocytes remained low for an extended period of time (Fuks et al. 1976). Consequently, the CD4/CD8 T-cell ratio remained markedly reduced for at least 5 years (Lauria et al. 1983). Decreased absolute lymphocyte counts returned to pretreatment levels 2 years post-TLI; however, at this time the percentage of T-cells was only half the pre-TLI value (Fuks et al. 1976).

The cells repopulating the blood after TLI exhibited different phenotypic characteristics from the peripheral blood T-lymphocytes prior to radiotherapy. A large disparity between CD3-staining T-lymphocytes and the sum of $CD4^+$ plus $CD8^+$ T-cells was observed and suggested that repopulating cells were immature, and not $CD4^+/CD8^-$ or $CD4^-/CD8^+$ but presumably either $CD4^+/CD8^+$, $CD4^+/CD3^-$ or $CD8^+/CD3^-$ (Haas et al. 1984). Two-color immunofluorescence analysis suggested that these lymphocytes were $CD4^+/CD3^-$ or $CD8^+/CD3^-$ (Haas et al. 1984). There was also increased CD38 reactivity of lymphocytes after therapy (Haas et al. 1984). No detailed phenotypic analysis of these cells has been performed to confirm their immaturity. The reduction of the pool of circulating lymphocytes was accompanied by impaired in vitro cell-mediated lymphocyte function. T-cell proliferative responses to mitogens, allogeneic cells and soluble antigens were profoundly diminished as was delayed hypersensitivity to dinitrochlorobenzene (Fuks et al. 1976).

In rheumatoid arthritis (RA) and systemic lupus erythematosus (SLE) patients, similar changes in T-lymphocytes occurred in response to TLI (Kotzin et al. 1981; Strober et al. 1987,1988). There was an increase in percent $CD8^+$ T-cells with only a slight reduction or no change in the number of CD8-bearing lymphocytes (Kotzin et al. 1981, 1983; Trentham et al. 1981). The CD4/CD8 T-cell ratio decreased markedly after therapy. The number of B cells declined in the TLI-treated RA patients (Kotzin et al. 1983). There have been no reports on the effect of TLI on the number of B cells in SLE patients or on the number of NK cells in RA and SLE. However, a detailed sequential monitoring of T-, B- and null-cell subset changes occurring early after TLI and throughout a long-term follow-up period has not been performed.

In animal studies, the most striking effects of TLI are the generation of nonspecific suppressor cells capable of abrogating both cellular and humoral immune responses and of inducing tolerance. Antigen nonspecific suppressors of the mixed lymphocyte response (MLR) are large, mononuclear cells, lacking surface markers of mature lymphocytes and are found in the absence of antigenic challenge (King et al. 1981; Okada and Strober 1982a; Oseroff et al. 1984). These "null" cells and neonatal suppressor cells have been called natural suppressor (NS) cells. NS cells are found transiently and can no longer be detected by about 1 month after birth or radiotherapy (Okada and Strober 1982b). Functional suppressor cells have been detected in a small number of TLI-treated RA patients but the cell surface phenotype of these cells was not determined (Kotzin et al. 1981). Additional studies are required to define precisely the NS cells that appear post-TLI in patients with autoimmune diseases.

Animals given TLI have been successfully tolerized to heterologous serum proteins and alloantigens and permanently accept skin and heart transplants following marrow transplantation (Slavin 1978; Zan-Bai et al. 1978). NS cells may be involved in the induction of tolerance to allogeneic tissues by inhibiting the generation of antigen-specific cytotoxic T lymphocytes and by enhancing the generation of antigen-specific suppressor cells (Okada and Strober 1982b). The reduced numbers of mature immunocompetent T and B cells and macrophages in TLI-treated animals may also facilitate tolerance induction.

In summary, the mechanism by which TLI exerts its immunosuppressive effects is unclear. Evidence suggests that the depletion of mature lymphocytes, the emergence of immature antigen-nonspecific suppressors which inhibit in vitro and possibly in vivo cell-mediated immune responses, the alteration in the lymphocyte maturation environment and the transient state of tolerance induction contribute to the overall immunosuppressive effects of this therapy. The precise interrelationship between these mechanisms in inducing remission of autoimmune conditions remains to be elucidated.

Total Lymphoid Irradiation in Intractable Rheumatoid Arthritis

Five centers have reported the use of TLI in patients with intractable RA unresponsive to immunosuppressive drugs (Tanay et al. 1987; Brahn et al. 1984; Nusslein et al. 1985; Hanly et al. 1987; Trentham et al. 1987; Scheinberg and Weltman 1985; Strober et al. 1985b). Results from all studies showed statistically-significant improvement in joint disease activity during a 6–12-month follow-up period. The controlled studies reported that patients receiving a total dose of 2000 rad were significantly improved as compared with those given 250 rad (Strober et al. 1985a), but in one study, the short-term efficacy of 750 rad was similar to that of 2000 rad (Hanly et al. 1987). In one study, long-term follow-up indicated that improvement after TLI persisted for at least 4 years in most patients (Tanay et al. 1987). A gradually increasing proportion of patients, however, developed active disease after 2 years, and required the use of adjuvant drug therapy such as corticosteroids or methotrexate in order to maintain improvement (Tanay et al. 1987). Moreover, the approximately 40% "important improvement" observed in the controlled trials is equal to or greater than that achieved with gold or methotrexate. This improvement and the associated suppression in number and function of the T-helper lymphocyte subset persist for many years.

Marked differences in the incidence and severity of side effects and complications following TLI have been reported. The incidence of herpes zoster varied from 0 to 36% and that of severe bacterial infections from 0 to 33% (Tanay et al. 1987; Brahn et al. 1984; Trentham et al. 1987). Interestingly, the study with the lowest incidence of patients with viral and bacterial infections used the lowest dose of irradiation (750 rad) and excluded the spleen from the field of irradiation (Hanly et al. 1987), whereas the study with the highest incidence of systemic staphylococcal infections used the highest dose (3000 rad including the spleen) (Brahn et al. 1984).

The mortality rates of patients in the RA studies also varied considerably from 0 to 36% (Nusslein et al. 1985; Trentham et al. 1987; Gaston et al. 1988). Overall, 13 deaths in 108 patients were reported in published studies from 1979 through 1987 (Tanay et al. 1987; Brahn et al. 1984; Nusslein et al. 1985; Hanly et al. 1987; Trentham et al. 1987; Scheinberg and Weltman 1985; Strober et al. 1985b; Gaston et al. 1988). Several factors contributing to the death rate have been identified. Recent studies have shown that age and severity of disease are important variables for determining mortality rates in RA unrelated to TLI (Pincus et al. 1984; Mitchell et al. 1986). Patients with pre-existing rheumatoid lung disease, amyloidosis, prosthetic joints, or receiving concomitant immunosuppressive drugs appear to be at risk of death from TLI. It may be possible to reduce mortality rates of TLI in RA by limiting TLI to subjects who are younger than 50 years of age and have earlier and milder joint disease. Excluding the spleen from the field of radiation when treating patients with RA may be as effective as TLI with splenic irradiation but may minimize the risk of serious bacterial infections, thereby improving the risk–benefit ratio (Hanly et al. 1987).

Total Lymphoid Irradiation in Lupus Nephritis

Seventeen patients, with severe lupus nephritis and nephrotic syndrome, whose disease was not adequately controlled with steroids alone or in combination with cytotoxic drugs, have been treated with TLI (total dose 2000 rad) (Strober et al. 1987, 1985a). Almost all of the patients fell into the poor-prognosis category based on pretreatment renal biopsies (Austin et al. 1983). Results of the outcome of 15 patients followed for 6 years have been reported (Strober et al. 1987). There was a statistically significant improvement in the mean levels of serum albumin, proteinuria, serum anti-DNA antibodies, and C3 during the first 3 years. The mean levels of serum creatinine did not significantly change. There was a substantial reduction in the mean daily dose of prednisone such that during the second and third years after radiotherapy the dose was less than or equal to 10 mg/day in all patients. However, as in RA, steroids could only be discontinued in 10% of patients without an exacerbation of nephritis occurring.

During the follow-up that ended in April 1987, 1 of the 17 patients died due to an apparent suicide and two progressed to renal failure. Three patients developed minor bacterial infections, 5 developed localized herpes zoster and 2 amenorrhea.

Table 13.1. Troiano Functional Status Scale

Gait	Activities of daily living	Transfers
0 Normal	0 Normal	0 Slight or no difficulty
1 Abnormal, independent	1 Independent with minimal dysfunction; may choose to use assistance or device for speed and efficiency	1 Uses arms to shift weight, sitting to standing, or sitting to sitting, from a straight chair or wheelchair; transfers are independent
2 Uses unilateral assistance device	2 Routinely uses partial human assistance for dexterity functions (writing, managing utensils, buttons, etc.) and dressing and bathing of lower body	2 Routinely uses assistance for most transfers; actively participates
3 Uses bilateral assistance device; may use wheelchair for longer mobility; walking is sufficient to serve various routine daily activities	3 Uses substantial human assistance for most activities, including bathing and dressing lower and upper body; actively participates	3 Dependent for all transfers; passive with no effective participation
4 Depends mainly on wheelchair for mobility; may stand and take some steps with bilateral assistance; walking not very useful for practical purposes, done largely for short transfers and excercise activity, preferably with supervision	4 Dependent for all activities; passive with no effective participation	
5 No standing or steps excluding active human support or rigid support such as Kim stander		

Total Lymphoid Irradiation in Chronic/Progressive Multiple Sclerosis

In 1982, based on the apparent safety and effectiveness of TLI in Hodgkin's disease, we began to use TLI for the treatment of patients with chronic/progressive MS. Our initial study was a prospective randomized double-blind trial in which 24 patients received TLI (1980 rad) and 21 sham TLI. All TLI patients had shielding of the spinal cord to limit irradiation to a maximum of 1000 rad. Subsequently 27 additional patients received TLI plus tapering doses of low-dose prednisone (≤30 mg/day) in an open pilot study. The last 15 of these patients received TLI without splenic irradiation in an attempt to reduce the possibility of subsequent infections due to functional hyposplenism. No significant differences existed among the patients who received TLI alone, the patients who received sham TLI, and the TLI-plus-prednisone treated patients, with regard to age, sex, duration of MS, or pretreatment Troiano Function Status Scale score (TFSS) (Table 13.1, Cook et al. 1986). Details of TLI administration and clinical evaluations have been published (Cook et al. 1986; Devereux et al. 1988; Troiano et al. 1988; Cook et al. 1987, 1990).

Effect of Total Lymphoid Irradiation on Blood Lymphocyte Counts and Lymphocyte Subsets

A significantly lower mean blood lymphocyte count was seen for 30 months following therapy when the TLI group was compared to the sham irradiated

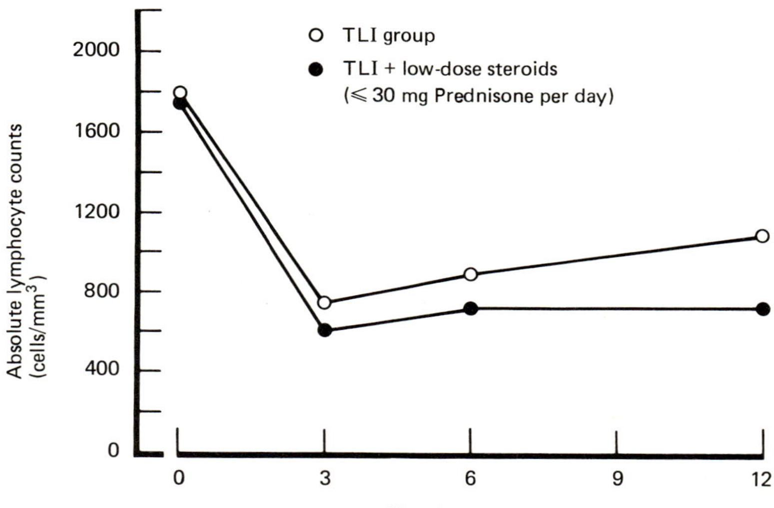

Fig. 13.1. Comparison of mean peripheral blood lymphocyte counts following TLI or TLI plus low-dose prednisone (≤30 mg per day).

group. An even greater mean blood lymphocytopenia was found in the 12 months after TLI in those CPMS patients receiving low-dose prednisone as compared to TLI alone ($p < 0.01$, Fig. 13.1). Thus TLI is markedly lymphocytopenic and TLI with low-dose prednisone induces a greater blood lymphocytopenia than TLI alone.

TLI plus low-dose prednisone also had a major effect on lymphocyte subsets (Rohowsky-Kochan et al. unpublished observation). There were significant decreases ($p < 0.001$) in the percent and absolute numbers of total $CD3^+$ T-cells, helper $CD4^+$ T-cells and suppressor-inducer $CD4^+CD45R^+$ T-cells (Figs. 13.2, 13.3) as compared to baseline values. The percent $CD8^+$ T-lymphocytes increased whereas the absolute number of CD8 carrying T-cells decreased. These changes resulted in a significantly lowered ($p < 0.001$) CD4/CD8 T-cell ratio. Likewise, we observed a drop in both percent and number of B-lymphocytes during this period. Preliminary results on a small number of these patients showed an increase in percent and number of $CD16^+$ NK cells.

In our double-blind study, the curve showing proportion of TLI patients stable on the Troiano Functional Status Scale at 6-month time-intervals post-TLI was not significantly different from sham-treated patients with chronic/progressive MS ($p = 0.144$) although significantly fewer TLI than sham patients progressed during the first 12 months post-therapy ($p \leqslant 0.05$; Cook et al. 1990). When all patients receiving TLI were considered, the curve showing the proportion of patients with stable function scores was significantly greater ($p \leqslant 0.05$) for the TLI-treated patients (including TLI alone and TLI plus prednisone groups) than the sham-irradiated patients (Fig. 13.4). Significantly fewer TLI patients than sham patients experienced progressive deterioration through 18 months of follow-up. To date, those patients receiving TLI plus low-dose steroids, with or without splenic irradiation, have had as good or better a clinical course as indicated by the Kaplan–Meier curve at 6, 12, and 18 months follow-up than patients who received TLI alone. In interpreting the biologic significance of these results, it should be noted that our patients with chronic/progressive MS were generally moderately to severely affected by their disease (mean entry TFSS, 5.2), and had MS for a mean duration of greater than 10 years. It is possible that, as with immunosuppression in other autoimmune disorders, better results might be obtained with TLI by treating less severely affected patients earlier in their course.

Relationship of Disease Course to Blood Lymphocyte Count

In our double-blind study, the subgroup of patients with chronic/progressive MS with mean peripheral blood lymphocyte counts below 850 per mm^3 in the 3- and 12-month periods post-TLI had a significantly better course than sham-irradiated patients or patients with higher mean lymphocyte counts. Significantly fewer of the TLI patients with a mean absolute lymphocyte count of less than 850 per mm^3 during the 3 months post-irradiation deteriorated by one point on the functional scale through 18 months of follow-up as com-

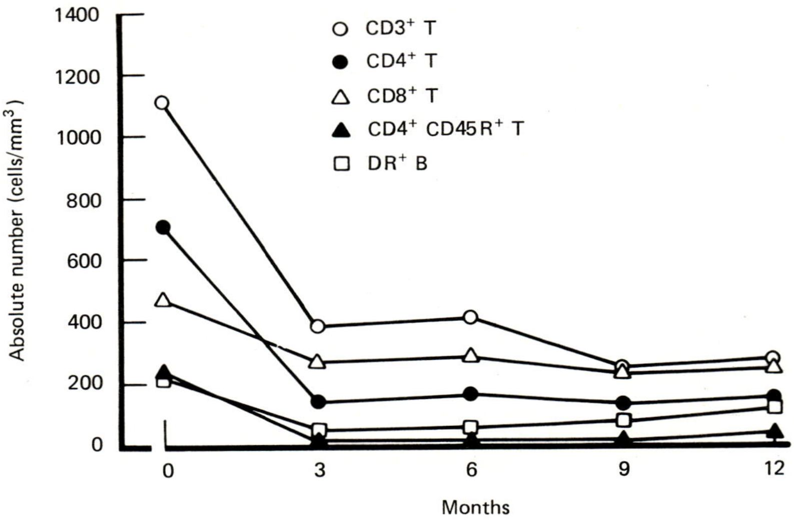

Fig. 13.2. Change in number of T- and B-cells following TLI and low-dose corticosteroids.

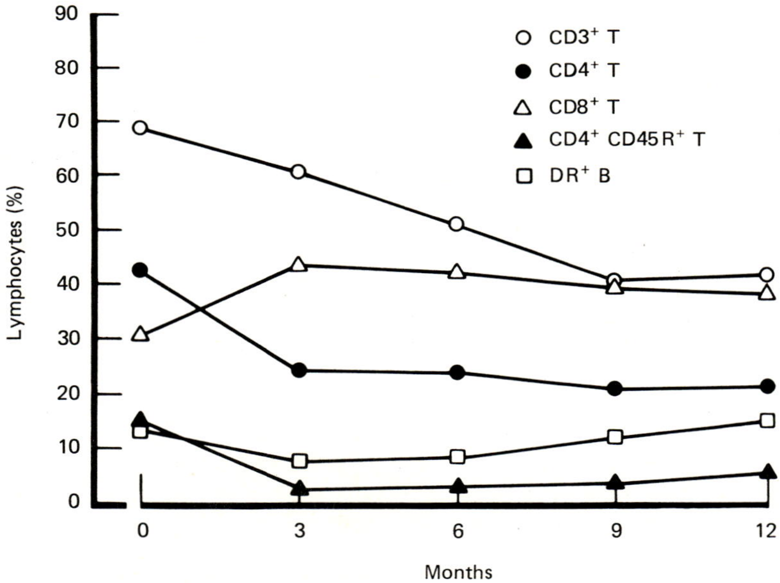

Fig. 13.3. Change in percentage of lymphocyte subsets following TLI plus low-dose corticosteroids.

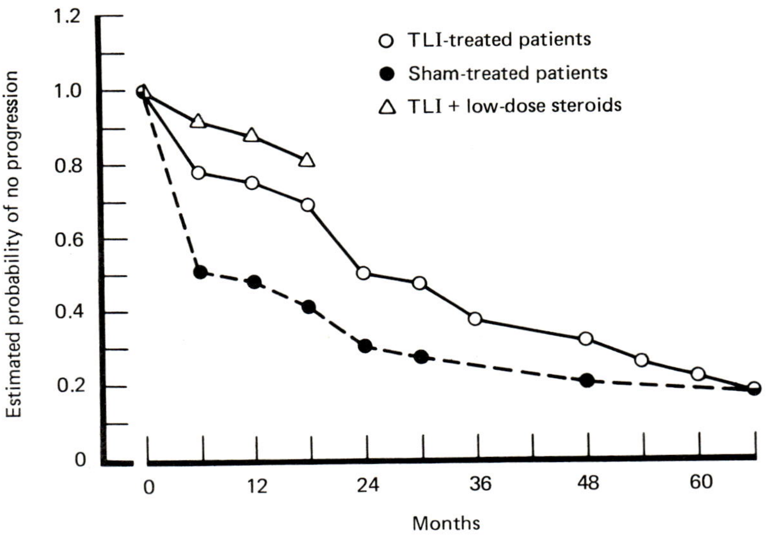

Fig. 13.4. Kaplan–Meier curves of estimated probability of no progression over time. Comparison of all TLI (including TLI plus low-dose corticosteroids) and sham-TLI chronic/progressive MS patients (*$p \leqslant 0.05$).

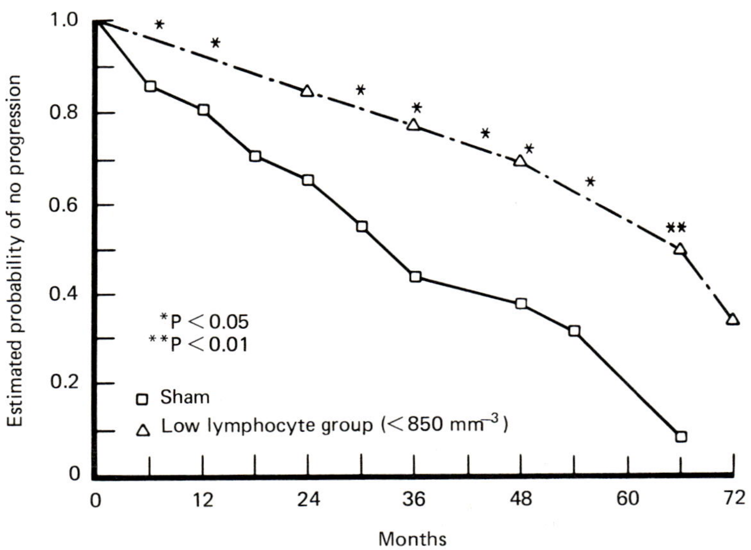

Fig. 13.5. Kaplan–Meier curves of estimated probability of no progression over time using 2-point decline in functional status scale as end point. Comparison of patients with chronic/progressive MS, with mean blood lymphocyte count below 850 per mm^3 during the 3 months post, TLI with sham-irradiated patients (*$p \leqslant 0.05$, **$p \leqslant 0.01$).

pared to sham-irradiated patients, and the Kaplan–Meier curve of functional stabilization was also significantly different from the sham curve through 66 months ($p = 0.054$). When functional stabilization curves were analyzed using a 2-point deterioration as the endpoint, even greater differences were noted between sham and TLI patients with low lymphocyte counts ($p = 0.016$), and significant differences were noted at every 6-month interval ($p \leq 0.05$ to 0.01) up to 66 months post-treatment (Fig. 13.5).

TLI patients with mean peripheral lymphocyte counts below 850 per mm^3 during the first 3 months post-TLI also had a significant difference in their Kaplan–Meier functional stabilization curve as compared to TLI-treated patients with higher lymphocyte counts ($p = 0.007$) (Fig. 13.6). When functional status at 6-month intervals was determined, patients with the lower lymphocyte counts also deteriorated significantly less through the entire 72 months of follow-up using a 2-point drop, as compared to patients with higher lymphocyte counts ($p \leq 0.05$ to 0.005).

In contrast, no difference in Kaplan–Meier curves or functional status at 6-month intervals was found when the TLI patients with high lymphocyte counts were compared to sham-treated CPMS patients, using either a 1- or 2-point drop in the functional scale as end points (Cook et al. 1990). Thus TLI appears not to adversely affect functional stabilitzation post-therapy, even in patients with high lymphocyte counts.

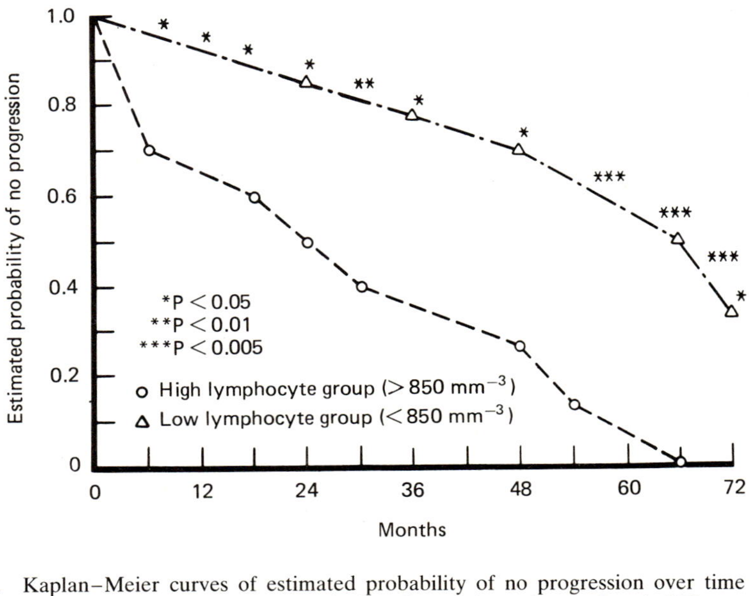

Fig. 13.6. Kaplan–Meier curves of estimated probability of no progression over time using 2-point decline in functional status scale as endpoint. Comparison of mean low (<850 per mm^3) and high blood lymphocyte groups ($*p \leq 0.05$, $**p \leq 0.01$, $***p \leq 0.005$).

Adverse Effects of Total Lymphoid Irradiation in Chronic/Progressive Multiple Sclerosis

Adverse effects of TLI in patients with chronic/progressive MS have generally not been severe. In fact, immediately post TLI or sham-TLI therapy, no significant difference was found in the proportion of patients who successfully identified which treatment they had received (Cook et al. 1986). However, significantly greater nausea, diarrhea, dyspepsia, dysphagia and axillary or inguinal hair loss were transiently seen following TLI as compared to sham irradiation (Cook et al. 1990). In addition, over 90% of premenopausal women in our study developed amenorrhea. No significant difference in mortality was seen between TLI and sham-treated patients, with 11% of TLI and 10% of sham-treated patients dying during the follow-up period of up to 6 years (Cook et al. 1990). Of the 5 patients who died after TLI, 3 had aspiration pneumonias, one a myocardial infarction and one bladder carcinoma. Two patients died in the sham group, one from cardiovascular disease and one from urosepsis.

Summary and Future Directions

A double-blind controlled study has shown significantly greater stabilization of patients with chronic/progressive MS receiving TLI than sham TLI, with a beneficial response limited to those patients with sustained mean peripheral lymphocyte counts below 850 per mm^3. Unfortunately, TLI alone has not been shown to be curative in any autoimmune disease. Following TLI in patients with chronic/progressive MS, a functional decline occurred in the low lymphocyte group as mean lymphocyte count normalized. However, this deterioration occurred at a slower rate than in the sham-irradiated group or the TLI group with a higher initial post-treatment lymphocyte level. Recently, in open pilot studies, we have found that giving low-dose prednisone with TLI, results in significantly greater and more protracted lymphocytopenia in patients than does TLI alone. Double-blind trials will be started shortly to determine if, as in lupus erythematosus and rheumatoid arthritis, the addition of low-dose prednisone will lead to longer duration of stability in chronic/progressive MS patients following TLI. These trials will be carried out without irradiating the spleen, which should diminish the risk of severe bacterial infections, although these were not seen at a significantly higher rate in TLI than control patients in our prior study. We hope that these trials may also give us better insight into subgroups of patients who might best respond to this therapy.

Our results with TLI in chronic/progressive MS also imply that the immune response is important in the genesis of MS lesions, and that lymphocytes derived from peripheral lymph nodes circulate and enter the brain to contribute in this regard.

Since beneficial effects of TLI in patients with chronic/progressive MS have not been confirmed by other groups as yet, we believe this treatment should be considered experimental at the present time, and its use limited to patients in controlled studies.

Acknowledgements. This work was supported in part by the Medical Research Service of the Department of Veterans Affairs and the National Multiple Sclerosis Society.

References

Austin HA, Muenz LR, Joyce KM et al. (1983) Prognostic factors in lupus nephritis. Contribution of renal histologic data. Am J Med 75:382–391

Bookman MA, Longo DL, Young RC (1988) Late complications of curative treatment in Hodgkin's disease. JAMA 260:680–683

British and Dutch Multiple Sclerosis Azathioprine Trial Group (1988) Double-masked trial of azathioprine in multiple sclerosis. Lancet 2:179–183

Brahn E, Helfgott SM, Belli JA et al. (1984) Total lymphoid irradiation therapy in refractory rheumatoid arthritis: fifteen to forty-month follow-up. Arthritis Rheum 27:481–488

Calin A (1985) X-radiation in the management of rheumatoid disease. Br J Hosp Med 33:261–265

Cook SD, Devereux C, Troiano R et al. (1986) Effect of total lymphoid irradiation in chronic progressive multiple sclerosis. Lancet i:1405–1409

Cook SD, Devereux C, Troiano R et al. (1987) Total lymphoid irradiation in multiple sclerosis: Blood lymphocytes and clinical course. Ann Neurol 22:634–638

Cook SD, Troiano R, Zito G et al. (1990) The treatment of patients with chronic progressive multiple sclerosis with total lymphoid irradiation. In: Cook SD (ed) The handbook of multiple sclerosis. Marcel Dekker, New York and Basel, pp 401–421

Devereux C, Troiano R, Zito G et al. (1988) Effect of total lymphoid irradiation on functional status in chronic multiple sclerosis: Importance of lymphopenia early after treatment: the pros. Neurology 38:32–37

Ellison GW, Myers LW, Mickey MR, Graves MC, Tourtellotte WW, Nuwer MR (1988) Clinical experience with azathioprine: the pros. Neurology 38 (suppl 2):20–23

Fuks Z, Strober S, Bobrove AM, Sasazuki T, McMichael A, Kaplan HS (1976) Long term effects of radiation on T and B lymphocytes in peripheral blood of patients with Hodgkin's disease. J Clin Invest 58:803–814

Gaston JSH, Strober S, Solovera JJ et al. (1988) Dissection of the mechanisms of immune injury in rheumatoid arthritis using total lymphoid irradiation. Arthritis Rheum 31:21–30

Haas GS, Halperin E, Doseretz D et al. (1984) Differential recovery of circulating T cell subsets after nodal irradiation for Hodgkin's disease. J Immunol 132:1026–1030

Hanly JG, Hassan J, Moriarty M et al. (1987) Lymphoid irradiation in intractable rheumatoid arthritis: a double-blind, randomized study comparing 750-rad treatment with 2000-rad treatment. Arthritis Rheum 30:980–987

Hauser SL, Dawson DM, Lehrich JR et al. (1983) Intensive immunosuppression in progressive multiple sclerosis: a randomized, three-arm study of high-dose cyclophosphamide, plasma exchange, and ACTH. N Engl J Med 308:173–180

Kaplan HS (1980) Hodgkin's disease, 2nd edn. Harvard University Press, Cambridge, pp 366–441

King DP, Strober S, Kaplan HS (1981) Suppression of the mixed leukocyte response and graft vs host disease by spleen cells following total lymphoid irradiation (TLI). J Immunol 126:1140–1145

Kotzin B, Strober S (1979) Reversal of NZB disease with total lymphoid irradiation (TLI). J Exp Med 150:371

Kotzin BL, Strober S, Engleman E et al. (1981) Treatment of intractable rheumatoid arthritis with total lymphoid irradiation. N Engl J Med 305:969–975

Kotzin BL, Kansas GS, Engleman E, Hoppe RT, Kaplan HS, Strober S (1983) Changes in T-cell subsets in patients with rheumatoid arthritis treated with total lymphoid irradiation. Clin Immunol Immunopath 27:250–260

Lauria F, Foa R, Gobbi M et al. (1983) Increased proportion of suppressor/cytotoxic (OKT8+) cells in patients with Hodgkin's disease in long-lasting remission. Cancer 52:1385–1388

Mitchell DM, Spitz PW, Young DY, Bloch DA, McShane DJ, Fries JF (1986) Survival, prognosis, and causes of death in rheumatoid arthritis. Arthritis Rheum 29:706–714

Nusslein HG, Herbst M, Manger BJ et al. (1985) Total lymphoid irradiation in patients with refractory rheumatoid arthritis. Arthritis Rheum 28:1205–1210

Okada S, Strober S (1982a) Spleen cells from adult mice given total lymphoid irradiation (TLI) or from newborn mice have similar regulatory effects in the mixed leukocyte reaction (MLR). I. Generation of antigen-specific suppressor cells in the MLR after the addition of spleen cells from adult mice given TLI. J Exp Med 156:522–538

Okada S, Strober S (1982b) Spleen from adult mice given total lymphoid irradiation (TLI) or from newborn mice have similar regulatory effects in the mixed leukocyte reaction (MLR). II. Generation of antigen-specific suppressor cells in the MLR after the addition of spleen cells from newborn mice. J Immunol 129:1892–1897

Oseroff A, Okada S, Strober S (1984) Natural suppressor (NS) cells found in the spleen of neonatal mice and adult mice given total lymphoid irradiation (TLI) express the null surface phenotype. J Immunol 132:101–110

Pincus T, Callahan LF, Sale WG, Brooks AL, Payne LE, Vaughn WK (1984) Severe functional declines, work disability, and increased mortality in seventy-five rheumatoid arthritis patients studied over nine years. Arthritis Rheum 27:864–872

Rudge P, Koetsier JC, Mertin J et al. (1989) Randomized double blind controlled trial of cyclosporine in multiple sclerosis. J Neurol Neurosurg Psychiatry 52:559–565

Scheinberg MA, Weltman E (1985) Plasmapheresis vs. total lymphoid irradiation in the treatment of severe rheumatoid arthritis. Clin Exp Rheum 3:127–130

Slavin S, Strober S, Fuks Z, Kaplan HS (1977) Induction of specific tissue transplantation tolerance by using fractionated total lymphoid irradiation in adult mice: long-term survival of allogeneic bone marrow and skin grafts. J Exp Med 146:34–48

Slavin S, Reitz B, Bieber CP, Kaplan HS, Strober S (1978) Transplantation tolerance in adult rats using total lymphoid irradiation: permanent survival of skin, heart and marrow allographs. J Exp Med 147:700–707

Strober S, Field RT, Hoppe BL et al. (1985a) Treatment of intractable lupus nephritis with total lymphoid irradiation. Ann Intern Med 102:450–458

Strober S, Tanay A, Field E et al. (1985b) Efficacy of total lymphoid irradiation in intractable rheumatoid arthritis: a double-blind, randomized trial. Ann Intern Med 102:441–449

Strober S, Farinas MC, Field EH et al. (1987) Lupus nephritis after total lymphoid irradiation: persistent improvement and reduction of steroid therapy. Ann Intern Med 107:689–690

Strober S, Farinas MC, Field EH et al. (1988) Treatment of lupus nephritis with total lymphoid irradiation. Observations during a 12–79 month followup. Arthritis Rheum 31:850–858

Tanay A, Field EH, Hoope RT, Strober S (1987) Long-term follow-up of rheumatoid arthritis patients treated with total lymphoid irradiation. Arthritis Rheum 30:1–10

The Multiple Sclerosis Study Group (1990) Efficacy and toxicity of cyclosporine in chronic progressive multiple sclerosis: a randomized, double-blinded, placebo-controlled clinical trial. Ann Neurol 27:591–605

Trentham DE, Belli JA, Anderson RJ et al. (1981) Clinical and immunologic effects of fractionated total lymphoid irradiation in refractory rheumatoid arthritis. N Engl J Med 305:976–982

Trentham DE, Belli JA, Bloomer WD et al. (1987) 2000-centiGray total lymphoid irradiation for refractory rheumatoid arthritis. Arthritis Rheum 30:980–987

Troiano R, Devereux C, Oleske J et al. (1988) T cell subsets and disease progression after TLI in chronic progressive multiple sclerosis. J Neurol Neurosurg Psychiatry 51:980–983

Zan-Bai I, Slavin S, Strober S (1978) Induction and mechanism of tolerance to bovine serum albumin in mice given total lymphoid irradiation (TLI). J Immunol 121:1400–1404

Chapter 14

Specific Immunotherapeutic Strategies: Lessons from Myelin Basic Protein-Induced Experimental Allergic Encephalomyelitis

Robert B. Bell and Lawrence Steinman

The progress of research on the pathogenesis and treatment of multiple sclerosis (MS), the principal human demyelinating disease of the central nervous system (CNS), has intensified in the past 3 years. In part, this is due to the application of advances in molecular biology, like polymerase chain reaction (PCR), and to developments in cellular immunology, like technology for the growth of T-cell clones. Many lessons that have been learned in an animal model of CNS demyelinating disease, experimental allergic encephalomyelitis (EAE), have been verified in the human disease MS. Indeed, certain successful approaches for treatment of EAE are being attempted in MS at the present time.

This review describes the strong parallels that exist between T-cell receptor (TCR) usage in the pathogenesis of EAE, TCR usage in myelin basic protein (MBP)-specific T-cells in the peripheral blood of MS patients (Wucherpfennig et al. 1990; Ota et al. 1990; Martin et al. 1991) and in T-cells in demyelinative plaques in MS brain (Oksenberg et al. 1990). Based on these similarities, selective immunotherapy that targets either class II molecules of the major histocompatibility complex (MHC) or TCR variable regions will be described in EAE, with consideration given to application of these principles in MS. These new therapeutic approaches involve monoclonal antibodies (mAbs) directed to either HLA class II molecules or TCR V region molecules, or peptides that compete with HLA class II molecules or vaccinate against TCR V regions.

Relevance of EAE to Multiple Sclerosis

It has become increasingly clear that MS is a disease in which immunologic factors play a major role in the demyelinative lesion. This is supported by a large body of evidence of immune dysfunction in this disease (Reder and Arnason 1985). In EAE, we have considerable knowledge of the encephalitogenic antigen MBP and how T-cell recognition of that antigen is influenced by genetic susceptibility to the disease. In MS, on the other hand, the precise nature of the antigen remains unclear and the genetic elements that determine susceptibility are less completely understood. EAE continues to be the model for MS, however, providing extensive information on the demyelinative process and allowing investigation into fundamental aspects of the autoimmune response, including providing a testing ground for new approaches to therapy which may potentially be extrapolated to demyelinating disease in man.

EAE is perhaps the best characterized model of an antigen-specific, T-cell-mediated autoimmune disease. It develops as a result of an immune response to the autoantigen MBP and can be induced in many species including rats and mice. It is characterized by the acute onset of paralysis subsequent to the inoculation of animals with either MBP or peptides of MBP in adjuvant, or by intravenous injection of T-cell clones. Perivascular infiltration by mononuclear cells in the central nervous system is seen with disease onset and demyelination can be clearly demonstrated. The disease is mediated by $CD4^+$ T-lymphocytes and susceptibility to the resulting demyelination is linked to genes of the MHC class II region (Paterson 1960). The inbred mouse species we have utilized for EAE study include PL/J, (PLSJ)F1, and SJ/L, restricted by the MHC haplotypes $H\text{-}2^u$, $H\text{-}2^{u/s}$, and $H\text{-}2^s$ respectively. Within the $H\text{-}2^{u/s}$ haplotype $H\text{-}2^s$ appears to be differentially expressed and is thus non-functional. Many parallels exist in the etiopathogenesis of EAE and MS and it is based upon these similarities that successful immunotherapeutic strategies in EAE may have application to the human condition.

The T-Cell Response

We understand the lesion development in EAE and in MS to be a result of the abnormal activation of autoreactive class II-restricted $CD4^+$ T-lymphocytes. The role for $CD8^+$ T-cells is less clear. The trigger for T-cell activation in EAE is exposure to encephalitogenic antigen together with an adjuvant, while the trigger in MS has been proposed to be the result of either a viral or environmental influence (McFarland and Dhib-Jalbut 1989). Although the immune system of a given host has a wide repertoire of antigens it can recognize, response to each antigen is specific. To understand how T-lymphocytes participate in autoimmune disease it is necessary to be familiar with the fundamentals of antigen recognition.

T-cells recognize antigen only in association with a product of the MHC, the class I and class II antigens. The resulting ternary interaction of antigen, MHC, and the clonally distributed antigen-specific T-cell receptor is referred to as the trimolecular complex (McFarland and Dhib-Jalbut 1989; Hohlfeld 1989; Bjorkman et al. 1987a,b; Zamvil and Steinman 1990; Acha-Orbea et al. 1989) (Fig. 14.1). Major histocompatibility complex class I molecules are cell surface proteins expressed on all nucleated cells. In man these are the HLA-A, B, C antigens. In mice the homologous proteins are H-2K, D, L antigens. Class II molecules are cell surface glycoproteins expressed constitutively by macrophages, B cells and dendritic cells. In the CNS, class II molecule expression can be induced upon CNS endothelial cells and astrocytes (Hohlfeld 1989). In man these molecules are HLA-DP, DQ, and DR antigens. In mice they are I-A and I-E with the homologs being I-A to HLA-DQ and I-E to HLA-DR. Class II molecule cell-surface glycoproteins are heterodimers composed of an

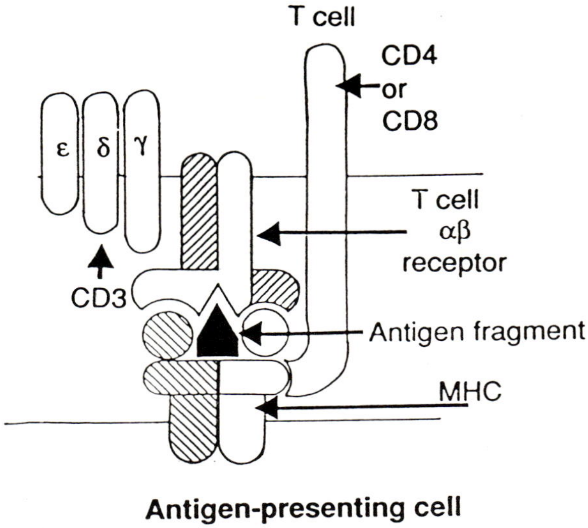

Fig. 14.1. The trimolecular complex. Reprinted with permission from *Science* (Blackman et al. 1990).

alpha and beta chain which fold to create an antigen-binding cleft formed by the polymorphic residues of the two chains. Of fundamental importance in the recognition of antigen is the requirement of binding of the peptide antigen to a specific allelic MHC molecule, for subsequent presentation to the T-cell. Control over how antigen is presented is exerted by the MHC composition of an individual. An isolated change in the MHC restricting element can have a dramatic influence on the T-cell response to similar antigenic proteins. In addition, the MHC is able to influence T-cell repertoire by both positive and negative selection during T-cell development.

Numerous associations exist between autoimmune disease in man and the MHC antigen, with the strongest linkages being to specific allelic class II HLA-D genes (Todd et al. 1988). Rheumatoid arthritis, insulin-dependent diabetes mellitus, pemphigus vulgaris, thyroiditis, systemic lupus erythematosus, myasthenia gravis, and multiple sclerosis all exhibit MHC associations. Susceptibility to both insulin-dependent diabetes mellitus and pemphigus vulgaris has been linked to a polymorphism at residue 57 in the DQ beta chain (Todd et al. 1987; Sinha et al. 1988). Modelling of the class II structure suggests this residue is located in the antigen-binding cleft and may be particularly important in determining the conformation of the cleft.

The presentation of antigen to T-helper cells requires the processing of antigen by class II expressing cells. This involves the enzymatic cleavage of protein antigen with the exposure of individual peptide antigenic epitopes. Common structural characteristics of these epitopes have been proposed by DeLisi and Berzofsky (1985) and by Rothbard and Taylor (1988) enabling, in some circumstances, the prediction of autoantigenic epitopes. The recognition of antigens in vivo is also influenced by competition by peptides for the class II restricting element, the nature of the enzymatic production of epitopes, and the available T-cell repertoire.

The T-cell receptor is a clonally distributed transmembrane heterodimer consisting of alpha and beta chains in association with the CD3 complex. These chains each contain a variable domain involved in antigen recognition and a constant region anchor domain. The genes encoding alpha and beta chains are encoded as variable (V), diversity (D) (beta chain only), joining (J), and constant (C) gene segments, located noncontiguously on chromosomes 7 and 14 in man. They undergo recombination and RNA splicing following transcription during T-cell development creating unique Vα-Jα-Cα and Bβ-Dβ-Jβ-Cβ RNA molecules that are subsequently translated into the expressed alpha and beta chains. Each T-cell expresses only one T-cell product. The potential T-cell repertoire is extremely large, the result of the potential participation of a large number of germline gene segments. There are approximately 100 germline Vα gene segments and 50–100 Jα genes in both humans and mice. The potential for somatic recombination of these gene segments and the combinatorial association of individual alpha and beta chain genes leads to a potential 10^7 unique T-cell receptor molecules that can be generated. Further heterogeneity can be generated post-translationally to give a potential number of unique T-cell receptor molecules as numerous as 10^{15} (Zamvil and Steinman 1990; Kronenberg et al. 1986).

In general, although the potential repertoire is very large, a restricted usage of T-cell receptor gene elements has been found among T-cell clones that share antigen fine specificity and MHC restriction. Although the molecular basis for antigen/MHC recognition by the T-cell is still unclear, some studies demonstrate that V gene usage may be influenced by the MHC type (Morel et al. 1987).

Multiple Epitopes of Myelin Basic Protein in Mouse and Man

The animal model of autoimmune demyelinative disease (EAE) has provided an extremely useful system for the examination of immune mechanisms, and the development of potential new therapeutic strategies for autoimmune disease. Short peptides of MBP may induce a monophasic, chronic or chronic/relapsing EAE, dependent upon the inoculation schedule (Zamvil and Steinman 1990; Acha-Orbea et al. 1989). Other peptide fragments of MBP are also immunogenic, but instead of inducing disease these fragments can protect mice from a single progenitor T-cell is referred to as a T-cell clone and of course all immunogenic epitopes of MBP are pathogenic.

Clones of T-cells may be derived from afflicted animals by harvesting draining lymph nodes, collection of lymphocytes and the subsequent growth in culture of those cells reactive to the inducing antigen. A growth of cells derived from a single progenitor T-cell is referred to as a T-cell clone and of course all of these cells will bear the same T-cell markers including TCR, and will have the same antigenic specificity. The isolation of MBP reactive T-cell clones which mediate EAE facilitated the identification of individual encephalitogenic epitopes. The encephalitogenic T-cell epitope within MBP peptide 1-37, in mice bearing the MHC haplotype H-2^u, was the first to be identified and has been characterized in greatest detail (Wraith et al. 1989a,b; Zamvil et al. 1986). In fact, the amino acids within this epitope that contact MHC and T-cell receptor have been deduced (Wraith et al. 1989a).

We had initially observed that separate forms of native (intact) MBP, varying in their N-terminal sequences, differed in their ability to stimulated individual MBP-derived clones that were encephalitogenic and responded to MBP fragment 1-37, restricted by I-A^u. In fact, bovine MBP, which is less encephalitogenic in PL/J mice, was less stimulatory than rat or mouse MBP. Because bovine MBP 1-37 differs from the mouse MBP 1-37 sequence at residues 2 and 17 only (Fig. 14.2), we predicted that the epitope recognized by these clones would include one of these two residues (Zamvil et al. 1986). Using overlapping synthetic peptides containing these two residues we identified the encephalitogenic epitope to be located within the first 11 residues. Peptides 1-11 and 1-16 were equipotent with intact rat or mouse MBP. Acetylation of the N-terminus (Ac1-11), as is found in native MBP, is necessary for the encephalitogenicity of p1-11 and p1-16. Shorter peptides, Ac1-7 and Ac1-9, were less stimulatory in vitro, although Ac1-9 remains encephalitogenic (Zamvil et al. 1986).

A few features of this T-cell epitope were intriguing. First we noted that Ac1-11(4A), with an alanine for lysine substitution at position 4, produced an exaggerated lymphocyte proliferative response compared to Ac1-11 in encephalitogenic T-cell clones reactive to the N-terminus (Wraith et al. 1989a). Using a photo-affinity probe to measure direct binding of I-A^u, Wraith, Smilek, McDevitt and our group showed that Ac1-11(4A) binds to I-A^u with at least a tenfold higher relative affinity when compared to Ac1-11 (Wraith et al. 1989a).

In contrast, peptides Ac1-11(3A) and Ac1-11(6A) with amino-acid substitution at the 3 and 6 positions, did not stimulate T-cell clones or T-cell hybridomas reactive to Ac1-11 (Wraith et al. 1989a). However, peptides Ac1-11(3A) and Ac1-11(6A) both significantly inhibited binding of the photo probe to I-A^u at 1000-fold molar excess. This implies that their inability to activate Ac1-11 reactive T-cells reflects a defect in TCR interactions rather than I-A^u binding.

It was then demonstrated that (PL/J × SJL/J)F1 ((PLSJ)F1) mice were able to generate T-cell responses to both Ac1-11(3A) and Ac1-11(6A), but that the majority of these responses were mutually non-crossreactive with the response to Ac1-11. They also explain why the substituted peptides failed to stimulate encephalitogenic T-cell clones even though they were able to bind to I-A^u. These observations strongly suggest that residues 3 and 6 of Ac1-11 determine TCR interactions rather than MHC interactions (Wraith et al. 1989a).

```
                          10        20        30
Rat/Guinea Pig MBP   Ac-A S Q K R P S Q R H G S K Y L A T A S T M D H A R H G F L P R H R D T G I
Mouse MBP            Ac-————————————————( )——————————————————————————————————
Bovine MBP           Ac-— A ————————————( )————— S ——————————————————————————
```

Fig. 14.2. N-terminal amino acid sequence of myelin basic protein from various species. Reprinted with permission from the *Journal of Experimental Medicine* (Zamvil et al. 1988a).

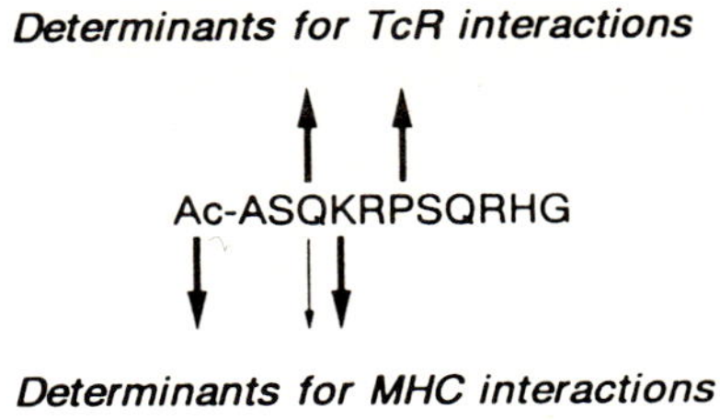

Fig. 14.3. Determinants for interactions. Arrows point from each amine acid residue of Ac1-11 to its role as either a T-cell or an MHC interaction determinant. Reprinted with permission from *Cold Spring Harbor Symposia on Quantitative Biology* (McDevitt et al. 1989).

MBP occurs naturally acetylated at its N-terminus. Acetylation of residue 1, Ac-ALA, was essential for stimulation of all encephalitogenic clones that recognize the N-terminus of MBP. Using a photoaffinity probe to measure the direct binding of peptides to I-A^u, Wraith, Smilek, McDevitt and we showed that unacetylated 1-11(4A) (peptide 1-11 with alanine substituted for lysine) bound to I-A^u weakly compared with Ac1-11(4A). However, despite its decreased binding to I-A^u, unacetylated 1-11(4A) effectively activated an encephalitogenic T-cell hybridoma reactive to Ac1-11 and restricted by I-A^u (Wraith et al. 1989a). Like the unacetylated peptide 1-11(4A), peptide 1-11 does not bind to I-A^u; however, unlike p1-11(4A) it fails to stimulate encephalitogenic T-cell clones reactive to the N-terminus of MBP (Wraith et al. 1989a). This implicates the N-acetyl group as a determinant important in interactions with I-A^u, but not absolutely necessary for effective TCR interactions. These data confirm the assignment of function to particular residues of Ac1-11. Thus, residue 1, Ac-alanine, contacts MHC, as does residue 4, lysine. Residues 3 (glutamine) and 6 (proline) interact with TCR (Fig. 14.3).

Other epitopes within the N-terminus of MBP have been identified. These include Ac9-20 which protects mice from EAE induced with Ac1-11 despite eliciting a strong proliferative response itself (Zamvil et al. 1987). The peptide Ac1-20 contains an I-A^u restricted encephalitogenic epitope, but when deacetylated, p1-20, loses its pathogenicity while retaining immunogenicity. Additional cryptic encephalitogenic epitopes have been identified in H-2^u mice. An epitope recognized by an encephalitogenic T-cell clone, restricted to a hybrid I-E rather than I-A MHC molecule was identified. This T-cell epitope, p35-47, also causes severe EAE in H-2^u mice (Zamvil et al. 1988a).

Thus, in I-A^u and in $A^{u/s}$ mice certain peptides within the N-terminus were encephalitogenic, and others were immunogenic and protective. It is not clear what features of certain peptides render them encephalitogenic. Some evidence suggests that lymphokine activity in T-cell clones may correlate with pathogenicity (Powell et al. 1990).

In other genetic strains of mice encephalitic fragments of MBP closer to the C-terminus have been identified to be encephalitogenic. In contrast with the encephalitogenic response to the N-terminus, in SJL/L mice there is more than one discrete population of I-A^s restricted T-cells which is encephalitogenic. In fact, several overlapping epitopes have been identified (Sakai et al. 1988; Kono et al. 1988; Padula et al. 1991) (Table 14.1).

Table 14.1. Multiple discrete T-cell epitopes of myelin basic protein. Several immunogenic epitopes of MBP were determined using pepsin-digested peptides and synthetic oligopeptides. Although these determinants induce strong T-cell immune responses in the context of a certain MHC class II molecule, not all the determinants are encephalitogenic. The ability of MBP epitopes to induce EAE, then MHC class II restriction and the nature of the variable region gene of the T cell receptor β chain (Vβ) elicited in response to the epitope are shown here

Peptide	Encephalitogenic potential	Class II restriction[a]	Va[b]	Vb[c]
pAc1-9	+	$A\alpha^u A\beta^u$	4.3[d] 4.2/2.3[e]	$8^+/4$[d] $8^+/13$[e]
pAc1-11	+	$A\alpha^u A\beta^u$	ND	8^+
pAc1-20	+	$A\alpha^u A\beta^u$	ND	ND
p1-20	–	$A\alpha^u A\beta^u$	ND	ND
p5-6	–	$A\alpha^u A\beta^u$, $A\alpha^s A\beta^u$	ND	8^+
pAc9-16	–	$A\alpha^u A\beta^u$, $A\alpha^s A\beta^u$	ND	ND
p17-27	?	$A\alpha^s A\beta^s$	ND	ND
p35-47	+	$E\alpha^u E\beta^u$, $E\alpha^u E\beta^s$	ND	8^-
p89-100	+	$A\alpha^s A\beta^s$	ND	ND
p89-101	+	$A\alpha^s A\beta^s$	ND	17_a
p96-109	+	$A\alpha^s A\beta^s$	ND	ND
p92-103	+	$A\alpha^s A\beta^s$	ND	4

[a] Aα, alpha chain of I-A; Aβ, beta chain of I-A; Eα, alpha chain of I-E; Eβ, beta chain of I-E.
[b] Vα, variable region of TCR alpha chain.
[c] Vβ, variable region of TCR beta chain.
[d] PL/J animals.
[e] B10PL animals.

In Table 14.1 we enumerate multiple immunogenic epitopes of MBP in just two strains of inbred mice. The implications of this diversity for outbred human populations are apparent. It should be noted that other myelin antigens, such as proteolipid, may also cause EAE. Several groups have now identified immunogenic epitopes of MBP in MS patients and in healthy human controls (Ota et al. 1990; Martin et al 1990a,b). Among MS patients and controls who were DR2DQw1 there was an increased frequency of peripheral blood T-cell lines from MS patients that proliferated to MBP 89-102 which, incidentally, includes the encephalitogenic epitope for H-2^s mice (Ota et al. 1990). Other peptide epitopes also elicited proliferation of T-cell lines but with equal frequency among patients and controls. The difficulty, of course, is knowing whether an epitope is necessarily pathogenic because pathogenic epitopes are not always the immunodominant ones by immunological assay and, even so, immunodominant epitopes may be protective as well as pathogenic. As Hafler and colleagues suggest: "To show that MS as a cell mediated autoimmune disease is analogous to EAE, certain criteria can be proposed. First, an association should exist between an immunodominant region of the presumed autoantigen and disease associated MHC haplotypes (like HLA-DR2, DQw1). Second, there should be an increase of T cells that react with this immunodominant epitope. Finally, the course of the disease must be altered by elimination of autoreactive T-cells or by inducing immune tolerance to the autoantigen identified in the first two criteria. This final condition implies that in vitro experiments on their own cannot prove the association of an autoantigen with a disease, and instead clinical trials are necessary." (Ota et al. 1990).

Martin and colleagues have obtained similar results in studies of cytotoxic T-lymphocyte lines that recognize MBP and its fragments in association with HLA class II molecules (Martin et al. 1990). Both MS patients and healthy controls responded to MBP p87-106 in association with HLA-DR2 and DR4. It was postulated that this peptide, which is encephalitogenic in some experimental animals and which may be presented by multiple HLA-DR molecules associated with MS, may be related to the pathogenesis of the disease. Because the peptide is also recognized by T-cells of healthy individuals, it seems evident that the presence of the peptide alone is necessary but not sufficient for induction of disease. Other factors including the available TCR repertoire and environmental or infectious factors may be necessary for disease development.

In Man and in Rodents T-cell Receptor Usage is Restricted in T-cells Responding to Specific Epitopes of Myelin Basic Protein

The identification of multiple encephalitogenic epitopes of MBP indicated that the potential repertoire of MBP-specific T-cells includes more than one population of T-cells. However, the T-cell response to each epitope appears limited to discrete populations of T-cells. For example, encephalitogenic N-terminal MBP-specific T-cell clones could not be distinguished from one another on the basis of their reactivity to peptides of MBP or class II restriction. Furthermore, there was a concordance between in vitro T-cell recognition and encephalitogenic potential after active immunization. Both of these results suggested that the TCR repertoire of encephalitogenic N-terminal MBP-specific T-cells in H-2^u was limited. Recent advances in molecular biology have made it possible to examine the T-cell receptor of individual T-cells. With this technology it is possible to examine TCR gene expression of T-cells mediating EAE, and to address whether T-cells that appear phenotypically similar in their Ag/MHC recognition express common TCR genes. TCR gene expression has been examined for the encephalitogenic response to MBP 1-9 and MBP 89-101.

T-cell Response to N-terminus Peptides

TCR gene expression of MBP p1-9 specific T-cells has been examined by three approaches: (a) cell surface staining with TCR Vβ-specific monoclonal antibodies; (b) Southern analysis; and (c) TCR gene sequencing.

Antibody staining of N-terminus Ac1-9 specific and H-2^u restricted T-cell clones from PL/J mice was conducted using a monoclonal antibody specific for TCR Vβ8. TCR Vβ8 is a 3-member family of TCR genes encoding TCR expressed by several strains including PL/J. A high percentage of clones (85%)

expressed this receptor type (Zamvil et al. 1988b). When lymph node cells from Ac1-9 primed mice were sorted into $CD4^+/V\beta8^+$ and $CD4^+/V\beta8^-$ populations and stimulated again in vitro, the majority of the response occurred in the $V\beta8^+$ population. Conversely, when the T-cell proliferative response to p35-47 was examined the response occurred primarily in the $V\beta8^-$ population. However, TCR Vβ8 usage in the response to MBP is not specific for MBP 1-19 as clones recognizing the nonencephalitogenic epitope p5-16 were also largely $V\beta8^+$ by antibody staining. It has been suggested that Vβ usage may correlate with class II restriction. If so, based on our results, Vβ8 expression may correlate with I-A restriction in PL/J mice.

Heterogeneity in the T-cell response to MBP 1-9 was further evaluated by molecular genetic techniques. By Southern analysis, Vβ8.2 was identified as the TCR Vβ gene used by $V\beta8^+$ T-cell clones. This was confirmed by the sequencing of TCR genes of eight MBP 1-9 specific T-cell clones (Acha-Orbea et al. 1988, 1989). Of these eight clones, seven utilized Vβ8.2; one encephalitogenic clone expressed Vβ4 (Table 14.2). There was less restrictive use of Dβ and Jβ, with four clones utilizing Jβ2.7, two using Jβ2.3, and two clones expressing Jβ2.5. Thus, the predominant Vβ-Jβ, expressed by 4 (50%) of these clones, was Vβ8.2-Jβ2.7. Even less heterogeneity was observed in α chain gene usage. All eight clones used the same Vα, Vα4.3, a new member of the Vα4 family (also referred to as VαPJR-25). Six of these clones utilized JαTA31, one used JαTT11, and one used JαF1-12. The predominant Vα-Jα, expressed by six (75%) clones was Vα4.3-JαTA31 (Table 14.2). Thus, there was a striking degree of restriction in the α and β chain TCR gene usage in response to the encephalitogenic N-terminus.

TCR gene expression for MBP 1-9 specific T-cells was examined in another $H\text{-}2^u$ strain, B10.PL (Urban et al. 1988; Kumar et al. 1989). This strain contains the same MHC, the $H\text{-}2^u$ haplotype, on a B10 background. As in PL/J mice, MBP Ac1-9 is encephalitogenic in B10.PL and p1-9 specific T-cells are restricted by $I\text{-}A^u$. Although β chain gene usage was very similar to that seen

Table 14.2. Summary of TCR sequences. The TCR α and β chain variable and junctional regions utilized by these eight encephalitogenic T-cell clones are demonstrated. A marked degree of restriction in α and β chain gene usage is present

Clone	Vβ[a]	Jβ[b]	Vα[c]	Jβ[d]	
PJB-20	8.2	2.7	4.3	TA31	Group 1
PJpR-2.2	8.2	2.7	4.3	TA31	
PJpR-6.2	8.2	2.7	4.3	TA31	
F1-21	8.2	2.7	4.3	TA31	
PJR-25	8.2	2.3	4.3	TA31	Group 2
PJB-18	8.2	2.3	4.3	TA31	
PJpR-7.5	8.2	2.5	4.3	TT11	Group 3
F1-12	4	2.5	4.3	F1-12	Group 4

[a] Variable region of TCR beta chain.
[b] Junctional region of TCR beta chain.
[c] Variable region of TCR alpha chain.
[d] Junctional region of TCR alpha chain.

for PL/J p1-9 specific T-cell clones, α chain gene expression was somewhat different. In contrast with the PL/J clones analyzed, all having used Vα4.3, of the B10.PL clones examined, 58% used Vα2.3 and 42% expressed Vα4.2.

Within PL/J and B10.PL mice, the expression of TCR genes in the MBP p1-9 specific response is quite strikingly limited. However, when comparing TCR gene expression between these two strains, certain differences were apparent. Even though Vβ8.2 is used to the same extent by both strains, it is unclear why Vα2.3, which was not expressed by any of the PL/J clones, was used more frequently than Vα4 in B10.PL mice. A potential explanation is that polymorphic differences in TCR gene expression may exist between these strains.

T-cell Response to C-terminus Peptides

TCR gene usage in the encephalitogenic T-cell response of SJL/J mice to the C-terminus has been examined, although not as extensively as for MBP p1-9. The T-cell response appears more complex. Four encephalitogenic peptides have been identified, p89-101, p89-100, p96-109 and p92-103 (Table 14.1). TCR Vβ expression has been examined for T-cells responsive to p89-101 and p92-103. Approximately 50% of T-cells which proliferate to p89-101 also respond to p89-100. The other 50% require Pro101 for stimulation. TCR Vβ gene expression for these two populations has been examined most closely with a monoclonal antibody that recognizes Vβ17, a single gene family, expressed by several I-A$^+$/I-E$^-$ strains, including SJL/J (Kappler 1987a,b). Interestingly, all clones that recognize p89-101, but not 89-100, use TCR Vβ17. All clones that proliferate to p89-100 are Vβ17$^-$ (Sakai et al. 1988). The TCR Vβ(s) expressed by Vβ17$^-$ clones is not known at this time. Examination of TCR α chain genes and further analysis of the β chain genes is currently in progress.

Recently, Padula and colleagues have identified a Vβ gene segment, Vβ4, used by encephalitogenic T-cells responsive to the C-terminal epitope p92-103. The utilization of this gene segment is intriguing. As demonstrated (Table 14.2) the alternate Vβ gene segment identified in (PLSJ)F1 mice was Vβ4. These clones were p1-9 specific and restricted by H-2^u. The identification of p92-103 specific, H-2^s restricted, Vβ4 bearing clones in SJL mice represents a Vβ correlation that crosses MHC/antigenic restriction barriers (Padula et al. 1991). As postulated by Acha-Orbea and Heber-Katz, the utilization of common variable regions (e.g., Vβ4) in the pathogenesis of EAE in these two murine genotypes may suggest that TCR V regions are mediators of EAE by mechanisms apart from MHC/antigen specificity (Heber-Katz and Acha-Orbea 1989).

Restriction in T-cell Receptor Usage in Patients with Multiple Sclerosis

Recently, several studies have attempted to extend to MS the identification of a restricted T-cell repertoire utilized in disease which has been identified in EAE. The TCR usage has been studied by Hafler and colleagues in T-cell clones derived from peripheral blood that respond to epitopes on MBP (Wucherpfennig et al. 1990). The Vβ gene usage in peripheral blood derived T cell lines reactive to either of the previously defined immunodominant regions of human MBP, residues 84-102 or 143-168, was studied. The Vβ17 and Vβ12 receptor types were used frequently, but not exclusively, in recognition of p84-102 by both patients and controls, but these same receptors were used infrequently in the recognition of p143-168. Reactivity to p84-102 was restricted most frequently by DR2, whereas reactivity to p143-168 was associated with DRw11. These findings suggest there may be a degree of shared Vβ gene usage in the recognition of immunodominant regions of the autoantigen MBP in humans. Contrary to this view, Martin and colleagues have examined the T-cell response to another MBP epitope which is frequently recognized by both patients and controls, p87-106. In patient-derived T-cell lines a similar core sequence was recognized in conjuction with four different HLA-DR molecules and with markedly heterogeneous Vβ usage (Martin et al. 1991).

In an attempt to elucidate the nature of the lymphocytic infiltration in the brains of MS patients, we undertook to examine expression of TCR genes at the site of disease (Oksenberg et al. 1990). The mRNA isolated from demyelinating brain plaques from 3 MS patients with chronic/progressive disease, and from 3 control brains (non-MS) was used to synthesize cDNA. These cDNAs were then subjected to enzymatic gene amplification by the polymerase chain reaction (PCR) method using specific primers for 18 different Vα families, pairing them with a common Cα primer. No Vα transcripts could be amplified from control brain cDNA and in each of the MS brains only 2-4 Vα segments were found to be expressed. The Vα 10 family was detected in all 3 MS samples, suggesting that this TCR might be responding to a major epitope of an antigen involved in pathogenesis of MS. Sequence analysis of the Vα transcripts encoded by Vα 12.1 showed rearrangements to a limited number of Jα region segments. The implication of these studies is that TCR Vα gene expression in MS brain lesions is restricted.

Further analysis of TCR Vα and Vβ transcripts has demonstrated a marked to moderate restriction for both chains (JR Oksenberg personal communication. 1991). In addition, there would appear to be some evidence that TCR Vβ genes may be preferentially rearranged in certain HLA haplotypes that are associated with an increased susceptibility to MS. These findings, of course, may have major therapeutic implications paralleling the success of targeted therapy in EAE of the TCR V genes or MHC class II molecules.

The Potential Strategies for Immuno-intervention in EAE and MS

The current therapies for autoimmune disease in general were developed without any clear knowledge of the immune mechanisms involved in the generation and perpetuation of the disease, particularly the importance of T-cell activation as an initiating factor. They are, thus, relatively nonspecific in their action and fail to differentiate abnormal from normal immune reactions. The

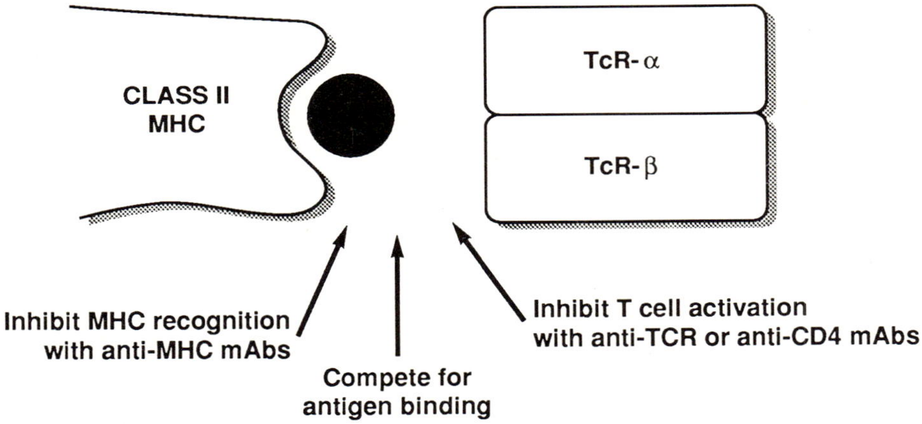

Fig. 14.4. Interfering with activation of auto-reactive T-lymphocytes. Reprinted with permission from *Cell* (Wraith et al. 1989a).

progress that has been made in understanding the immune response in EAE has enabled the development of immunotherapeutic strategies that are increasingly specific. The trimolecular complex of MHC, T-cell, and antigen affords multiple potential sites at which to intervene in the autoimmune process (Fig. 14.4).

Antibodies to Accessory Molecules

A variety of accessory molecules are involved in T-cell activation. The CD4 molecules are T-cell expressed antigens which bind to invariant regions of MHC class II and play a role in generating signals leading to T-cell proliferation and differentiation following the recognition of an antigen peptide by the TCR-CD3 complex. Monoclonal antibodies to CD4 inhibit T-cell activation both in vivo and in vitro, and may allow the induction of tolerance to antigens introduced during the course of therapy. This has been established in model systems by the generation of tolerance to grafted tissue. Potentially this may allow for the reinduction of self-tolerance to an autoantigen in circumstances like MS. Anti-CD4 antibody therapy has been demonstrated to be very effective in reversing and preventing demyelination in EAE (Waldor et al. 1985). Currently, early phase trials are evaluating its safety in rheumatoid arthritis and MS patients.

Antibodies to HLA Class II Molecules

A common feature of many human autoimmune diseases is the increased frequency of some class II alleles in affected individuals. In animal models of autoimmune disease, susceptibility is frequently strain- and MHC-specific. It appears likely that MHC alleles associated with susceptibility participate in the presentation of antigen to the autoreactive T-cell. Blocking antigen presentation should, therefore, interfere with disease induction or perpetuation. Approximately a decade ago it was shown that EAE could be prevented by injection of anti-I-A antibodies prior to MBP immunization (Sriram and Steinman 1983). In addition, early disease could be rapidly reversed following this therapy and the number and severity of relapses in chronic/progressive EAE could be reduced. Success has also been achieved in induced demyelinating disease in rhesus monkeys.

This therapy is only partially specific, however, blocking responses restricted by a given class II isotype. Although anti-I-A blocks EAE, experimental myasthenia gravis and thyroiditis, in each of these diseases responses to PPD were left intact. Like other monoclonal antibody therapy, it remains complicated by the immunogenicity of the antibody itself, particularly with prolonged administration.

Peptide Blockade of MHC

It has been demonstrated that peptide fragments of antigenic proteins directly bind to the MHC class II molecule to be recognized by T-cells. It has been suggested that a given MHC molecule has a single functional antigen-binding site. Peptides from unrelated antigens can compete with one another for T-cell activation. Extending these observations, the possibility has been proposed that the relative immunodominance of an epitope might be determined in part by its affinity for the MHC class II molecule.

Based on these findings we have attempted to see whether in vivo competition betweeen pathogenic and nonpathogenic self-peptides can be applied to prevention of autoimmune disease. We first predicted which competitor peptides might be efficacious in vivo by screening their ability to block in vitro the stimulation of an encephalitogenic T-cell clone that recognizes Ac1-20 with I-A^u.

Peptides p1-20 and Ac9-20 were shown to inhibit proliferative responses to the encephalitogenic peptide Ac1-11 both in vitro and in vivo (Sakai et al. 1989). The demonstration that peptide p1-20 can compete in the in vivo induction of Ac1-11-primed T-cells suggested that this nonpathogenic peptide might be able to reduce the induction of autoaggressive T-cells and thereby prevent EAE. Thus, the preventive effect of the competitor peptide p1-20 on induction of EAE with Ac1-11 was tested. Neither p1-11 nor Ac2-11 could prevent disease even at a 6:1 ratio relative to Ac1-11, whereas injection of p1-20 significantly prevented the clinical development of EAE at a 3:1 ratio. In addition, Ac9-20 had a preventive effect on EAE at a 3:1 or 6:1 ratio. Injection of p1-20 at a 3:1 or 5:1 ratio did not prevent EAE induced with the I-A^s-restricted peptide p89-101 in SJL/J mice. In reviewing representative sections of 20 mice treated with competitors (p1-20 and Ac9-20), which did not show any clinical signs of EAE, no perivascular cuffs or submeningeal cell infiltrates were evident.

Further experiments with peptide inhibition have been performed. Peptide Ac1-11(4A) binds with greater affinity than Ac1-11 to I-A^u. Mice co-immunized with Ac1-11(4A) and Ac1-11 were protected from EAE (Kumar 1989). In a first experiment to test the protective effect of Ac1-11(4A) on EAE induction with Ac1-11, Ac1-11(4A) completely inhibited disease induction with 0 of 14 mice paralyzed, compared with 8 of 13 control mice who were paralyzed. In a second experiment, the protective effect of co-immunization with peptide Ac1-11(4A) was confirmed. The overall incidence of disease was substantially reduced with 3 paralyzed out of 15 co-immunized mice, versus 14 of 15 paralyzed control mice. The onset of disease was significantly delayed in the co-immunized group.

By analogy, it is worth noting that Sela, Arnon and colleagues have treated EAE with a random copolymer termed Cop I of tyrosine, alanine, lysine and glutamate. This peptide blocks MHC binding of MBP and is currently employed in the therapy of relapsing/remitting MS.

Antibodies to TCR V Region Molecules

The definition of a marked restriction in the T-cell repertoire in sensitized lymph nodes from animals with EAE raised the possibility of immunospecific therapy by ablation of the T-cell subset bearing that receptor subtype. This was accomplished using a monoclonal antibody to Vβ8 (F23.1) which is effective in depleting the T-cells bearing this receptor from the peripheral blood. T-cells reactive with mAb F23.1 constitute 25% of the T-cells in lymph nodes of normal PL/J mice. In the (PLSJ)F1 mouse this percentage is 14%. The depletion of T-cells reactive with mAb F23.1 is 98% complete 3 days after intraperitoneal (IP) administration of a dose of 0.5 mg.

EAE was first induced with T-cell clone PJR-25. This clone is fully encephalitogenic, capable of inducing paralysis and demyelination. PJR-25 expresses the epitope recognized by mAb F23.1. Therapy was begun 24 h after the mice first developed paralysis. In two experiments (PLSJ)F1 mice were randomly divided into two groups, with 16 mice each receiving two 100 μg injections of F23.1 ip at 72-h intervals, while 16 mice received mAb Leu 5b (S5.2), an isotype-matched control reactive with the CD2 antigen (a pan T-cell marker on human but not on mouse T-cells). Within 2–4 days mice receiving F23.1 showed a marked reversal in their paralysis and 13 out of 16 were completely free of disease 10 days after therapy started. Only one relapse with tail weakness was seen, on day 35, in the animals given mAb F23.1 (Acha-Orbea et al. 1988).

Next we tested whether EAE induced with p1-11 in complete Freund's adjuvant (CFA) in (PLSJ)F1 mice could be prevented with mAb F23.1 (Table 14.3). Immunization with MBP peptide p1-11 in CFA can induce clones which

Table 14.3. Prevention of MBP peptide p1-11 induced EAE with mAb F23.1. Monoclonal antibody to the TCR β chain variable region (F23.1) may be effective in preventing peptide induced EAE under circumstances where TCR gene usage is highly restricted

Monoclonal antibody[a]	Incidence[b]	Clinical disease mean onset (day)
F23.1	1/19	20
S5.2	9/20	15[c]

[a] mAbs F23.1 or S5.2 were given ip (500 μg) on days −1, 1 and 9, where immunization with p1-11 was on day 0.
[b] The ratio of number of paralyzed mice to the total number of mice. All mice were examined through day 40.
[c] The standard deviation was 1.7 days.

are both F23.1-positive and negative, and which are fully encephalitogenic. Successful prevention of disease with F23.1 would indicate that the F23.1-positive T-cell clones predominate in the development of disease and that the depletion of these T-cell clones in vivo would not simply result in an escape to F23.1-negative T-cell clones that would cause disease. Results shown in Table 14.3 indicate that whereas 1 of 19 mice receiving mAb F23.1 developed EAE, 9 out of 20 mice given mAb S5.2 became paralyzed: a significant difference. These results serve to indicate that the Vβ8-expressing clones *function* in the induction of EAE.

(PLSJ)F1 mice were immunized with guinea-pig MBP. In (PLSJ)F1 mice there are at least two distinct encephalitogenic epitopes for MBP, p1-11 and p35-47. The response to p35-47 is restricted to I-E^u and involves mostly Vβ8-negative T-cells. After paralysis was present, mice were given 0.2 mg IP of the mAb F23.1 or $KJ23_a$, a monoclonal antibody specific for the product of the TcR $V\beta17_a$ gene product. $KJ23_a$ prevents EAE induced with T-cell lines responsive to MBP p89-101 in the SJL mouse. Of 19 (PLSJ)F1 mice given F23.1, 12 returned to normal within 72 h, while 21 of 22 mice given $KJ23_a$ had moderate to severe paraplegia after 72 h (Table 14.4). Relapses were seen in 5

Table 14.4. Reversal of guinea-pig MBP-induced EAE with mAb F23.1. Reversal of EAE using Vβ specific monoclonal antibodies may also be effective when multiple encephalitogenic epitopes are present. Treatment failures may be due to Vβ8 negative T-cells mediating disease

Treatment[a]	Number of mice with clinical symptoms 72 h after treatment[b]			Number of mice with clinical symptoms 14 days after treatment			
	None	Mild	Severe	None	Mild	Severe	Deaths
F23.1	12	5	2	14	3	1	1
$KJ23_a$	1	12	9	9	2	7	4

[a] Treatment was begun 24 h after mice exhibited EAE. At this time the mice were separated randomly into two groups. Mice in each group received one 200-μg IP injection of F23.1 or S5.2. Nineteen mice received F23.1 and 22 mice received $KJ23_a$.
[b] Clinical status was graded as follows: none, no neurologic symptoms; mild, flaccid tail and/or mild paraparesis; severe, severe paraparesis or complete paraplegia.

of 19 F23.1-treated mice in the next 14 days. Thus, treatment with F23.1 reversed EAE in a situation where multiple encephalitogenic epitopes were present. Vβ8-negative T-cells capable of responding to MBP p1-11 or p35-47 may have accounted for the relapses seen in the F23.1-treated mice.

In contrast, the SJL (I-A^s) mouse strain recognizes a peptide from the C terminus of MBP with several overlapping epitopes. There is evidence for limited TcR gene usage in recognition of two of these epitopes. However, depletion of a single subset of T-cells did not prevent antigen-induced EAE. Elimination of one Vβ subset, in a polyclonal autoimmune disease such as this, may not be sufficient to prevent or reverse disease.

Vaccination to TCR V Regions

For some time it has been apparent that autoaggressive T cells mediating disease could also provide resistance to disease if reinfused following manipulation of the same cells after one of several mechanical treatments such as irradiation or high-pressure treatment. T-cell vaccination may take one of two forms. Firstly, it may involve the transfer of attenuated pathogenic T-cells which elicit clonotype-specific regulatory cells that behave like anti-idiotype suppressors. This was first demonstrated by Cohen and associates, who showed it was possible to use autoimmune T-cell clones or lines as vaccines to prevent or reverse autoimmune disease (Lider et al. 1988). Animals thus treated remained free of disease for a prolonged time and EAE could not be induced with T-cell lines, T-cell clones, or with MBP in adjuvant. The second approach has involved active immunization of rats with peptide sequences from the V-D-J region of Vβ8, expressed in three fourths of T-cell clones recognizing the encephalitogenic MBP peptide 72-86 (Howell et al. 1989). Similarly, Vandenbark and colleagues protected against EAE by vaccinating with a peptide from the CDR2 region of Vβ8 (Vandenbark et al. 1989). The applicability of these therapies in man is dependent upon an increased knowledge of the molecular nature of the T-cell receptor repertoire utilized by pathogenic T-cells.

Conclusion

Relatively specific immunotherapy utilizing antibodies or peptides directed at single or multiple sites of the trimolecular complex appears to be feasible in the treatment of autoimmune disease. Growing knowledge of the disease relationship to the MHC and of TCR utilization may allow for increasingly selective interventions. Because multiple antigenic epitopes and a spectrum of T-cell receptors that are utilized may be a feature of the autoimmune response, several therapeutic avenues or several V-region antibodies in each patient may be required. As demonstrated by Hood, Zaller and colleagues, cocktails of anti-T-cell receptor V region antibodies may improve the results of this therapy even though one particular TCR has a dominant influence on pathogenesis

(Zaller et al. 1990). In multiple sclerosis there are multiple potential antigens including not only MBP but also PLP and other myelin structural antigens. Customizing therapy based upon an individual's MHC and TCR repertoire may be a rational and feasible approach given the ease with which it may be possible to produce monoclonal antibodies to TCR V regions and to humanize or chimerize them as necessary. The development of peptide-based vaccines is also amenable to a patient-specific approach whereby the physician could choose from a set of peptides from all of the human Vα and Vβ regions. Finally, the design of pharmaceuticals that interfere with TCR-MHC interactions should be pursued vigorously in the light of the success obtained thus far with peptides that block TCR-MHC interactions in MHC. Further examination of the autoimmune demyelinating process in EAE will likely continue to provide valuable lessons which may aid in the future approach to the immunotherapy of MS.

References

Acha-Orbea H, Mitchell DJ, Timmermann L et al. (1988) Limited heterogeneity of T cell receptors from lymphocytes mediating autoimmune encephalomyelitis allows specific immune intervention. Cell 54:263–273

Acha-Orbea H, Steinman L, McDevitt HO (1989) T cell receptors in murine autoimmune diseases. Annu Rev Immunol 7:371–405

Bjorkman PJ, Saper MO, Samraoui B, Bennett WO, Strominger J, Wiley DC (1987a) Structure of the human class I histocompatibility antigen, HLA-A2. Nature 329:506–512

Bjorkman PJ, Saper MA, Samroui B, Bennett WS, Strominger JI, Wiley DC (1987b) The foreign antigen binding site and T cell recognition regions of class I histocompatibility antigens. Nature 329:512–518

Blackman M, Kappler J, Marrack P (1990) The role of T cell receptor on positive and negative selection of developing T cells. Science 248:1335–1341

DeLisi C, Berzofsky JA (1985) T cell antigenic sites tend to be amphipathic structures. Proc Natl Acad Sci USA 82:7048–7052

Hohlfeld R (1989) Neurological autoimmune disease and the trimolecular complex of T-lymphocytes. Ann Neurol 25:531–538

Heber-Katz E, Acha-Orbea H (1989) The V-region disease hypothesis: Evidence from autoimmune encephalomyelitis. Immunol Today 10:164–169

Howell MD, Winters ST, Olee T, Powell HC, Carlo DJ, Brostoff SW (1989) Vaccination against experimental allergic encephalomyelitis with T cell receptor peptides. Science 246:668–670

Kappler JW, Roehm N, Marrack P (1987a) T cell tolerance by clonal elimination in the thymus. Cell 49:273–280

Kappler JW, Wade T, White J et al. (1987b) A T cell receptor Vβ segment that imparts reactivity to a class II major histocompatibility complex product. Cell 49:263–271

Kono DH, Urban JL, Horvath SJ, Ando DG, Saavedra RA, Hood L (1988) Two minor determinants of myelin basic protein induce experimental allergic encephalomyelitis in SJL/J mice. J Exp Med 168:213–227

Kronenberg M, Siu G, Hood L, Shastri N (1986) The molecular genetics of the T cell antigen receptor and T cell antigen recognition. Annu Rev Immunol 4:529–591

Kumar V, Kono DH, Urban JL, Hood LE (1989) The T cell receptor repertoire and autoimmune diseases. Annu Rev Immunol 7:657–682

Lider O, Reshef T, Beraud E, Ben-Nun A, Cohen IR (1988) Anti-idiotypic network induced by T cell vaccination against experimental autoimmune encephalomyelitis. Science 239:181–183

Martin R, Jaraquemada D, Flerlage M et al. (1990) Fine specificity and HLA restriction of MBP-specific cytotoxic T cell lines from MS patients and healthy individuals. J Immunol 145:540–548

Martin R, Howell MD, Jaraquemada D et al. (1991) A myelin basic protein peptide is recognized by cytotoxic T-cells in the context of four HLA-DR types associated with multiple sclerosis. J Exp Med 173:19–24

McDevitt HO, Wraith DC, Smilek DE, Lundberg AS, Steinman L (1989) Evolution, function and utilization of major histocompatibility complex polymorphism in autoimmune disease. In: Cold Spring Harbor symposia on quantitative biology, vol. LIV, Immunological recognition. Cold Spring Harbor Press, pp 853–857

McFarland HF, Dhib-Jalbut S (1989) Multiple sclerosis: Possible immunological mechanisms. Clin Immunol Immunopath 50:S96–S105

Morel PA, Livingstone AM, Fathman CG (1987) Correlation of T cell receptor Vβ gene family with MHC restriction. J Exp Med 166:583–588

Oksenberg JR, Stuart S, Begovich AB et al. (1990) Limited heterogeneity or rearranged T-cell receptor V alpha transcripts in brains of multiple sclerosis patients. Nature 345:344–346

Ota K, Matsui M, Milford E, Mackin G, Weiner HL, Hafler DA (1990) T cell recognition of an immunodominant myelin basic protein epitope in multiple sclerosis. Nature 346:183–187

Padula SJ, Lingenheld EG, Stabach PR, Clou CJ, Kono DH, Clark RB (1991) Identification of encephalitogenic Vβ4 bearing T cells in SJL mice. J Immunol 146:879–883

Paterson PY (1960) Transfer of allergic encephalomyelitis in rats by means of lymph node cells. J Exp Med 111:119-135

Powell MB, Mitchell D, Lederman J et al. (1990) Lymphotoxin and tumor necrosis factor-alpha production by myelin basic protein. Int Immunol 2:539–544

Reader AT, Arnason BG (1985) Immunology of multiple sclerosis. In: Vinken PJ, Bruyn GW, Klawans HC (eds) Handbook of clinical neurology. Elsevier, Amsterdam, 47:337–396

Rothbard JB, Taylor WR (1988) A sequence pattern common to T cell epitopes. EMBO J 7:93–100

Sakai K, Sinha AA, Mitchell DJ et al. (1988) Involvement of distinct murine T-cell receptors in the autoimmune encephalitogenic response to nested epitopes of myelin basic protein. Proc Natl Acad Sci USA 85:8608–8612

Sakai K, Mitchell D J Hodgkinson SJ, Zamvil S.S, Rothbard JB, Steinman L (1989) Prevention of experimental encephalomyelitis with peptides blocking T cell-MHC interaction. Proc Natl Acad Sci USA 86:9470–9474

Sinha AA, Brautbar C, Szafer F et al. (1988) A newly characterized HLA DQ beta allele associated with pemphigus vulgaris. Science 239:1026–1029

Sriram S, Steinman L (1983) Anti I-A antibody suppresses active encephalomyelitis: treatment model for diseases linked to IR genes. J Exp Med 158:1362–1367

Todd JA, Bell JI, McDevitt HO (1987) HLA-DQβ genes contribute to susceptibility and resistance to insulin dependent diabetes mellitus. Nature 329:599–604

Todd JA, Acha-Orbea H, Bell JI et al. (1988) A molecular basis for MHC class II-associated autoimmunity. Science 240:1003–1009

Urban JL, Kumar V, Kono DH et al. (1988) Restricted use of T cell receptor V genes in murine autoimmune encephalomyelitis raises possibilities for antibody therapy. Cell 54:577–592

Urban J, Horvath S, Hood L (1989) Autoimmune T cells: immune recognition of normal and variant peptide epitopes and peptide-based therapy. Cell 59:257–271

Vandenbark AA, Hashim G, Offner H (1989) Immunization with a synthetic T-cell receptor V-region peptide protects against experimental autoimmune encephalomyelitis. Nature 341:541–544

Waldor MK, Sriram S, Hardy R et al. (1985) Reversal of experimental allergic encephalomyelitis with monoclonal antibody to a T-cell subset marker. Science 227:415–417

Wraith DC, Smilek DE, Mitchell DJ, Steinman L, McDevitt HO (1989a) Antigen recognition in autoimmune encephalomyelitis and the potential for peptide-mediated immunotherapy. Cell 59:247–255

Wraith DC, McDevitt HO, Steinman L, Acha-Orbea H (1989b) T-cell recognition as the target for immune intervention in autoimmune disease. Cell 57:709–715

Wucherpfenning K, Ota K, Endo N et al. (1990) Shared human T cell receptor Vβ usage to immunodominant regions of myelin basic protein. Science 248:1016–1019

Zaller D, Osman G, Kanagawa O, Hood L (1990) Prevention and treatment of murine EAE with TcR Vβ-specific antibodies. J Exp Med 171:1943–1955

Zamvil SS, Steinman L (1990) The T lymphocyte in experimental allergic encephalomyelitis. Annu Rev Immunol 8:579–621

Zamvil SS, Nelson PA, Mitchell DJ, Knobler RL, Fritz RB, Steinman L (1985) Encephalitogenic T cell clones specific for myelin basic protein. An unusual bias in antigen recognition. J Exp Med 162:2107–2124

Zamvil SS, Mitchell DJ, Moore AC, Kitamura K, Steinman L, Rothbard JB (1986) T-cell epitope of the autoantigen myelin basic protein that induces encephalomyelitis. Nature 324:258–260

Zamvil SS, Mitchell DJ, Moore AC et al. (1987) T cell specificity for class II (I-A) and the encephalitogenic N-terminal epitope of the autoantigen myelin basic protein. J Immunol 139: 1075–1079
Zamvil SS, Mitchell DJ, Powell MB, Sakai K, Rothbard JB, Steinman L (1988a) Multiple discrete encephalitogenic epitopes of the autoantigen myelin basic protein include a determinant for I-E class II-restricted T cells. J Exp Med 168:1181–1186
Zamvil SS, Mitchell DJ, Lee NE et al. (1988b) Predominant expression of a T cell receptor V beta gene subfamily in autoimmune encephalomyelitis [published erratum appears in J Exp Med 1988 Jul 1; 168(1):455]. J Exp Med 167:1586–1596

Chapter 15

Experimental Approaches to Specific Immunotherapy in Multiple Sclerosis

David A. Hafler, Staley A. Brod and Howard L. Weiner

Introduction

There is increasing evidence that multiple sclerosis (MS) is an autoimmune disease where a small number of activated, white matter-reactive T-cells specifically migrate into the myelinated central nervous system leading to inflammation, and eventually demyelination (McFarlin and McFarland 1982; Waksman and Reynolds 1984). It appears that one necessary component to MS and in fact other autoimmune diseases is lack of immune regulation (Hafler and Weiner 1987; Hafler et al. 1989). A second component in MS may be the capability of a patient's T-cells to recognize white matter structures such as myelin basic protein and proteolipid protein, which have been postulated to be the immune targets in the disease's initial induction (Ota et al. 1990). Thus there must be very careful regulation of the ability of autoreactive T-cells to become activated with their potential to mediate inflammatory, destructive processes in the nervous system.

In designing specific immunotherapies for a presumed autoimmune process, one could direct attention to two major avenues of intervention. First would be an attempt to correct the lack of proper immune regulation which may allow for the activation of autoreactive T-cells. As is discussed in this book (see Chap. 14), there are a number of immune regulatory abnormalities that have been described in MS which are linked to decreases in subpopulations of immunoregulatory T-cells. It may be possible to correct these defects by forms of immunotherapy which correct these natural immunoregulatory abnormalities which allow for the activation of autoreactive T-cells. The second, and potentially most specific means for the eventual immunotherapy of autoimmune disease, would be specifically to suppress or tolerize the autoreactive T-cells. The elegance of such an approach would be that T-cells reactive to other antigens, which may be important for immune defenses, would not be altered in such a process.

In this review, potential methods to alter both antigen non-specific abnormalities of the immune system, and methods to specifically alter antigen reactive T-cells will be discussed (Fig. 15.1). An important caveat for this discussion is that we do not know with certainty that MS is mediated by autoreactive T-cells. It is still possible that an as yet unidentified infectious agent exists in the nervous system and that the inflammatory responses observed in MS represent

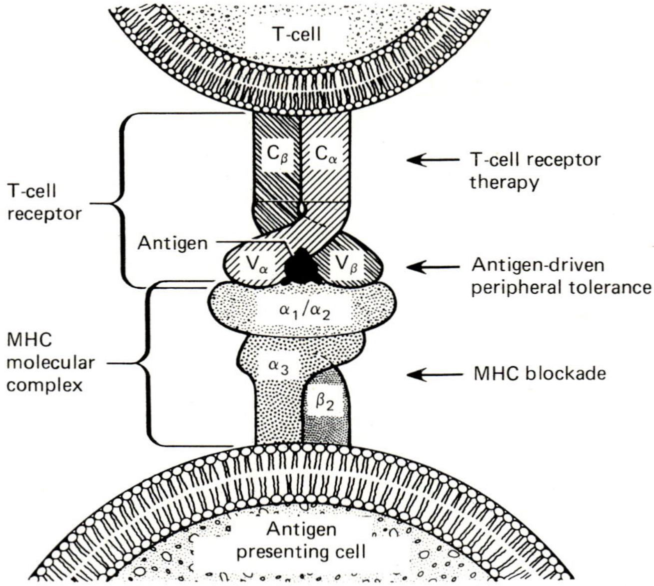

Fig. 15.1. Potential mechanisms to target the tri-molecular complex of T-cell receptor, antigen, and MHC molecular complex in relationship to antigen specific manipulation of the immune system. T-cell receptor therapy can include: T-cell vaccination, where antigen specific T-cells are injected (Cohen 1986); injection of peptides derived from the structure of the T-cell receptor (Vandenbark et al. 1990); or anti-T-cell receptor monoclonal antibodies targeted against specific T-cell receptors (Hafler et al. 1988). Antigen driven peripheral tolerance includes: oral tolerance (Higgins and Weiner 1988; Lider et al. 1989; Zhang et al. 1990; Brod et al. 1991; Khoury et al. 1990); antigen coupled to mononuclear cells (Kennedy et al. 1988); and IV injection of soluble antigens. MHC blockade involves approaches that block the ability of MHC molecules to present antigen to T-cells.

an attempt by the immune system to destroy or inactivate such an organism. However, as will be discussed at the end of this review, proof that MS is an autoimmune disease will rest with clinical trials that can specifically alter a particular immune function with subsequent amelioration of the disease. Thus, it may be more proper to view clinical trials as clinical experimentation in order to define the etiology and pathogenesis of the disease.

Antigen Nonspecific Immune Alteration

Anti T-cell Monoclonal Antibodies

With increasing evidence that MS is mediated by activated T-cells, a logical approach for immunotherapy would be specifically to alter the T-cells in some fashion. This could be accomplished by reagents that (1) inhibit the normal cell-to-cell contact necessary for T-cell function or (2) specifically signal the T-cell to be turned off or (3) lyse and destroy specific subpopulations of T-cells. Monoclonal antibodies, which represent immortalized antibody-secreting B-cells, present a potentially ideal reagent for targetting T-cells. Once a particular monoclonal antibody-secreting B-cell is isolated, that B-cell can potentially grow forever and be used as an unlimited source of reagent for treatment of disease.

We have been involved in phase I studies in subjects with MS to study the effectiveness of anti T-cell monoclonal antibody infusions in humans (Hafler et al. 1988). To date, we have studied the immunologic affects of three anti T-cell monoclonal antibodies: anti CD2, anti CD4, and anti T12 monoclonal antibodies. We have specifically asked whether there is selective elimination of T-cell subpopulations with the monoclonal antibody infusions. Secondly, we have asked whether there is immunosuppression using in vitro measures of immune function after infusions of the anti T-cell monoclonal antibodies. Thirdly, we have asked what is the host immune response to repeated infusions of these murine antibodies. We found that anti T-cell monoclonal antibody infusions specifically suppress in vitro measures of the human immune response. Specifically, an anti CD2 monoclonal decreased T-cell activation by phytohemagglutinin, and anti CD4 monoclonal antibody infusions abolished pokeweed mitogen-induced immunoglobulin synthesis without lysis of the CD4 positive T-cell populations. Thus, we were able to demonstrate for the first time in humans that monoclonal antibodies specifically directed against T-cell surface structures could be immunosuppressive (Hafler et al. 1988). More recently it has been learned that many cell surface structures are involved in cell-to-cell contact such as the CD4 determinant which recognizes invariant structures of Class II MHC and CD2 which binds to LFA-3. In particular, CD2-LFA-3 interactions are involved in T–T-cell signalling which may be important for amplification of the immune response (Brod et al. 1990). These results would indicate that anti T-cell monoclonal antibodies, which were used without any side effects in patients with MS, might be useful to alter non-specifically the immune system. However, with repeated infusions of the monoclonal antibody, human anti-mouse antibodies were found in the circulation. Although most of the human anti-mouse antibodies were not immunoglobulin isotype-specific, significant anti-idiotypic activity was observed after repeated infusions (Hafler et al. 1988). These human anti-mouse antibodies blocked the binding of the mouse anti-T-cell monoclonal antibodies to the T-cell surface.

Though the clinical usefulness of currently available anti-T-cell murine monoclonal antibodies in chronic diseases such as MS is hampered by human anti-mouse antibodies, there are a number of potential approaches which may get around this problem. First is the use of humanized monoclonal antibodies (Mayforth and Quintans 1990, Reichman et al. 1990). That is, one could potentially use monoclonal antibodies with a human Fc and mouse Fab region. A second approach would be to attach a toxin to the murine monoclonal antibody, which would result in a greater elimination of targetted T-cell populations in addition potentially to preventing human anti-mouse antibodies (Vitetta et al. 1987). In summary, monoclonal antibodies offer the potential of a non-toxic form of immune therapy for MS. However, technical problems as yet prevent their use for chronic autoimmune disease processes such as MS.

Cytokine Regulation

Besides direct T–T-cell contact which is involved in immunoregulation, activated T cells also secrete hormones called cytokines which regulate the immune response. We have found that the autologous mixed lymphocyte response, one in vitro measure of immune function that is decreased in MS, can be specifically corrected by interleukin-1 (IL-1) (Hafler et al. 1991). These and other clinical trials in progress with other cytokines such as α and β interferon suggests the potential utility of direct cytokine manipulation of immune response. Again one is left with the issue that any in vitro observation in a disease such as MS may be secondary rather than primary to the disease process. Clinical experimentation where cytokines are used in the treatment of the disease may allow the differentiation between primary and secondary immunologic events. The use of interferons is specifically discussed in more detail in Chap. 11 of this volume.

Another means of directly manipulating the immune system in an antigen non-specific fashion would be with pharmacologic agents that specifically alter T-cell function. One such example is cyclosporine-A, which is discussed in Chap. 10. Cyclosporine-A specifically decreases the secretion of IL-2 and the expression of IL-2 receptors on T-cells, which allows for the specific manipulation of T-cell function. Another approach in the future may be the development of drugs that specifically alter T-cell-specific tyrosine kinases. For example, $p56^{lck}$ is a T-cell-specific tyrosine kinase which plays a major role in T-cell immune regulation. The development of specific reagents to alter the function of a T-cell-specific kinase in such a fashion may allow for the development of specific immunotherapies in the future.

Antigen-specific Immune Alteration

The second major category of immunotherapies involve antigen-specific modalities which would be the best theoretical approach for the treatment of autoimmune disease. The difficulty with any antigen-specific therapy is the presumption that one knows which antigen the T-cells are directed against. Although there is accumulating data from both animal models and work in humans with MS that both myelin basic protein and proteolipid apoprotein may well be the target antigens in MS, only specific modulation of the immune system with amelioration of disease activity will allow us to know whether these molecules are T-cell targets in the disease. In this regard, we have recently proposed certain criteria to demonstrate that MS is a cell-mediated autoimmune disease analogous to EAE (Ota et al. 1990). First should be the demonstration of an association between an immunodominant region of a presumed autoantigen and disease-associated major histocompatibility haplotypes such as DR2 in MS. Second, there should be an increase in frequency of T-cells that react with this immunodominant epitope. Finally, as mentioned in the introductory paragraph, the course of the disease must be altered by elimination of autoreactive T-cells or by inducing immune tolerance to the autoantigen identified in the first two criteria. Thus the following discussion of

Table 15.1. Criteria for defining MS as a T-cell-mediated autoimmune disease

1. Association between an immunodominant region of a presumed autoantigen and disease associated major histocompatibility haplotypes such as DR2 in MS
2. Demonstration of in vivo activated and/or clonally expanded T-cell populations specific for the target antigen in peripheral blood and the target organ of affected individuals
3. Effective treatment of the disease by tolerance induction to the target antigen or by specific elimination of autoreactive T-cells

antigen-specific immunotherapy should be viewed as necessary to prove that the association of a particular autoantigen is associated with the actual disease process.

T-Cell Vaccination

Inoculation of attenuated T-cell clones recognizing the inciting autoantigen can specifically prevent the induction of experimental autoimmune diseases including EAE, adjuvant arthritis, and spontaneous diabetes (Cohen 1986). It has been shown that the mechanism for this protection involves both an "anti-activated T-cell" response which is short lived, and anti-clonotypic T-cell responses, which are longer lived. Moreover, animal experimentation has suggested the safety of T-cell vaccination using either fixed or irradiated T-cell clones. We have recently been engaged in phase I investigation of T-cell vaccination therapy in humans with the following objectives: (1) to examine the feasibility of innoculating T-cell clones into humans and to determine how such clones should be selected, expanded and attenuated; (2) to study whether there are associated toxicities with inoculation into humans; (3) to define the immunologic responses to the inoculation of attenuated T cell clones using simple measures of immune activation.

To date, 4 subjects with progressive MS have been treated with a total of 7 inoculations with attenuated, autologous T-cell clones isolated from the cerebrospinal fluid. We found there are no untoward side effects with the T-cell vaccination. The results of immunologic study suggested that the inoculation of autologous T-cell activated clones was associated with partial, short term immunosuppression as evidenced by downregulation of subsequent stimulation via the CD2 pathway of activation. In addition, we observed that the autologous mixed lymphocyte response (AMLR), which is reduced in about half of the patients with multiple sclerosis, could be enhanced for a short period of time after the T-cell vaccination. These results indicate the injection of attenuated autoreactive T-cell clones appears to be feasible for further clinical trials in humans.

In this first series of clinical trials with T-cell vaccination, T-cells were grown by single cell cloning directly from the spinal fluid of patients with MS. Clones were chosen on the basis of using common T-cell receptor gene rearrangements indicating clonal expansion in the spinal fluid for use in the vaccination protocol. Other T-cell clones could potentially be used for T-cell vaccination. For example, we have recently identified an immunodominant region on myelin basic protein associated with the DR2 MHC phenotype (Ota et al. 1990).

The T-cell receptor used to recognize these dominant peptides is restricted (Wucherpfennig et al. 1990), suggesting the potential efficacy of T-cell vaccination approach with myelin basic protein reactive T-cell clones. Besides using T-cell clones to vaccinate, it may be possible to inoculate subjects with immunogenic regions of the T-cell receptor itself that recognizes these presumed immunodominant regions of myelin antigens in the context of major histocompatibility antigens. Such an approach has been reported to be of use in the treatment of EAE (Vandenbark et al. 1990).

Tolerization with Antigen

An alternative response to using activated, antigen reactive T-cells to manipulate the immunoresponse is to bind myelin antigens directly to autologous mononuclear T-cells. This approach has been used in the EAE model of multiple sclerosis where whole myelin antigen, in addition to myelin basic protein had been non-covalently attached to lymphocyte surface injected into animal (Kennedy et al. 1988). Such approaches may specifically alter immune responses by the ability of T-cells to present antigen to other T-cells and thus manipulate the immune response (LaSalle et al. 1991).

An alternative means to cell therapy in the treatment of multiple sclerosis is the use of antigens to directly tolerize the immune system. It is well known that intravenous administration of soluble antigen can lead to tolerogenic signals to the immune system. In fact a number of years ago, phase I trials using injections of porcine myelin basic protein in humans was attempted with negative results. An alternative approach to the parenteral injection of autoantigens is the technique of oral tolerance. There appear to be very strong suppressor signals generated with oral feeding of antigens (Higgins and Weiner 1988). Teleologically, this may relate to the need of ingesting many different proteins without generating immune responses. Very strong suppressor signals are generated to antigens that are taken by the oral route. Work from this and other laboratories have demonstrated that the EAE can be prevented by the oral ingestion of myelin antigens prior to or in fact after the induction of disease (Higgins and Weiner 1988; Lider et al. 1989; Zhang et al. 1990; Brod et al. 1991; Khoury et al. 1990). This effect is due to the generation of T-cells that can be transferred to naive animals and subsequently suppress disease activity. This has led to phase I clinical trials in patients with early relapsing/remitting multiple sclerosis. Development of synergist which may potentiate the effect of oral ingestion of myelin antigens prior to or in fact after the induction of disease (Higgins and Weiner 1988; Lider et al. 1989; Zhang et al. 1990; Brod et al. 1991; Khoury et al. 1990). This effect is due to the generation of T-cells that

References

Brod SA, Purvee M, Benjamin D, Hafler DA (1990) Autologous T-T cell activation mediated by cellular adhesion molecules. Eur J Immunol 20:2259–2268

Brod SA, al-Sabbagh A, Hafler DA, Sobel RA, Weiner HL (1991) Suppression of relapsing

experimental allergic encephalomyelitis in Lewis rats and Strain 13 guinea pigs by oral administration of myelin antigens. Ann Neurol (in press)
Cohen IR (1986) Regulation of autoimmune disease – physiology and therapeutics. Immunol Rev 94:5–21
Hafler DA, Weiner HL (1987) T cells in multiple sclerosis and inflammatory central nervous system disease. Immunol Rev 100:307–333
Hafler DA, Ritz J, Schlossman SF, Weiner HL (1988) Immunologic responses to anti-CD4 and anti-CD2 murine monoclonal antibody in humans. J Immunol 141:131–138
Hafler DA, Brod SA, Weiner HL (1989) Immunoregulation in multiple sclerosis. Res Immunol 140:233–239
Hafler DA, Chofflon M, Kurt-Jones E, Weiner HL (1991) Interleukin-1 corrects the decrease in the autologous mixed lymphocyte reaction in multiple sclerosis. Clin Immunol Immunopath 58:115–125
Higgins P, Weiner HL (1988) Suppression of experimental autoimmune encephalomyelitis by oral administration of myelin basic protein and its fragments. J Immunol 140:440–445
Kennedy MK, Dal Canto MC, Trotter JL, Miller SD (1988) Specific immune regulation of chronic-relapsing experimental allergic encephalomyelitis in mice. J Immunol 141:2986–2993
Khoury SJ, Lider O, Al-Sabbagh A, Weiner HL (1990) Suppression of experimental autoimmune encephalomyelitis by oral administration of myelin basic protein. III. Cell Immunol 131:302–310
LaSalle J, Ota K, Hafler DA (1991) Presentation of autoantigen by human T cells. J Immunol 147: 774–780
Lider O, Santos LMB, Lee CSY, Higgins PJ, Weiner HL (1989) Suppression of experimental autoimmune encephalomyelitis by oral administration of myelin basic protein II. Suppression of disease and in vitro immune responses is mediated by antigen-specific CD8+ T lymphocytes. J Immunol 142:748–752
Mayforth RD, Quintans J (1990) Designer and catalytic antibodies. N Engl J Med 323:173–178
McFarlin D, McFarland H (1982) Multiple sclerosis. N Engl J Med 307:1183–1188
Ota K, Matsui M, Milford E, Mackin G, Weiner HL, Hafler DA (1990) T cell recognition of an immunodominant myelin basic protein epitope is linked to DR2 in multiple sclerosis. Nature 346:183–187
Reichman L, Clark M, Waldmann H, Winter G (1990) Reshaping human antibodies for therapy. Nature 332:323–327
Vandenbark AA, Hashim G, Offner H (1990) Immunization with a synthetic T-cell receptor V-region peptide protects against experimental autoimmune encephalomyelitis. Nature 341:541–543
Vitetta ES, Fulton RJ, May RD, Till M, Uhr JW (1987) Redesigning nature's poisons to create anti-tumor reagents. Science 238:1098–1104
Waksman B, Reynolds WE (1984) Multiple sclerosis as a disease of immune regulation. Proc Soc Exp Biol Med 175:282–294
Wucherpfennig KW, Ota K, Endo N, Seidman JG, Rosenzweig A, Weiner HL, Hafler DA (1990) Shared human T cell receptor V_β usage to immunodominant regions of myelin basic protein. Science 248:1016–1019
Zhang ZJ, Lee C SY, Lider O, Weiner HL (1990) Suppression of adjuvant arthritis in Lewis rats by oral administration of type II collagen. J Immunol 145:2489–2493

Subject Index